UNDER THE SAFETY NET

THE EDITORS

PHILIP W. BRICKNER, M.D.

LINDA KEEN SCHARER, M.U.P.

BARBARA A. CONANAN, R.N., M.S.

MARIANNE SAVARESE, R.N., B.S.N.

BRIAN C. SCANLAN, M.D.

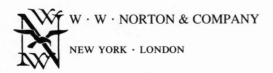 W · W · NORTON & COMPANY

NEW YORK · LONDON

UNDER THE SAFETY NET

The Health and Social Welfare

of the Homeless in the United States

A UNITED HOSPITAL FUND BOOK

First published as a Norton paperback 1992

The text of this book is composed in Times Roman, with the display set in Modern No. 20 and Blado. Composition and manufacturing by the Maple-Vail Book Manufacturing Group. Book design by Marjorie J. Flock.

Library of Congress Cataloging-in-Publication Data

Under the safety net: the health and social welfare of the homeless
    in the United States / Philip W. Brickner . . . [et al.], editors.
    p.   cm.
    "A United Hospital Fund book."
    Includes bibliographical references.
    1. Homeless persons—Health and hygiene—United States.
    2. Homeless persons—Medical care—United States. 3. Homeless
persons—Social aspects—United States. 4. Homeless persons—
Government policy—United States. I. Brickner, Philip W., 1928–

RA654.9.H63U53   1990   90-30578
362.1'0425—dc20

ISBN 0-393-30875-8

W.W. Norton & Company, Inc., 500 Fifth Avenue, New York, N.Y. 10110
W.W. Norton & Company Ltd, 10 Coptic Street, London WC1A 1PU

2 3 4 5 6 7 8 9 0

Contents

P A R T   I I CLINICAL CONCERNS

PART III PROGRAMS AND PARTNERSHIPS

DREW ALTMAN

BRUCE C. VLADECK

Preface

THIS BOOK RECORDS the many lessons learned from a truly extraordinary national experiment. The Health Care for the Homeless Program mobilized forces in nineteen big cities to reach out and bring critically needed services to homeless persons.

When it was first developed, those of us involved had high hopes for this program. We hoped that through it we could demonstrate new ways to deliver health and social services to homeless persons. We hoped to demonstrate better ways to link the homeless with public benefits for which they are eligible. We hoped to encourage a broad cross section of groups in our big cities to bury their hatchets and work together in a common cause. We hoped that the program would provide an opportunity for learning, leading to further action down the road. And we hoped, of course, that the program would make a difference for the homeless people it served and that the projects themselves, having proved their worth, would survive.

Because of extraordinary commitment and energy of all those in the nineteen cities who rose to this challenge and because of the hard work of new partners (such as Comic Relief) picked up along the way, these goals have, in the main, been realized.

At the same time the very existence of the Health Care for the Homeless Program reflects the major failure of our nation's health care system, the failure to provide basic health coverage to more than thirty-five million of our citizens. It reflects the failures in mental health services and the broken promises of "deinstitutionalization." It reflects failures in housing, in welfare, and elsewhere across the spectrum of human services.

Virtually everybody involved in the Health Care for the Homeless Program believed the effort to have been a worthwhile one but understood as well its obvious limitations. People often asked the question, "Isn't this just a Band-Aid approach after all?" The answer to that question is no. We have by now learned enough about the homeless to know that services, not just roofs over people's heads, are essential. How homeless people enter the service system may be much less important than having them enter at all. We should no longer be squeamish about saying that substance abuse, mental illness, family violence, poor education and skills, and many other problems, in addition to physical illness, are dimensions of homelessness that must be met head-on. At the same time housing and jobs remain the fundamental concerns, and these are issues that the Health Care for the Homeless Program could not address, except through the most indirect means.

That a commitment of twenty-five million dollars by two private foundations received so much attention reflects also the failure of leadership in Washington during the Reagan years to confront the burgeoning problems of homelessness. Had it been launched in the middle of the war on poverty, we doubt that this program would have received so much attention.

If we are honest with ourselves, however, we would also recognize that the absence of national policy leadership reflects more than just the philosophical predispositions of a particular administration. It also reflects the fact that we, as a society, have serious difficulties confronting big social problems like homelessness.

Most Americans understand that homelessness is a serious problem. But while many believe government must do more, many also believe that government often does more harm than good, and they prefer that the private sector lead the way. While there is substantial consensus that the biggest need in mental health is for community-based services, demonstrative citizens want the homeless off their streets and out of their neighborhoods—even back in big state institutions, if that's what it takes.

Given an inability to confront the root causes of homlessness head-on, health care offered a sort of neutral turf on which all sides could meet and agree. Indeed, this realization was later incorporated into federal legislation, when dollars were provided through the Stewart McKinney Act to support these and similar health care projects around the country, a classic case of a foundation-funded program leveraging government support later on.

While much remains to be done, the preparation of this book marks an appropriate occasion to render some credit when it is due. Both the Pew Charitable Trusts and the Robert Wood Johnson Foundation not only developed and supported the Health Care for the Homeless Program but have made homelessness a continuing programmatic concern. The Robert Wood Johnson Foundation also provided support for development of this book, as a way of helping collect and disseminate many of the lessons learned in the program.

Support for development of this book was also provided by the United Hospital

Fund of New York, a philanthropic, educational, and research organization which seeks to improve health care through a range of activities, including a publications program—which this book is part of—and which also administers the New York City Coalition for Health Care for the Homeless, a part of the national program, on behalf of a broad coalition of public and private agencies.

The United Hospital Fund supported publication of the first scholarly survey of health services for the homeless, edited by Philip Brickner, M.D., and his colleagues at St. Vincent's Medical Center. Their work first inspired the involvement of the fund and both foundations in the issue of homelessness, and it is thus especially appropriate that they have again taken the lead in preparing this book.

Indeed, this volume was written almost entirely by people who have been individually engaged, on the front lines, in providing hands-on care to homeless persons. What they have learned is instructive, informative, insightful. But what they have done, their commitment and their contribution, is the most important point to emphasize here. We hope their light shines through.

PHILIP W. BRICKNER

LINDA KEEN SCHARER

BARBARA A. CONANAN

MARIANNE SAVARESE

BRIAN C. SCANLAN

Acknowledgments

THOSE WHO HAVE brought us together as authors, editors, and readers of this work are the homeless human beings of the United States. We acknowledge them and the privilege and duty of serving and helping them.

The support and venture of this book are in large part the responsibility of the United Hospital Fund of New York, and we wish to record that fact with gratitude. Much of the material we consider here stems from the experiences since 1984 of the Health Care for the Homeless Program, supported in nineteen cities across the nation by the Robert Wood Johnson Foundation and the Pew Charitable Trusts. The laudable creative intent and courage of these two major philanthropies in engaging with the challenging issue of homeless health care deserve strong recognition here.

The United States Conference of Mayors has developed significant analyses of the extent of homelessness across the country. The conference also cosponsored the Johnson/Pew program and is credited here.

The National Association of Community Health Centers (NACHC), through the Stewart B. McKinney Homeless Assistance Act, has become involved in recent years with extending health services to the homeless well beyond the range of the programs sponsored initially by the two foundations. We acknowledge NACHC as a noteworthy sharer in this work.

St. Vincent's Hospital and Medical Center of New York, our own institution, has been a major force in developing health care programs for the homeless. Since 1969 St. Vincent's nurses, physicians, social workers, and other staff members have been at work in Manhattan's shelters and single room occupancy hotels.

These efforts stem logically from the founding mission of our hospital in 1849, to care for the sick poor.

We greet and appreciate as partners all those who have devoted their lives to work in service for the homeless, in the national Health Care for the Homeless Program, at community health centers, and through St. Vincent's Hospital in New York. It gives us particular pleasure to thank the following individuals who have been integral to the development of work in this field and to the creation of this book. We apologize to those many others whose names, omitted here, could well have been noted: Drew Altman, then of the Robert Wood Johnson Foundation, who crafted the idea in 1982 and fought for the creation of the national program in 1983 and 1984; Bruce Vladeck, president of the United Hospital Fund, long a significant innovator in health care design and a major supporter of this work; Andrew Greene and Stephen Somers of the Robert Wood Johnson Foundation and David Rogers, Linda Aiken, and Rolando Thorne, formerly of the foundation; Rebecca Rimel and Nadya Shmavonian of the Pew Charitable Trusts; Laura Waxman and Lilia Reyes of the United States Conference of Mayors; Freda Mitchem of the National Association of Community Health Centers, Inc.; Sally Rogers of the United Hospital Fund; Honorable Charles Royer, Honorable Henry Maier, Andreas Schneider, Jack Raba, John Noble, Don Hammersley, Karen Lamb, David Rosenbloom, John B. Waller, Ted Wilson, Torrey Brown, John R. Colemen, Sister Rosemary Donley, and Norman Marshall of the national program's advisory committee; Bob Zmuda and Dennis Albaugh of Comic Relief.

At St. Vincent's Hospital: Sister Evelyn Schneider, Sister Margaret Sweeney, Sister Marian Catherine Muldoon, Sister Karen Helfenstein, Sister Eileen Hawkey, Lambert King, Tom McGourty, Jane Connorton, Joe Brown, Debra Oryzysyn, Paulette Ortiz, Roger Weaving, Ray Scardapane, Gary Zuar, Herman Muller, Mary Ann Maisonet, Frank Scheets, Al Elvy, Andy Portelli, Joe English, Ted Druhot, Sister Margaret Murphy, Anthony Lechich, Arthur Kaufman, Mary Hart, Laura Starita, Sue Post, and Bara Swain.

Steve Wobido who, from 1984 through 1989, served as deputy director of the Health Care for the Homeless Program; Richard Moss, whose fine and persevering efforts to produce the actual text of this volume, and other services to the program, are deeply appreciated; Robert J. Markel of Markel Enterprises for agenting; and Mary Cunnane of W. W. Norton & Company for editing.

We also thank the authors who shared in the writing of this book. These people put forth great effort, often under considerable pressure of time, to prepare their work for this purpose.

The Editors

PHILIP W. BRICKNER, M.D., is a graduate of Columbia University College of Physicians and Surgeons. He is an internist and has been director of the Department of Community Medicine at St. Vincent's Hospital and Medical Center of New York since 1974. The Department of Community Medicine has among its goals the seeking out and assisting of medically unreached people in New York City, including the homeless, the frail, homebound aged, and immigrant children. Dr. Brickner is the author of numerous articles on these subjects in the professional literature.

LINDA KEEN SCHARER, M.U.P., received her master's degree in urban planning from New York University. She is presently assistant director of the Department of Community Medicine at St. Vincent's Hospital and Medical Center of New York. In addition to her work with the homeless, Ms. Scharer has written extensively on home health care issues and serves on the editorial board of the PRIDE Institute's *Journal of Long-Term Home Health Care*.

BARBARA A. CONANAN, R.N., M.S., is director of the SRO/Homeless Program within the Department of Community Medicine at St. Vincent's Hospital and Medical Center of New York. She has served in this capacity since January 1983. In addition, Ms. Conanan gives direct patient care as a community health nurse. Prior to her employment at St. Vincent's, she worked at the Manhattan Bowery Corporation as supervisor in an outpatient clinic that provided services to chronic alcoholics.

MARIANNE SAVARESE, R.N., B.S.N., is the supervisor of nurses within the Department of Community Medicine at St. Vincent's Hospital and Medical Center of New York. She is a graduate of St. Vincent's Hospital School of Nursing and received her bachelor's degree from Adelphi University. Since 1979 she has worked among homeless individuals and families as the community health nurse member of an interdisciplinary team. Ms. Savarese has written and lectured about the value of teams in providing health care to homeless persons.

BRIAN C. SCANLAN, M.D., is a graduate of New York Medical College. Trained in internal medicine, he spent from 1984 to 1989 as an attending physician in the Department of Community Medicine at St. Vincent's Hospital and Medical Center of New York with a concentration of interest on emotionally disabled homeless persons. Dr. Scanlan is the author of several papers related to the health of the homeless. He is now practicing medicine in Amherst, Massachusetts.

The Contributors

Dennis Albaugh
Vice-president
Comic Relief
Los Angeles, California

Rita Altamore, M.D., M.P.H.
Director
Extended Degree Program
School of Public Health,
University of Washington
Seattle, Washington

Drew Altman, Ph.D.
Director
Health and Human Services
Pew Charitable Trusts
Philadelphia, Pennsylvania

Marc Arkovitz
Medical student
New York University School of Medicine
New York, New York

Robin Avery, M.D.
Attending physician
Boston Health Care for the Homeless
Boston, Massachusetts

Deirdre Bastible, M.D.
Attending physican
Department of Community Medicine
St. Vincent's Hospital and Medical Center of New York
New York, New York

Tom Bennett, M.D.
Project physician
Health Care for the Homeless
Boston City Hospital, HealthLink
Boston, Massachusetts

Deborah Benton, N.P.
Associate director of health services
Health Care for the Homeless Project
Chicago, Illinois

Barry Blackwell, M.D.
Professor and chairman
Department of Psychiatry
University of Wisconsin Medical School
Milwaukee, Wisconsin

Gary L. Blasi
Directing attorney
Homeless Unit of Legal Aid Foundation
of Los Angeles
Los Angeles, California

Penthea Bouma, N.P.
Philadelphia Health Management Corporation
Philadelphia, Pennsylvania

Sharon Brammer, F.N.P.
Birmingham Health Care for the Homeless
Birmingham, Alabama

William Breakey, M.D.
Director
Division of Social and Community Psychiatry
Johns Hopkins Medical Institute
Baltimore, Maryland

Ron Burris
Program director
Health Care for the Homeless
United Way
San Antonio, Texas

Jennifer Burroughs, M.S.N.
Boston Health Care for the Homeless
Program
Boston, Massachusetts

Randall Byrd, M.D.
Former medical director
Downtown Clinic
Nashville, Tennessee

Edward Cagan, M.D.
Attending physician
Department of Community Medicine
St. Vincent's Hospital and Medical Center of New York
New York, New York

Marsia Canto, M.S.W.
Project social worker
Philadelphia Health Management Corporation
My Brother's House—Shelter
Philadelphia, Pennsylvania

Michael R. Cousineau
Executive director
Los Angeles Homeless Health Care
Project
Los Angeles, California

John Crocco, M.D.
Director of Medicine, Jersey Shore Medical Center
Neptune, New Jersey

Robert W. Deisher, M.D.
Professor
Division of Adolescent Medicine
Department of Pediatrics
University of Washington School of Medicine
Seattle, Washington

Tom Detrano, C.S.W.
Department of Community Medicine
St. Vincent's Hospital and Medical Center of New York
New York, New York

Pat Doherty, R.N.
Department of Community Medicine
St. Vincent's Hospital and Medical Center of New York
New York, New York

Amy E. Duff, M.H.S.
Robert Wood Johnson Medical School
New Brunswick, New Jersey

Jed Emerson, M.S.W.
Executive director
Larkin Street Youth Center
San Francisco, California

Bob Erlenbush, Ph.D.
Program director
Los Angeles Homeless Health Care Project
Los Angeles, California

Almeta Fant
Project director
Health Care Project
Department of Health and Human Services
Newark, New Jersey

Camille Ferdinand, B.S.W.
SRO/Homeless Program
Department of Community Medicine
St. Vincent's Hospital and Medical Center of New York
New York, New York

Elaine Fox, M.A.
Project director
Philadelphia Health Management Corporation
Philadelphia, Pennsylvania

Tena Frank, M.S.W., D.C.S.W.
Director
Outreach Services to the Homeless
Lenox Hill Neighborhood Association, Inc.
New York, New York

Jacquelyn Gaines, M.S., C.R.N.P.
Executive director
Health Care for the Homeless, Inc.
Baltimore, Maryland

Mary Ann Gleason
Project director
Health Care for the Homeless
Colorado Coalition for the Homeless
Denver, Colorado

Hope Burness Gleicher
Former executive director
Health Care for the Homeless, Inc.
Baltimore, Maryland

Janelle Goetcheus, M.D.
Medical director
Christ House
Washington, D.C.

Andrew R. Greene
Vice-President for financial monitoring
Robert Wood Johnson Foundation
Princeton, New Jersey

Janet L. Groth
Public health nurse
Boston City Hospital, HealthLink
Boston, Massachusetts

Donald Hammersley, M.D.
Former deputy medical director
American Psychiatric Association
Bethesda, Maryland

Roger Hammond, M.D.
Psychiatrist
Albuquerque Health Care for the Homeless
Albuquerque, New Mexico

Karen Haught, M.D.
Attending physician
Department of Community Medicine
St. Vincent's Hospital and Medical Center of New York
New York, New York

Joan Haynes
Program coordinator
Health Care for the Homeless
Seattle King County Department of Health
Seattle, Washington

Richard W. Heim
Former senior vice-president
St. Joseph Healthcare Corporation
Albuquerque, New Mexico

Mary Hennessey, R.N.
Clinical instructor
University of Massachusetts College of Nursing
Boston, Massachusetts

Pauline Heslop, M.D.
Staff pediatrician
Covenant House
New York, New York

Tom Hickey
Project manager
Health Care for the Homeless Program
Coalition for Community Health Care
Milwaukee, Wisconsin

Mandy Johnson
Program director
Venice Family Clinic
Venice, California

Herman Joseph
Research scientist
Bureau of Research and Evaluation
New York State Division of Substance
  Abuse Services
New York, New York

Lawrence I. Kameya
Director of research
United Way Services
Cleveland, Ohio

F. Russell Kellogg, M.D.
Attending physician
Department of Community Medicine
St. Vincent's Hospital and Medical Cen-
  ter of New York
New York, New York

Mike Kelly
Staff member
Cleveland Health Care for the Homeless
  Program
Cleveland, Ohio

Angela Kennedy, Ph.D.
Director
Detroit Wayne County Community Men-
  tal Health Board
Detroit, Michigan

James T. Kennedy, M.D.
Former medical director
Covenant House and
Associate professor of clinical medicine
New York University School of Medi-
  cine
New York, New York

Stacy Kiyasu, R.N.
Nursing coordinator
Downtown Emergency Service Center
Seattle, Washington

Jill Koproski, R.N.
Formerly of the Department of Commu-
  nity Medicine
St. Vincent's Hospital and Medical Cen-
  ter
New York, New York

Mary Ann Lee, M.D.
Attending physician
Department of Community Medicine
St. Vincent's Hospital and Medical Cen-
  ter of New York
New York, New York

Armand H. Levin
Senior vice-president
Trust Division
Signet Bank Maryland
Baltimore, Maryland

Ada Lindsey, R.N., Ph.D.
Dean
University of California, Los Angeles
  School of Nursing
Los Angeles, California

John N. Lozier
Former project director
Health Care for the Homeless
Metro Health Department
Downtown Service Center
Nashville, Tennessee

John M. McAdam, M.D.
Attending physician
Department of Community Medicine
St. Vincent's Hospital and Medical Cen-
  ter of New York
New York, New York

Karen McGee
Project director
Birmingham Health Care for the Home-
  less
Birmingham, Alabama

Marsha McMurray-Avila
Project director
Albuquerque Health Care for the Home-
  less
Albuquerque, New Mexico

Bill Merritt
Outreach services coordinator
Health Care for the Homeless
United Way
San Antonio, Texas

Max Michael, M.D.
Medical director
Birmingham Health Care for the Homeless
Birmingham, Alabama

Maureen M. Mitchell, Ed.D., R.N.
Director of nursing and personal health care services
Bureau of Clinical Services
Cleveland Health Department
Cleveland, Ohio

Freda Mitchem
Coordinator
National Association of Community Health Centers, Inc.
Washington, D.C.

Susan Neibacher, C.S.W.
Project director
Health Care for the Homeless
United Hospital Fund of New York
New York, New York

James J. O'Connell, M.D.
Project director
Boston Health Care for the Homeless
Boston, Massachusetts

Eileen O'Connor, F.N.P.
New York Health Care for the Homeless Program
New York, New York

Sandra Orlin, N.P.
Philadelphia Health Management Corporation
Philadelphia, Pennsylvania

Donald W. Parsons, M.D.
Kaiser-Permanente Clinic
Denver, Colorado

Brenda Pelofsky
Vice-president
Swope Parkway Comprehensive and Mental Health Center
Kansas City, Missouri

Joseph Petrone, M.D.
Staff psychiatrist
Covenant House and
Department of Psychiatry
St. Vincent's Hospital and Medical Center of New York
New York, New York

Olga Piantieri, R.N.
SRO/Homeless Program
Department of Community Medicine
St. Vincent's Hospital and Medical Center of New York
New York, New York

Maria Pitaro, M.D.
Physician
Boston Health Care for the Homeless Program
Boston, Massachusetts

Robert Prentice, Ph.D.
Project director
Health Care for the Homeless
San Francisco Department of Public Health
San Francisco, California

Larry Prisco
Service center coordinator
Metro Health Department
Downtown Clinic
Nashville, Tennessee

John M. Raba, M.D.
Medical director
Cook County Jail
Cermak Health Services
Chicago, Illinois

Irwin Redlener, M.D., F.A.A.P.
Chief
Division of Ambulatory Pediatrics
New York Hospital-Cornell Medical Center
New York, New York

Lilia M. Reyes
Principal associate
United States Conference of Mayors
Washington, D.C.

William Vicic, M.D.
Attending physician
Department of Community Medicine
St. Vincent's Hospital and Medical Center of New York
New York, New York

Bruce C. Vladeck, Ph.D.
President
United Hospital Fund of New York
New York, New York

John B. Waller, Jr., Dr.P.H.
Associate professor and chairman
Department of Community Medicine
Wayne State University School of Medicine
Detroit, Michigan

Laura D. Waxman
Assistant executive director
United States Conference of Mayors
Washington, D.C.

Carol Martinez Weber, M.D.
Attending physician
Department of Community Medicine
St. Vincent's Hospital and Medical Center of New York
New York, New York

Dan Wlodarczyk, M.D.
Medical director
Health Care for the Homeless
San Francisco Department of Public Health
San Francisco, California

Stephen L. Wobido, C.S.W.
Coordinator
Homeless Service Training Program
Brookdale Center on Aging of Hunter College
New York, New York

Phyllis B. Wolfe
Project director
Health Care for the Homeless
Washington, D.C.

James D. Wright, Ph.D.
Favrot professor of human relations
Department of Sociology,
Tulane University
New Orleans, Louisiana

Catherine Zandler, B.A.
Executive director
Advocates for the Disabled
Phoenix, Arizona

Beth Zeeman, M.D.
Physician
Boston Health Care for the Homeless Program
Boston, Massachusetts

Bob Zmuda
President
Comic Relief
Los Angeles, California

PART I

THE CHALLENGE

MARSHA MCMURRAY-AVILA

Sleepin' in the Streets

Well, it's a '62 Chevy, it's a home for four
With a dog and two kids and another at the door
They were robbed last night on Central when the car broke down
Now they're sleepin' on a side street near downtown

Chorus
What can be done about this problem
They all say and wring their hands
It's a scar across the face of this land
Let's move 'em out, let's move 'em on
Let's keep it quiet, don't let on
That they are sleepin' in the streets
In the good ol' USA

Well, there's a bridge over the river, it's a home for four
Maybe seven maybe eight, and tonight maybe three more
With just a blanket between them and the hard cold graveled ground
They will wake up in the morning to this sound

Chorus

Well, she's twenty years and pregnant for the third time in a row
She was beat up by her husband, now she's got no place to go
She's too sick now to be workin' and too tired to even try
For the little help she'd get if she could only qualify

Chorus

Well he's an oilman from Texas, never knew the food stamp line
Till he lost his job last year and then his house and then his mind
Now he's traveled town to town to find some work in what he knows
But there's no job for a man without a home

Chorus

Well, there's a fella down the street who says he doesn't understand
Why those people live like that and no one wants to lend a hand
Give 'em food, give 'em shelter, give 'em jobs, it's not so hard
Just as long as it is not in my backyard

Chorus

Well, there's a president back east who says
It's plain for all to see
That those people live like that because that's where they want to be
And besides, there's no money in the budget for the poor
'Cause it's military aid we're voting for

Chorus

PHILIP W. BRICKNER

BRIAN C. SCANLAN

1

Health Care for Homeless Persons: Creation and Implementation of a Program

Introduction

Caring for homeless persons, protecting their health, treating them when they are ill, demands that we recognize and appreciate the inherent dignity of each as an individual human being. We must understand their goals for today and for the future, be sensitive to their needs, and comprehend the peculiarities of their life situations.

For human beings, shelter is essential for sustaining good health. If it is reasonable to believe that inadequate housing creates a threat to life and safety, and surely this is so, then it is a stark truth that those persons without shelter are at grave risk. Analyses of health status among homeless persons over the last several years[1–9] show, in fact, that indices for many diseases are far higher for them than for those who are housed.[10]

The medical disorders of the homeless are all the ills to which flesh is heir, magnified by disordered living conditions, exposure to extremes of heat and cold, lack of protection from rain and snow, bizarre sleeping accommodations, and overcrowding in shelters.[11]

Certain subgroups of the homeless, considered in further detail below, are especially at risk. Among these are children, pregnant women, and the mentally ill. The elderly are strikingly vulnerable. According to demographic studies of over 220,000 homeless persons examined at shelter clinics in nineteen cities across the United States through the Robert Wood Johnson Foundation/Pew Charitable Trusts (RWJF/Pew) National Health Care for the Homeless Program (HCHP) in the period 1985–89,[12] 3 to 4 percent are age sixty-five and older. This is a remarkable figure. For the population of our country at large, about 12 percent are in that age-group. Why is the percentage of the elderly homeless so low? What happened to the remainder? As James Wright points out in his 1989 book *Address Unknown: The Homeless in America*,[13] the shortfall among the elderly homeless may be explained in part by the fact that a number of entitlements become available at age sixty-five. These include Medicare and Social Security. These benefits may help some older persons leave the streets. Wright indicates, however, that premature mortality is likely as well. He notes: "Among 88 deaths occurring among clients seen in the HCHP, the average age of death was 51. Based on these findings, we can conclude that homeless men die some 20 or so years earlier than they should given normal life expectancies." One can only believe that while lack of shelter has a markedly harmful effect on human health, the elderly homeless are in double jeopardy.

One reason is that on the streets and in shelters, any person displaying weakness is a target. The elderly are often the first to go to the wall. More than twenty years ago, in 1969, staff members of one of the first free clinics for the homeless recognized this. The Greenwich Hotel in lower Manhattan, then a twelve-hundred-cubicle single room occupancy (SRO) building, housed young drug addicts (about five hundred of them, recently released from Rikers Island prison), some five hundred middle-aged chronic alcoholics, and about two hundred older men.

[The addicts] depended upon welfare payments as their only legitimate source of income and preyed upon the elderly . . . for money to support their addiction. The hotel management attempted to keep these groups separated . . . but access to all floors was easy. Consequently the younger, more aggressive men freely abused the others. At night the hotel became a jungle in which the aged and disabled barricaded themselves in their rooms or were subject to assault.[11]

Infection is a representative health problem in homeless persons. Infection may be defined accurately as a transmissible disorder caused by a virus, bacterium, parasite, or other agent. All people may be equally at risk of an infectious disorder by this simple definition. For homeless persons, however, other elements must also be considered causative. For instance, the physical settings in which the homeless may gather, such as large congregate shelters, allow the easy spread of disease vectors such as respiratory viruses, scabies and lice, and the tubercle bacillus. The physical deterioration that results from trauma, inadequate nourishment, exposure, and the inability to remain clean creates a bodily environment that allows infection to occur more easily. We all recognize as well that depression and anxiety alter the human biological balance, causing a receptivity to disease.

There is a remarkable parallel between the situation of homeless persons in the United States now and that of slaves in the pre-Civil War South:

The state of slave health depended not only on disease immunities and susceptibilities but also on living and working conditions. In the latter two matters, the South stood apart from the rest of the nation. Nowhere else did one group exert such great control over most aspects of their workers' lives as slaveowners and overseers had over the daily routines of their black slaves.

Most slaves on plantations or farms lived in a well-defined area known as the quarters. Here was a setting ideal for the spread of disease. At the slave quarters, sneezing, coughing, or contact with improperly washed eating utensils and personal belongings promoted transmission of disease-causing micro-organisms among family members. Poor ventilation, lack of sufficient windows for sunshine, and damp earthen floors added to the problem by aiding the growth of fungus and bacteria on food, clothing, floors, and utensils, and the development of worm and insect larvae. Improper personal hygiene (infrequent baths, hair-brushings, and haircuts, unwashed clothes, unclean beds) led to such nuisances as bedbugs, body lice (which also carried typhus germs), ringworm of skin and scalp, and pinworms.[14]

Creators of a health care program for the homeless must comprehend the virtues of providing this service and the resources required. They must develop an appreciation of the diversity among the homeless and define a pertinent taxonomy. They must also understand the nature of the prevalent clinical disorders, organize the physical setting, and recruit staff members appropriate to the needs of the persons served.

Who Are the Homeless?

Our definition of the homeless in this discussion includes:

- Skid row people, primarily men
- Patients discharged from mental hospitals
- The new homeless, purportedly without shelter because they are economic casualties
- Homeless youth
- Homeless women
- Homeless families
- The elderly homeless

People leading isolated lives in SRO hotels should be included. Where gentrification is taking place, SRO residents are at risk of being displaced to the streets. Furthermore, the similarities of personal conduct and illness between truly homeless individuals and those in marginal housing are striking.[11]

Skid Row

The most pervasive stereotype of the homeless person is the denizen of skid row. The term is derived from early Seattle's Skid Road, the saloon-lined thoroughfare down which logging teams slid their loads to a mill.[15] Skid row became an apt metaphor for the downhill course of the lives and health of its inhabitants. Alcoholism, trauma, and self-neglect are predominant characteristics of this largely male group.[16] Rough estimates suggest that the skid row population accounts for about 20 percent of the nation's homeless.[17,18] There is evidence that the classical profile of the skid row inhabitant is changing. For instance, in the early 1960's the typical client at New York City's Third Street Men's Shelter was a fifty-five-year-old white alcoholic.[16,19] Fifteen years later more than one-half of the shelter's population was under forty, nonwhite, and not alcoholic. A more recent retrospective study of the medical records kept by the men's shelter clinic[20] confirms the trends of decreasing age, decreasing prevalence of alcoholism, and increasing minority component.

Uncertainty exists regarding the growth trends of the skid row population. From the end of the Second World War until the mid-1960's, some observers noted a decrease in the numbers of people living on skid row.[21] The changes in philosophy and policy guiding the care of the mentally ill which have occurred over the past three decades, however, may have reversed this trend.[22] A study of clients at a Toronto mission shelter, based on information gathered in interviews and psychiatric evaluations, revealed that the younger men were significantly more likely to have received psychiatric care than those older.[21] Alcoholism may be a secondary diagnosis in an increasing proportion of primarily mentally ill younger men who have either been discharged from psychiatric facilities to the streets or have eluded formal diagnosis and treatment. Skid row may now indeed be "a microcosm of the former state hospital system."[19] If the trend toward youth and psychiatric disturbance continues, planning for health care services at skid row shelters will require additional emphasis on psychiatric treatment and attention to the medical problems of younger men, including adolescents.

Patients Discharged from Mental Hospitals

Deinstitutionalization of the mentally ill has had a tremendous influence on the numbers of homeless persons. The community mental health movement,[23–25] civil rights advocacy, and the revolution in psychopharmacology all contributed to the development of a belief among policy makers that institutional care of the chronically mentally ill could be replaced by more humane models based in the community. The concept of deinstitutionalization was embraced by policy makers as well, and by the mid-1960's federal legislation mandated the development of community mental health centers and initiated economic assistance to the psychiatrically disabled.[22] The development of a new philosophy of treatment, coupled with sweeping public policy decisions, set the stage for the return of large numbers of chronically ill patients to the community. In 1955 an estimated 560,000 people resided in psychiatric institutions; by 1984 this number had dropped to about 132,000.[26] The numbers also reflect the blocking of the road back to the state institutions; state judicial and legislative decisions[22] have since made the process of involuntary commitment more arduous.

However, comprehensive community-based psychiatric and medical care has not been implemented for most discharged mentally ill patients. Of the two thousand community mental health centers proposed, only eight hundred were ever funded, often without providing the full range of clinical services required of them by law.[27] Community resistance and hostility often posed political obstacles to the establishment of proposed centers, and patients became disaffiliated, beset with economic hardship, as the result of inadequate subsidies from federal, state, and local sources.

Shifting the locus of care to the community was prompted by well-documented excesses and failures of the state hospital system, but in the process the important function of asylum was lost for those incapable of caring for themselves. Reports from a number of urban centers suggest that the asylum function has in part been assumed by shelters for the homeless, which house large numbers of previously institutionalized patients, as well as mentally ill individuals who have eluded formal diagnosis and treatment.[28,29] The aberrant care-seeking behavior and withdrawal of many mentally ill persons, whether a feature of their illness or a product of the institutional experience,[22] pose significant challenges to care providers.

Irony abounds.[30] Manhattan State Hospital on Wards Island in New York City discharged many of its chronic patients to the streets during the past twenty years. It became an underutilized facility with empty buildings. At the same time the government of New York City lacked shelter space for a growing number of homeless persons. "Logic" prevailed, and the state leased the empty space to the city for a nominal sum. Now this city shelter, previously part of the state mental hospital system, houses in substantial number the same people who were previously wards of the state.[11]

The only essential distinction is that now they are labeled "homeless" rather than "mentally ill."

The New Homeless

The skid row inhabitants and the deinstitutionalized mentally ill are elements of virtually every urban population, but observers also describe numbers of homeless persons who do not fit the traditional models. Among the new homeless are those whose life on the streets or need for shelter in public facilities is primarily due to economic upheaval. The following case history from the Phoenix Health Care for the Homeless Program is illustrative:

———————

JR, a handsome fifty-five-year-old rugged-looking widowed Anglo male from Michigan, was asked on a number of occasions to consent to an interview. He repeatedly refused, citing numerous motives for the "real" purpose of the interviews, and despite reassurances, could not be persuaded until finally, one evening in the shelter TV room, he did tell his story. It went like this:

"I went through the Great War almost from the start in the South Pacific . . . in the navy. I worked for International Harvester as a machinist for thirty-five years. I had about three years to go to retirement and the company went bankrupt. You see, a few years ago I won a transfer to a new division of the company that made special parts. And it was the first to go. Some of the younger guys got other jobs, but I guess I was too old to retrain.

"My wife died five years ago, God rest her soul. She was sick for many years. I sold the big house and divided the dollars among three children. They're married and have children of their own . . . no, I can't impose on them . . . yes, I got unemployment, but I never went back to reapply. It just wasn't worth it. The hassle they put you through. As if you never worked and only sat home reading . . . all those people . . . always crowding . . . anyway, it wasn't enough to pay the rent on my small apartment. My kids wanted to help, but they're trying to make it, too, and I can't impose. Times are hard for them, too. When one of my sons found out that I was evicted, he was going to come and get me, so I took off. I just left. Oh, I drop them a line frequently, but I don't want them to know where I am till I get a job.

"Today I went out to work in the fields for a "short" hoe. My hands are all blisters, and my back has never hurt so much. I don't know if I can do that again. I can't sell. I never been able to sell anything. I just like to work, making things. . . . I don't mind being alone. In fact, I like it . . . if only I had a job."

The recession of the early 1980's, with its attendant unemployment reaching 10.8 percent in December 1982,[31] probably has contributed to homelessness, particularly in cities that experienced the permanent loss of unskilled and semi-skilled jobs with the closing of heavy industrial plants.[32] A trend toward longer duration of unemployment has also been cited as a potential influence on the pattern of homelessness, but exactly how any recent economic shift translates to homelessness is unclear.

Despite the well-publicized economic growth of the mid-1980's, including the addition of thousands of new jobs, the question remains whether the urban poor and the long-term unemployed have benefited.[33] Coupled with an occupancy rate for low- and middle-income housing stock that remains high, and no hint of improvement in the near future, joblessness and inadequate income may be expected to continue to contribute to homelessness. The possibility of a new recession adds to the threat.[34]

One particularly important aspect of the housing crisis is the loss of SRO hotels in virtually every major urban center. One million, or 50 percent, of the SRO units available in the United States at the beginning of the 1970's were lost by the end of that decade. In the same period New York City lost 81 percent of its SRO units to fire, demolition, new construction, and gentrification, and by July 1989 there remained only 52,000 such rooms,[35] of the approximately 250,000 that had existed two decades earlier. Previously it had been observed that roughly 10 percent of clients at New York City shelters had spent the previous night in an SRO hotel.[11,36]

Homeless Youth

There were an estimated 250,000 to 500,000 homeless youths, age twenty-one and under, in the United States in 1982. More current guesses are that up to 2 million youths may be homeless,[37,38] but the number is impossible to confirm.

The largest estimates include not only young people who run from home but also those who are kicked out (throwaways) and those whose homes evaporated because they grew too old for foster care placements. Homeless youths, in general, are alienated from their families and lack education and job skills. They are often ignored when the problem of homelessness is considered.

The health needs of homeless youth are sparsely documented, but to some extent this group reflects the general adolescent population, in that sexually transmitted disease, substance abuse, and nutritional disorders are frequently encountered. Trauma, including that associated with rape, sexual abuse, suicide, and attempted suicide, is frighteningly common among homeless youths. Homeless homosexual adolescents are subjected to rape and venereal disease and may be at particularly high risk for human immunodeficiency virus (HIV)-related disease. High rates of teenage pregnancy and aberrant parenting behavior similarly are the products of the failure to identify those at risk and to implement prevention strategies. Without intervention, many homeless youths surviving the violence of the streets are destined to homelessness in adulthood.[39]

Homeless Women

Women make up 20 to 27 percent or more of the total homeless population.[18,31] Factors that have led to a rise in the numbers of women seen in shelters and on the streets include deinstitutionalization, the loss of inexpensive housing, spouse abuse, and economic hardship resulting from sex and age discrimination.

While they share the risks to health experienced by their male counterparts, women living on the streets or in municipal shelters manifest distinctive problems. They are generally more easily victimized, assaulted, or raped;[40] both peripheral vascular disease and severe emotional illness appear to be more prevalent among women;[18,29,41] and homeless women often face pregnancy and child rearing alone.

Homeless Families

The "homeless family" is a euphemism for a woman with two to three children on average,[18,42] displaced from home by fire, abuse, or eviction. She is often pregnant. Sometimes the children are pregnant as well, but most are usually very young.

The families often suffer from an absolute absence of health services, despite the fact that many are Medicaid recipients. This is because they have been displaced to an unfamiliar area of their city into a form of shelter often lacking the requirements for family survival. The fear, anxiety, and confusion that result may drastically influence care seeking.

The consequences are pernicious. Many of the children lack immunizations, suffer from diverse skin infections, are poorly nourished and clothed. They are at substantial risk of victimization by predators in their hotel buildings. Those who are pregnant receive inadequate prenatal care. The result is often a low-birthweight baby who has decreased chances for survival and normal health.

The Elderly Homeless

Elderly homeless persons are perhaps less noticeable than other undomiciled individuals. The few relevant demographic analyses[18,37,43] reveal a marked diversity. Groups working with the elderly homeless have often chosen a definition based on age fifty-five and up. While this may seem peculiarly young, this choice of age for definition may reflect biological fact: Homelessness accelerates the process of aging. Older homeless persons include the few survivors of a life on skid row; men and women with chronic mental illness who lack access to asylum; economic casualties of job loss, no pensions, and no family supports; those whose low-income housing has fallen to gentrification; persons released from jail; and demented wanderers.

Access to Care

An elementary point demands notice in the development of programs of health care for the homeless: Health workers and patients must meet in order for care to be given. Many of the homeless do not seek attention at standard locations. For some, alienation, anger, anxiety, depression, or confusion creates barriers. For others, care of disease is of lower priority than obtaining a meal, looking for housing, or hunting for a job. Some homeless persons are so disabled by mental illness, alcoholism, or drug abuse that they are unable to keep appointments. The lack of money for transportation to a clinic or hospital is an effective bar to help for others.

To be frank, many medical institutions and staff members do not welcome the homeless. Hospitals and clinics must deal with financial considerations; in addition, some of the homeless are perceived to be objectionable patients for reasons of hygiene or conduct. As a result, individuals may find that their only recourse is at a county or municipal institution financed by the government, and usually the first contact is in an emergency room, a situation often doomed to failure. Picture this:

A homeless man with severe cellulitis of the legs, skin breakdown, and bilateral leg ulcers makes his way to the local hospital emergency room. Because he is not a genuine emergency, he waits for five hours. He loses his opportunity for lunch at a soup kitchen. He loses a bed for the night because he wasn't standing in line at the right time. He finally is examined by a physician and given a prescription for antibiotics, told to stay supine for a week with his legs elevated and soaked in warm dressings, and given a return appointment for clinic. The realities of his life prohibit him from carrying out any portion of this treatment plan.[44]

The frustration engendered by an emergency room visit is commonly experienced by patients, whether or not they are domiciled. For the homeless, however, the act of seeking health care at the only available site can, ironically, threaten their health and chance for survival.

If it is our true intention to give health care to the homeless, staff must go to where they are: shelters, soup kitchens, flophouses, public parks, train and bus stations, church basements. We must be prepared to offer solid, basic primary care services at these locations insofar as feasible and to take our patients to other sites of care and fight for fulfillment of their needs when that is indicated.

Access to services for the homeless through a health care program requires the following as a minimum:

- Professional health workers—usually a physician-nurse-social worker team—placed where the homeless are, willing to engage actively in case finding at these sites
- A hospital prepared to back up the program with a full set of services, including emergency room, clinics, psychiatric and medical inpatient care, laboratory and X-ray facilities, and a pharmacy
- Care given without regard to ability to pay
- Transportation to health service sites
- Sensitivity training for staff members[45]

Project Direction and Staffing

The Project Director

Here is the description of an impossible job: One individual is given the responsibility of hiring a diverse staff of health professionals to run a health care program, persons well qualified by experience and motivation to work with the poor. Work sites in deteriorated and unpleasant surroundings are the norm, situated in run-down sections of town. The staff members are to be kept happy and fulfilled despite the fact that many of their patients are recalcitrant, emotionally ill, drug-abusing, or alcoholic. Governance and oversight of this individual come from a broad range of community activists who have mixed agendas that may lead them to regard the needs of the health care program as secondary; the staff members may choose to bypass the project director and go directly to the governing board members to complain about personnel decisions. Local politicians, responsive to demands of the voting public, may be antagonistic to the presence of the project, its staff, and its clientele in the neighborhood.

These characteristics define the project director's job, and each of them has influenced the fate of project directors in the HCHPs. A project director must have a vision of the program and the ability to articulate it, through advocacy and dissemination of information. An understanding of the tasks and duties of each employee allows a director to facilitate direct service to patients.

Project directors have the toughest of jobs. Their success requires substantial interpersonal skill, stamina, courage, political savvy, and a sense of humor. The fatal bind—responsibility without authority—must be avoided.

The Staff

We assume that all program employees meet acceptable professional standards of education, experience, and licensure. The qualities that distinguish effective workers in HCHPs from those in other settings are usually maturity, motivation, and emotional balance. This opportunity for service demands as well an understanding of ourselves. Why did we choose to perform this work? What are our goals? What rewards can we expect?

Attitudes of health workers can interfere with the job, even when all other obstacles to care are cleared away. Most of the homeless are utterly destitute, and many are not able to present attractive appearances. In many instances the homeless are physically unclean or infested with lice, the result of living on the streets or moving from shelter to shelter. Physicians, nurses, and social workers, on the other hand, are likely to share life-styles and class values notably distinct from those of the homeless. Attitudes generated by differences between providers and clients tend to cause negative stereotyping of patients and can be harmful.

It takes an unusual degree of human understanding to remain engaged in this form of service when the commonplace measures of success are often absent. Patients may fail to follow through on therapeutic plans, miss important appointments, conduct themselves with anger toward staff. Gratitude is often in short supply. Boosting morale and providing positive feedback are, therefore, largely the responsibility of project directors and supervisors of the primary care givers.

Connecting the Program to a Full Range of Services

An effective HCHP defines its tasks broadly. To meet preventive and therapeutic goals, access to mental health and substance abuse services may be critically important. Obtaining dental, podiatric, and optometric care is also of great value. In addition, programs benefit from the establishment of strong connections to government agencies for obtaining entitlements and from effective contacts with general care hospitals.

Entitlements

The benefits of various entitlement programs may be essential to foster the hopes of homeless persons entering the mainstream of life in the United States. Medicaid purportedly gives access to health care for the poor. Does Medicaid work for the homeless? Often not.

In order for a person to receive Medicaid, two major obstacles must be overcome. He or she must have a stable address and proper documentation. The usual application process for Medicaid in New York, perhaps the least restrictive program in the country, requires an applicant to provide the following:

- Identification
- Current or past address
- Proof of citizenship
- Social Security card
- Evidence of disability, if any
- Indication of previous support by family or friends
- Past employment record
- Current income and financial resources, if any[45]

Requests for extensive documentation virtually guarantee noncompliance since few homeless persons carry or maintain timely records. Securing documents may be difficult for the homeless, estranged from families and out of touch with agencies able to replace lost or misplaced items. Entitlements may be out of reach for homeless persons unless they are assisted by savvy and aggressive advocates in the pursuit of documentation or unless standard documentation requirements are waived.

In order to overcome obstacles of this nature for their homeless patients, staff members must engage the personnel of government agencies. Employees of local Medicaid programs have proved willing to make regular site visits to a shelter in order to avoid the delays and intimidation inherent to the local government office. It has proved helpful in some instances to invite a high-level county or federal official of the social services or welfare agency to accept membership on the governance board. It pays to remember that government employees have personal qualities beyond their bureaucratic appearances and are often empathetic and eager to serve the homeless.

Working with Hospitals

When homeless persons require treatment at hospitals, problems relating to admission, compliance, length of stay, and payment for service often follow. Successful resolution of these matters varies with the individual patient's condition, the hospital chosen, and communication among all those involved in the care required. A review of the hospital's function and discussions with administrators and workers at shelter sites, hospitals, and government offices reveal the dimensions of the issues and provide specific suggestions for improving care of the homeless.[46]

An ideal hospitalization of a homeless person occurs when the need is evident, the hospital has a prior commitment to the homeless, financial arrangements are clear, the patient is compliant, the case is medically interesting, and a place exists for the patient to return to upon discharge. Most often, however, hospitalization for the homeless is problematic. The disgruntled house officer who wishes to avoid admissions, the nurse who dislikes caring for unappreciative patients, the trustee worrying about the reputation of the institution, and the administrator concerned about the financial life of the hospital all can present barriers to care for the homeless patient.

"Hospitals are composed of many types and levels of personnel."[46] To assure the best outcome for the homeless patient, the professional staff, admitting clerks, nurses, house officers, aides, utilization review committees, and business office administrators must work together. The task of establishing harmony among the diverse interest groups within the hospital is the shared responsibility of primary care givers and the HCHP governing body. Primary care givers can serve as advocates and case managers, but without the hospital's prior commitment to care for the homeless, frustration and neglect are likely to prevail.[46]

Conclusion

Relationship to Government and Long-Term Viability

All health services in our country swim in a government sea. HCHPs are no exception. Federal, state, and local governments control funds, license professional staffs, regulate premises, and mandate reporting requirements. This remains true despite the fact that much of the monies raised in support of this work may derive from private philanthropy.

Program staff and governance must therefore develop an effective working relationship with health and social services departments, entitlement officers, and elected officials to promote program viability. The passage of the Stewart McKinney Homeless Assistance Act, in 1987, is a noteworthy example, at the highest level, of effective working relationships between community agencies interested in the homeless and the legislative and executive branches of our national government.

Less dramatic local connections are fully as important. In regard to the ultimate test, long-term program viability, city and county health departments have been significant partners. For example, two of the nineteen Johnson/Pew programs, those in Nashville and San Francisco, have been integrated with their local health departments and appear to have gained permanent status.

Innovative Medicaid regulations in Arizona and Pennsylvania have given financial benefits to the HCHPs in Phoenix and Philadelphia. There geographical areas or specific zip codes where the poorest persons are congregated have been designated as beneficial targets for funding.

Examples of cooperation with government extend beyond cash. Personnel from relevant city, county, state, and federal agencies have been engaged—co-opted in a positive sense—by most of the Johnson/Pew projects to assist patients. They have helped ease registration for entitlements, entry into acute care hospitals, placement in long-term care facilities, participation in job-training programs, and finding permanent housing.

Negative consequences of relationships with government agencies must also be considered. The dead hand of regulation, complex and cumbersome documentation, arbitrary and pernicious changes in cash flow all have been known to occur. Government is an unreliable partner that one cannot do without.

In the face of stereotyping and easy negative generalizations about homeless persons, it is well to demand recognition of the individuality and character of each as a human being.[47,48] The possibilities of courage, determination, and grit—a sense of humor and spirit in the face of adversity—are noteworthy:

RR, a forty-eight-year-old black man with a past history of chronic alcoholism and schizophrenia, managed to find a room in the Keller Hotel in Manhattan, where a HCHP team grew to know him. This grim SRO is unclean and foreboding. Its stairwells are occasionally lit by twenty-watt bulbs. The residents tend to remain locked in their eight-by-eleven-foot rooms, afraid of drug-addicted predators. The manager surveys the entrance from behind wire, protected by two German shepherds.

RR, in contrast, managed to find some white paint and redecorated his room. He obtained a scrap of rug for the floor. He kept an Alaskan husky, impeccably groomed and well-trained, as a pet and for protection. He had crocheted a motto which he had framed and hung on the wall. It read: CUBICLE SWEET CUBICLE.

JAMES D. WRIGHT

2

The Health of Homeless People: Evidence from the National Health Care for the Homeless Program

Introduction

When the Robert Wood Johnson Foundation funded its national Health Care for the Homeless (HCH) demonstration program in 1985, it simultaneously contracted with the Social and Demographic Research Institute (SADRI) of the University of Massachusetts to undertake a four-year program of research on the health aspects of homelessness. The intent was not primarily to evaluate the HCH demonstration program; indeed, it was obvious even at the design stage that HCH was probably not evaluable in conventional "impact assessment" terms.[1] The intent, rather, was to exploit the research opportunity provided by the existence of HCH to address a range of unanswered questions. Here we summarize the principal findings from the ensuing research effort; a more complete account of methods and findings than is possible here may be found in the reference in Note 2.

The recent report of the Institute of Medicine[3] and the research summarized in that report[2,4,5] have made it clear that health and homelessness are linked together in three important ways. First, ill health, physical as well as mental, can be a cause of homelessness in many cases. Secondly, homelessness indisputably causes a great deal of physical illness. Thirdly, whatever the paths of cause and effect, the material conditions of homelessness greatly complicate the delivery of adequate primary health services. I touch on each of these in the following pages, but my focus is principally on the second, on homelessness as a risk factor in physical illness.

Poor physical health is not the most important or pressing problem homeless people face, falling at least behind shelter and nutrition on the agenda of human concerns. It is nonetheless obvious that many homeless people have severe, largely unmet primary health care needs and, moreover, that attention to physical health may play an important role in attempts to address many other problems. Many homeless people are simply too ill to be placed in employment or other counseling programs, too ill to stand in line while their applications for benefits are being processed, too ill to search for housing within their means. The extreme poverty of the homeless[6-8] also severely limits their access to conventional health care, as do their general disaffiliation and estrangement from society and its institutions. Thus, no comprehensive program of services to the homeless can be indifferent to health care needs.

Prior Research

Relevant research on health aspects of homelessness up through about 1984 is summarized in the reference in Note 4: "The information base about health problems of the homeless is rudimentary. . . . Studies of derelicts have produced many a Ph.D. thesis. In all this work, however, there is rarely a comment about health or disease. The same vacuum exists in the 957 pages of the 1982 *Congressional Hearings on Homelessness in America.*"[4]

The information base has developed impressively since 1984, and it now consists of perhaps a half dozen major studies and several scores of journal articles. In nearly all cases these more recent researches have only confirmed earlier, tentative conclusions: The homeless are subjected to uncertain and often inadequate provisions for simple acts of daily hygiene, communal bathing and eating facilities, unsafe, unsanitary shelters, exposure to the social environment of the streets, general debilitation and susceptibility to infection, inadequate diet, no access to a home medicine cabinet with its usual stock of palliatives, no place to go for bed rest, too much smoking and drinking, and absence of family networks and other support groups to fall back on in times of illness, crushing poverty, and no health insurance. But the basic conclusion remains intact. It is, indeed, a safe assertion that no aspect of homelessness is actually *good* for a person's health. Most of the material and existential conditions of homelessness are, in one or another way, strongly detrimental to physical well-being.[9-27]

Research Design and Procedures

A detailed account of the methods and procedures of the HCH research effort is given in Chapter 3 of the reference in Note 2. For technical reasons, data from two of the nineteen HCH cities are not included in the present analysis.* Program-wide, between start-up and the end of data collection in December 1987, nearly a hundred thousand homeless and destitute clients were seen in HCH clinics a total of three hundred thousand times. The data presented here are based on about sixty-three thousand clients seen in seventeen project cities.

Most encounters with most clients generated information about health and related problems that was recorded on contact forms and submitted to the research team for coding, entry, and analysis. The contact forms were, in essence, medical progress notes. Extraction of medical information from these notes was done exclusively by registered nurses. The HCH client population is in the first instance a *clinical* population, consisting of homeless and destitute persons who, for what-ever reason, sought health attention in the HCH clinics; thus, our clients may well differ from homeless people in general in any number ways. There are, however, no gross differences between homeless people in general and HCH clients specif-ically on any variable we have been able to examine.[2] We therefore treat the health problems of HCH clients as characteristic (if not strictly representative) of the health problems of the larger homeless population.

Table 2.1 shows the distribution of contacts with clients over the course of the demonstration program. Although data were collected for almost three years, the average client was seen in only one of those years; moreover, while the average client was seen altogether a bit more than three times, a large number (46 percent) were seen once and only once.† Many of these one-time contacts occurred in large-scale screening efforts (as, for example, when an entire shelter population was screened for hypertension in a single evening). In other cases, clients pre-

Table 2.1 PATTERNS OF CLIENT CONTACTS
(*N = 17 cities, adults only*)

NUMBER OF CONTACTS	TOTAL	MEN	WOMEN
One	45.6	45.6	45.7
Two	19.9	20.0	19.4
Three	9.7	10.0	9.0
Four	6.1	6.2	5.9
Five or More	18.7	18.1	20.0
N =	61,238	43,356	17,882

*Three of the HCH cities were computerized independently of SADRI's data system. In two cases the medical problem codes used for data processing were very different from the codes used by SADRI, so that translation from one set of codes to the other is possible only with the grossest of categories. Translation at the level of detail utilized in this report is *not* possible; hence the two cities are omitted from this analysis.

†The pattern of contact mirrors the transitory nature of homelessness itself. Contrary to popular imagery, most homeless people are not chronically homeless; the majority are episodically homeless, with periods of occasional homelessness punctuated by stretches of a more or less stable housing situation. See reference to Note 2, page 54, for data.

sented minor health problems requiring over-the-counter palliatives (e.g., cough syrup) or simple first aid (minor cuts, abrasions). In these and other similar cases, extensive probing about other, more serious health issues was often inappropriate, even counterproductive.

The ability of care providers to engage homeless clients in a system of continuous health care depends crucially on establishing rapport and trust, this in a population that by nature tends to be suspicious and disaffiliated. To the extent that extensive, detailed probing about health issues would interfere with the building of an appropriate relationship with a client, it is naturally and understandably avoided.* The point is that there are strict limits to the amount of health information likely to be obtained from a client in a brief, one-time encounter.

The methodological implication of these points is that most, if not all, disorders would normally be underdiagnosed in the first few visits with a client. We have examined this issue in considerable depth. In fact, the rates of occurrence of every disorder we have examined increase with the number of client contacts.[2] In order to provide a reasonably reliable and complete health picture, we therefore restrict all that follows to the subset of clients, about half, who were seen at least more than once.

Continuity of Care

The statistically average client was seen about three times in one year; that is an impressive achievement in continuity of care for a traditionally hard-to-reach population. Among the "more stable" client base, those seen at least twice, the average number of contacts was approximately 4.4 per year. This compares favorably with (indeed, is somewhat higher than) the U.S. adult average; among U.S. adults seen at least once by a doctor in a year, the average number of visits is about 3.[28]

The HCH research design specified a number of "tracer" conditions that were to be given special attention, among them tuberculosis, hypertension, diabetes, pregnancy, seizure disorders, and peripheral vascular disease (PVD). The average number of contacts is higher among clients afflicted with any of the tracer pathologies than among the remaining clients. Among those with hypertension or seizure disorders, the average is about five contacts per client (per year), and for those with tuberculosis, PVD, or diabetes, about six per client (per year). The average for pregnant patients is relatively low, only about four, but this is because pregnant clients were referred very quickly to other, more appropriate systems of care. (Indeed, the average elapsed time between first and last contact for pregnant women was barely a month.)

Clients with any of the tracer disorders were also much more likely than other clients to be referred to outside health facilities and in some cases—diabetes, pregnancy, and TB, in particular—the referral rates were very close to 100 per-

---

* As one homeless woman put it, "I just came here for the doctor to look at my eyes. What does that have to do with where I was born or my mother's name before she got married?" The case is reported in the reference in Note 27.

cent. We have no direct evidence on how many of these referral appointments were kept or on their outcomes. For what it is worth, care providers assessed clients with the tracer disorders as being more compliant with treatments on the average than other clients.

How any of these patterns compare with the larger population is hard to say. Among the "more stable" client base, somewhat more than half were given at least one referral in the average year; about 80 percent of these referrals were medical (as opposed to social or mental health) referrals. In the 1985 National Ambulatory Medical Care Survey (NAMCS), roughly 6 percent of the office visits recorded in the data were effectuated by referrals from another physician or health care facility; in turn, about 5 percent of the office visits were resolved by referral to another physician or by hospitalization. These results suggest that the use of referral services was *much* more widespread in HCH than in customary ambulatory practice.

Social and Demographic Characteristics of the Client Population

A detailed social and demographic analysis of the HCH client population has been published in the reference in Note 29. Perhaps the most consistent demographic finding in the recent literature is that the homeless are quite young, in contrast with a common stereotype. All recent studies have reported an average age somewhere in the thirties; in the HCH data the median age is about thirty-three.[30] Nearly 15 percent of the clients were children and youth aged nineteen or less; a tenth were dependent children under the age of twelve.

A second demographic fact of some significance is the proportion of women, amounting to 27 percent of all adults. Most recent studies[30-33] have also reported sizable numbers of homeless women, many of them with dependent children. Many of these women are victims of physical or sexual abuse; many likewise have lengthy psychiatric histories. Indeed, the rate of psychiatric disorder among HCH women, about 40 percent, is nearly twice that of the men (about 20 percent).

The racial composition of the HCH client base varied widely from city to city, reflecting underlying true differences in the racial composition of each city's poverty population. Across all projects and years, the clients split nearly fifty-fifty between whites and nonwhites, but in some projects the proportions of nonwhites exceeded 80 percent. About 38 percent of all clients were black, 12 percent were Hispanics, and 3 percent were American Indians. The corresponding percentages for the national population are 11.7, 6.4, and 0.6 respectively, so racial and ethnic minorities are heavily overrepresented. This, too, is a widely reported finding.[6]

Two additional and somewhat unexpected findings of some apparent significance are, first, that more than half the clients over twenty-five had at least a high school education (nearly 20 percent had one or more years of college) and, second, that only about half received any form of entitlement, welfare benefit, or other governmental assistance.[34] Many of the homeless have truly "fallen between the cracks" of the American welfare state.

Alcohol, Drug Abuse, and
Mental Health (ADM) Disorders

Alcoholism and mental illness have come to figure prominently in discussions of homelessness and in common stereotypes about homeless people.[35–37] Indeed, many accounts make it seem that nearly all homeless people are alcoholic or psychiatrically disabled, or both. This is unquestionably an exaggeration, but it is undeniable that alcohol abuse and mental illness are among the leading health problems homeless people face.

How many homeless people are alcoholic? Drug-abusive? Mentally ill? Our ability to answer these questions is compromised by the underdiagnosis problem discussed earlier.* It is easy to show the proportion of clients actually diagnosed with these disorders. But what can then be inferred about their true rate of occurrence within the homeless population?

Details on the methodology used to correct our estimates for underdiagnosis are published elsewhere.[2,14] The basic approach was to sort out all clients who had been seen at least five times *and* were known to be alcoholic, drug-abusive, or mentally ill and then to reconstruct the visit history for each of those clients, noting the actual contact at which the ADM diagnosis was first made. To illustrate, among 1,625 clients who were known to be mentally ill and who were seen five or more times in the first year of the program, only 43.7 percent were diagnosed as mentally ill *on the first visit;* 58.7 percent were diagnosed as mentally ill on *either the first or second visit;* nearly a quarter went undiagnosed until the fifth or later visit.

In view of these findings, it is then an easy step to a "best guess" about the true occurrence rates. Among all clients seen only once, for example, 11.2 percent were diagnosed as mentally ill. Since only 43.7 percent of the mentally ill are diagnosed as such on their first visit, our best guess about the rate of mental illness among clients seen just once is therefore 11.2 percent divided by 0.437, or 25.6 percent. Similar calculations may be made for clients seen twice, three times, and so on. Averaging estimates across visit groupings then produces a "best guess" about the population as a whole.

Results of these calculations suggest that 38 percent of the HCH clients are alcohol-abusive, 13 percent abuse drugs other than alcohol, and 33 percent are mentally ill. The rates differ significantly by gender. Thus 47 percent of the adult men but only 16 percent of the adult women are alcoholic; conversely, psychiatric illness is about twice as common among the women as among the men. Rates of drug abuse other than alcohol were nearly identical.†

Differences in the rates of ADM disorders by background characteristics other than gender were largely inconsequential. Alcohol abuse is curvilinear with age, being lowest among the young and old and highest among those of middle age.

---

*The underdiagnosis of various medical disorders in the early visit history with a client is apparently well known in the medical literature and is by no means confined to homeless clients. See Note 35.

†The same is largely true of the general population; among U.S. adults as a whole, alcoholism is more common among men, and psychiatric morbidity is more common among women.[36,37]

Drug abuse is most common (by far) among younger homeless persons (both sexes) and falls off rapidly with age. Of perhaps some interest, mental illness among homeless women is lowest among the young and increases with age, whereas among men the opposite pattern obtains.

As might be expected, the rates of most physical disorders are elevated among the alcohol- and drug-abusive and likewise among the mentally ill.[9,10,38] Further compounding the problem is a substantial overlap among all three of the ADM disorders; most of the drug abusers also abuse alcohol, rates of alcoholism are higher among the mentally ill than among the mentally healthy, etc.[39]

Physical Health Status

Basic epidemiological data on the health status of HCH clients is shown in Table 2.2 (acute physical disorders), Table 2.3 (chronic physical disorders), and Table 2.4 (infectious and communicable diseases relevant to the question of public health). The format of each table is the same: Cell entries show the percentages of HCH clients who have been diagnosed with the various disorders listed in the rows. The first column shows these percentages for the total adult sample regardless of number of contacts; the second column shows the corresponding percentages for adult clients seen more than once. Columns three and four present the data separately for men and women; columns five and six compare whites and nonwhites; columns seven through ten show the differences by age. For comparison, the right-most column shows the corresponding percentages for urban adults in NAMCS.[40]

Three general points about these tables require emphasis:

1. As mentioned above, the measured rate of *every disorder* shown in these tables is higher among clients seen more than once than among the total adult client base. I have already stated the reasons why the results for clients seen more than once are probably more representative, but it must also be acknowledged that this is mainly a judgment, not an empirical necessity.

2. In most cases, the rates at which these disorders appear in the HCH data are higher than the rates at which they appear in the NAMCS data; this tends to be true whether the comparisons are with the HCH totals or for those seen more than once. The homeless, in short, are generally more ill than the "normal" adult ambulatory population more or less across the board.

3. Observed differences across HCH subgroups reproduce well-known epidemiological patterns. Chronic disorders known to increase with age (diabetes, cardiac disorders, hypertension, chronic obstructive pulmonary disease, arthritis, etc.) do increase with age in the HCH data; likewise, disorders known to be linked to gender (diabetes, obesity, hypertension, traumas) or to ethnicity (hypertension, tuberculosis) show the expected patterns.

Acute Physical Disorders

Consistent with expectation, prior research, and the informal sense of many HCH care providers, the most common acute ailments presented by HCH clients

Table 2.2 RATES OF OCCURRENCE OF ACUTE PHYSICAL
DISORDERS IN THE HCH CLIENT POPULATION
(*N = 17 cities, adult clients only*)

| | | | | | | ADULTS SEEN MORE THAN ONCE | | | | | |
| | ALL | | | | | NOT | | AGE-GROUP | | | |
	ADULTS	TOTAL	MEN	WOMEN	WHITE	WHITE	I	II	III	IV	NAM
(N =)	63079	33682	23575	9711	16048	17634	10722	16941	4999	1020	499
Percent diagnosed with:											
INF	0.4	0.5	0.5	0.6	0.5	0.6	0.7	0.5	0.5	—	(
NUTDEF	1.5	2.3	2.1	2.8	2.4	2.2	1.9	2.3	2.8	4.1	(
OBESE	1.4	2.1	1.3	4.0	2.4	1.8	1.7	2.3	2.5	1.2	1
MINURI	24.4	32.9	32.6	33.5	35.3	30.7	33.0	33.4	33.2	20.8	5
SERRI	2.5	3.7	3.9	3.3	4.4	3.1	3.1	4.0	4.3	2.9	(
MINSKIN	10.6	15.3	15.2	15.4	16.5	14.1	15.7	15.2	14.7	14.0	(
SERSKIN	3.9	5.9	6.6	4.1	7.2	4.7	5.7	6.3	5.2	4.0	(
TRAUMA											
ANY	18.9	25.1	28.2	18.0	26.8	23.6	24.3	26.2	24.5	20.0	8
FX	3.9	5.5	6.6	3.1	6.1	5.0	4.5	5.8	6.9	4.9	2
SPR	4.8	6.8	7.1	6.2	7.3	6.4	6.8	7.2	6.3	4.3	3
BRU	4.5	6.2	6.7	5.3	6.6	5.9	6.6	6.2	5.8	5.0	1
LAC	6.8	9.4	11.4	4.9	9.7	9.2	9.1	10.0	8.8	7.5	(
ABR	2.2	3.3	3.7	2.4	4.0	2.6	3.3	3.3	3.4	3.0	(
BURN	1.0	1.5	1.7	1.1	1.8	1.2	1.5	1.6	1.5	1.2	(

Note • For explanation of columns and abbreviations, see *Notes*, Table 2.4.

are upper respiratory infections (33 percent), followed by traumas (25 percent) and minor skin ailments (15 percent).* More serious skin ailments are also very common (4 percent). All these health problems are very much more widespread among HCH clients than among NAMCS patients (in part, because many of them are ailments that a domiciled individual would self-treat) and are almost certainly referable to exposure to the environment inherent in a homeless existence.

Upper respiratory infections (URIs) of varying severity are endemic to homelessness and are observed among all subgroups in nearly equal proportions. The true rate of these disorders among the homeless is probably higher than shown, since many homeless people would not bother to go to clinic for minor ailments of this sort. In most cases, minor URIs are treated with over-the-counter palliatives that a person with disposable income would purchase in any drugstore. In these cases it is extreme poverty more than illness itself that causes homeless people to come to the HCH for treatment.

Lacerations and wounds are the most common of the traumas (9 percent), followed by sprains (7 percent), bruises (6 percent), and fractures (6 percent).

* All of the overall percentages given in the text throughout the following sections are for clients seen more than once.

Table 2.3 RATES OF OCCURRENCE OF CHRONIC
PHYSICAL DISORDERS IN THE HCH CLIENT POPULATION
(*N = 17 cities, adult clients only*)

	ALL ADULTS	\multicolumn{9}{c}{ADULTS SEEN MORE THAN ONCE}	NAMCS

	ALL ADULTS	TOTAL	MEN	WOMEN	WHITE	NOT WHITE	I	II	III	IV	NAMCS
(=)	63079	33682	23575	9711	16048	17634	10722	16941	4999	1020	49903
rcent diagnosed with:											
ANYCHRO	28.1	37.0	37.2	36.5	37.5	36.6	22.6	38.0	59.8	59.8	26.7
CANC	0.5	0.7	0.7	0.9	1.0	0.5	0.3	0.6	1.8	1.9	3.8
ENDO	1.4	2.2	1.5	4.0	2.6	1.8	1.7	2.2	2.9	3.9	1.5
DIAB	2.3	3.0	2.8	3.5	2.8	3.1	1.0	3.2	6.1	5.7	3.0
ANEMIA	1.3	2.0	1.4	3.5	1.8	2.2	2.1	1.8	2.4	3.1	0.7
NEURO	1.3	1.9	1.9	1.9	2.2	1.7	1.4	2.1	2.5	2.6	2.4
NEUROSYM	4.5	6.7	6.0	8.4	6.6	6.8	6.3	6.8	7.0	7.8	NA
SEIZ	3.9	5.1	5.5	4.1	5.2	5.0	3.7	5.9	6.1	2.6	0.1
EYE	6.4	9.5	10.0	8.2	9.2	9.7	7.5	9.1	13.8	15.0	15.4
EAR	3.7	5.4	5.2	6.0	6.7	4.3	5.8	5.1	5.3	6.9	2.0
HTN	10.9	14.4	15.2	12.4	12.0	16.5	4.6	15.4	29.0	27.4	6.5
CVA	0.5	0.7	0.7	0.5	0.8	0.5	0.1	0.6	1.7	2.5	0.6
COPD	4.3	6.0	6.0	6.1	7.7	4.6	3.9	5.3	12.1	11.9	2.5
GI	6.1	8.9	9.4	8.1	10.3	7.7	7.7	9.2	10.7	9.0	4.2
GISYM	4.8	7.4	6.4	9.8	7.8	7.0	7.3	7.0	8.5	7.5	NA
TEETH	8.6	11.5	11.8	11.1	11.3	11.7	12.0	12.3	9.0	6.0	0.4
LIVER	1.7	2.5	2.9	1.5	2.2	2.7	1.5	3.0	3.0	1.7	0.2
GENURI	4.3	6.6	4.5	11.9	6.9	6.4	8.8	5.6	5.1	9.2	3.6
MALEGU	1.7	2.6	2.6	—	2.2	2.8	3.5	2.0	2.5	4.3	6.4
FEMGU	11.5	16.7	—	16.7	17.6	15.9	21.2	15.9	7.9	2.0	5.8
PREG	10.1	12.2	—	12.2	11.0	14.4	23.4	5.9	0.3	—	7.1
PVD	3.2	4.8	5.0	4.3	5.6	4.0	2.0	4.9	8.7	11.9	1.1
ARTHR	3.6	5.3	5.2	5.8	5.5	5.2	1.8	4.7	13.5	13.4	4.0
OTHMS	6.2	9.4	9.9	8.1	10.7	8.1	7.4	9.6	12.8	10.4	7.0

Note • For explanation of columns and abbreviations, see *Notes,* Table 2.4.

Trauma of all types is more common among men than among women and slightly more common among young than old, patterns that are in turn no doubt linked to age and gender differences in aggressive behavior. While some of the traumas shown here are minor injuries of the sort that a domiciled individual would choose to self-treat, most are fairly serious injuries requiring medical attention in any case.

Nutritional deficiencies (mainly malnutrition and vitamin deficiencies) are

Table 2.4 RATES OF INFECTIOUS AND COMMUNICABLE DISORDERS IN THE HCH CLIENT POPULATION
(N = 17 cities, adult clients only)

| | ALL ADULTS | ADULTS SEEN MORE THAN ONCE | | | | | | | | | |
		TOTAL	MEN	WOMEN	WHITE	NOT WHITE	I	II	III	IV	NAM(
(N=)	63079	33682	23575	9711	16048	17634	10722	16941	4999	1020	4990
Percent diagnosed with:											
AIDS	0.2	0.2	0.3	0.1	0.2	0.2	0.2	0.3	0.1	—	0
HIV+	0.1	0.2	0.2	0.1	0.1	0.2	0.2	0.2	—	—	N
ACTTB	0.6	1.0	1.2	0.4	1.0	1.0	0.5	1.1	1.5	1.3	0.
ANYTB	3.5	5.7	7.1	2.6	4.5	7.0	3.2	6.0	9.6	7.9	N
VDUNS	1.3	1.9	1.0	4.1	1.9	1.9	3.5	1.5	0.6	0.5	1.
SYPH	0.2	0.4	0.3	0.5	0.1	0.6	0.4	0.4	0.2	0.2	0.
GONN	0.6	0.8	0.7	1.2	0.7	1.0	1.8	0.5	0.1	—	0.
ANYSTD	1.9	2.9	1.9	5.4	2.6	3.3	5.2	2.2	0.8	0.6	1.
INFPAR	0.4	0.5	0.5	0.6	0.5	0.6	0.7	0.5	0.5	—	0
ANYPH	14.4	21.1	22.6	18.6	22.7	19.9	20.5	21.4	21.7	20.0	3

1. COLUMNS

The first column shows data for all adult clients ever seen (N = 17 cities), regardless of number of contacts.

The next nine columns show data for adult clients seen more than once (N = 17 cities), first for the total, then by gender, then by race, then by age. Age-groups are as follows: I = 16–29; II = 30–49; III = 50–64; IV = 64+.

The last (right-most) column shows corresponding data for adult respondents in urban areas from the National Ambulatory Medical Care Survey.

NA = not available.

2. ROWS

The top row in each table gives sample sizes for each relevant group. Acronyms and abbreviations for the remaining row entries follow:

Acute disorders
INF	Infestational ailments (e.g., scabies, lice)
NUTDEF	Nutritional deficiencies (e.g., malnutrition, vitamin deficiencies)
OBESE	Obesity
MINURI	Minor upper respiratory infections (common colds and related symptoms)
SERURI	Serious respiratory infections (e.g., pneumonia, influenza, pleurisy)
MINSKIN	Minor skin ailments (e.g., sunburn, contact dermatitis, psoriasis, corns and calluses)
SERSKIN	Serious skin disorders (e.g., carbuncles, cellulitis, impetigo, abscesses)
TRAUMA	Injuries
ANY	Any trauma
FX	Fractures
SPR	Sprains and strains
BRU	Bruises, contusions
LAC	Lacerations, wounds
ABR	Superficial abrasions
BURN	Burns of all severities

Chronic disorders
ANYCHRO	Any chronic physical disorder

CANC	Cancer, any site
ENDO	Endocrinological disorders
DIAB	Diabetes mellitus
ANEMIA	Anemia and related disorders of the blood
NEURO	Neurological disorders, not including seizures (e.g., Parkinson's disease, multiple sclerosis, neuritis, neuropathies)
NEUROSYM	Symptoms of neurological disorder without firm diagnoses
SEIZ	Seizure disorders (including epilepsy)
EYE	Disorders of the eyes (e.g., cataracts, glaucoma, decreased vision)
EAR	Disorders of the ears (e.g., otitis, deafness, cerumen impaction)
HTN	Hypertension
CVA	Cerebrovascular accidents/stroke
COPD	Chronic obstructive pulmonary disease
GI	Gastrointestinal disorders (e.g., ulcers, hernias)
GISYMP	Symptoms of GI disorders without firm diagnoses
TEETH	Dentition problems (predominantly caries)
LIVER	Liver diseases (e.g., cirrhosis, hepatitis, ascites, enlarged liver or spleen)
GENURI	General genitourinary problems common to either sex (e.g., kidney, bladder problems, incontinence)
MALEGU	Genitourinary problems found among men (e.g., penile disorders, testicular dysfunction, male infertility)
NOTE:	Data on MALEGU shown in the table are for *men only* in all cases.
FEMGU	Genitourinary problems found among women (e.g., ovarian dysfunction, genital prolapse, menstrual disorders)
PREG	Pregnancies
NOTE:	Data on FEMGU and PREG shown in the table are for *women only* in all cases.
PVD	Peripheral vascular disease
ARTHR	Arthritis and related problems
OTHMS	All musculoskeletal disorders other than arthritis

Infectious and communicable disorders

AIDS	Autoimmune deficiency syndrome
HIV+	HIV positivity without an AIDS diagnosis
ACTTB	Active tuberculosis infection, any site
ANYTB	Active tuberculosis, history of TB, prophylactic TB therapy without a TB diagnosis, or unresolved positive PPD (tuberculin) test
VDUNS	Unspecified venereal disease, herpes
SYPH	Syphilis
GONN	Gonorrhea
ANYSTD	VDUNS or SYPH or GONN, or any combination
INFPAR	Infectious and parasitic diseases
ANYPH	Either AIDS or TB or ANYSTD or INFPAR or SERURI or INF or SERSKIN or any combination of these

observed in about 2 percent of the clients (vs. 0.1 percent of the NAMCS patients). These disorders tend to increase slightly with age. Obesity is a bit less common than malnutrition (in these data) and is more widespread among women than men.

Programwide, the daily project work load was heavily dominated by the treatment of the above and related acute disorders. The contact form asked HCH care providers to characterize the client's primary medical problem as either chronic or acute. Among the primary problems for which we have these data, two-thirds were judged acute and the remaining one-third was chronic. This is apparently similar to the situation in regular ambulatory medical practice.*

---

*In the 1979 NAMCS the "major reason for visit" was treatment of a chronic condition in 37.6 percent of all cases.[40]

Chronic Physical Disorders

Among all clients regardless of number of contacts, 28 percent have at least one chronic physical disorder; among clients seen more than once, the figure is 37 percent; and among NAMCS patients, 27 percent. We infer from these data that chronic physical disease, like chronic alcohol abuse and chronic mental illness, is also more common among the homeless than among the domiciled population.

Chronic disorders (all types combined) are about equally common among HCH men and women and are also about equally common among nonwhites and whites. In contrast, the prevalence of these disorders increases sharply with age, reaching about 60 percent among those over fifty.

The principal chronic disorders treated in the HCH projects are hypertension, arthritis and other musculoskeletal disorders, problems with dentition, gastrointestinal ailments, peripheral vascular disease, neurological disorders, eye disorders, genitourinary problems, musculoskeletal ailments, ear disorders, and chronic obstructive pulmonary disease. In most cases the HCH rate exceeds the NAMCS rate, usually by a substantial margin.

Hypertension is more common among men than women, is more common among nonwhites than whites, and increases sharply with age.[41] The disorder is also very much more common among alcohol abusers than nonabusers. In NAMCS 6.5 percent are hypertensive; thus, the homeless are two to four times more likely to suffer the disorder than the domiciled population.

The elevated incidence of hypertension in the HCH population is not exclusively a function of the high rate of alcohol abuse, although that is certainly a major contributory factor. Among *non*-alcohol-abusing HCH men, the rate of hypertension is over 12 percent and thus exceeds the NAMCS rate by an approximate factor of two.

Gastrointestinal Disorders include a wide-ranging mixture of chronic and acute disorders and symptoms. Differences across subgroups are minor. Here, too, there is an obvious link to alcohol abuse, but the rates for nonabusing HCH clients still exceed the NAMCS rate (data not shown). In short, even if we set aside the alcoholics, the homeless are two to three times more likely to suffer these disorders than the domiciled ambulatory population.

Peripheral Vascular Disease is perhaps *the* characteristic chronic physical disorder associated with a homeless existence.[42] Again, the category contains a wide range of specific disorders (varicosities, phlebitis, thrombosis, chronic edema, cellulitis of the extremities, gangrene), each sharing a common origin—namely, venous or arterial deficiencies in the extremities. In the HCH data these disorders are somewhat more common among men and whites than among women and nonwhites and, like most chronic disorders, increase regularly with age. Compared with the NAMCS data, PVD is four to five times more common among the homeless than among the population at large.

Although alcohol abusers are more prone to PVD than nonabusers, the differences are relatively slight. The inordinately high rate of PVD among the homeless is not primarily the result of alcohol abuse but can be traced directly to life-style considerations.

Poor Dentition is observed in more than a tenth of the HCH clients.* These problems, unlike most, appear to decline with age (presumably because the teeth are lost and therefore no longer a problem); differences by gender and race are minor. With only a few exceptions, dental services are not directly available to HCH clients but must be handled via referrals to other facilities.

Neurological Symptoms and Disorders range from migraine headaches and neuritis to Parkinson's disease, peripheral neuropathy, multiple sclerosis, and quadriplegia. The most common neurological disorders in this population are seizures, but these are treated as a separate category. If we exclude seizures, we find these disorders are about equally widespread across all subgroups.

Seizure Disorders are strongly linked to patterns of alcohol abuse, being about three times more common among homeless alcoholics than nonalcoholics. Still, the rates of seizure disorders among the nondrinking homeless are much higher than the rate in the general ambulatory population (0.1 percent).

Other Chronic Disorders that seem considerably more widespread among the homeless than among NAMCS patients include anemia, ear disorders, liver disease, chronic obstructive pulmonary disease, and genitourinary problems. The difference in liver disease is solely a function of alcohol abuse; among nondrinking homeless, the rate is not substantially higher than that observed in NAMCS.

Finally, the rate of *pregnancy* among homeless women is surprisingly high. Among all adult women ever seen programwide, 10.1 percent were pregnant at or since their first contact with HCH; among women seen more than once, the figure is 12.2 percent; in NAMCS the figure is 7.1 percent (the physician sampling frame for NAMCS includes physicians in gynecological and obstetrical practice). A more detailed analysis of pregnancies among HCH women is given in the reference in Note 43.

The major conclusion to be derived from these data is that the homeless suffer from most chronic physical disorders at an elevated and often exceptionally elevated rate. Some share of the effect is no doubt due to the unique demographic characteristics of the homeless (compared with the domiciled population); an even larger share results from the high rates of alcohol and drug abuse and mental illness. These points granted, the largest share of the difference results from the conditions of homelessness itself: first, the extreme poverty that characterizes this population and, second, the life-style factors enumerated earlier. Persons denied adequate shelter, in short, not only lose the roofs over their heads but are also thereby exposed to a range of risk factors that are uniquely and strongly destructive of physical health.

From the viewpoint of national health policy, it would therefore be justifiable to look on homelessness as a remediable condition of the environment that places a numerically large and growing portion of the urban poverty population at high health risk. Indeed, it is hard to conceive of a socially defined risk factor that is of greater consequence for a person's physical well-being. Yet current national health policy with respect to the homeless is strongly oriented toward amelioration, not prevention. Through the auspices of the McKinney Act, we now have Health Care

*Since dentists are not included in the NAMCS physician sampling frame, any comparison with NAMCS is meaningless.

for the Homeless clinics in operation in 108 cities across the nation. What we do not have is a set of policies or programs to prevent homelessness in the first place. And no matter what we do in the way of amelioration, the fact remains that one cannot be physically, mentally, or socially healthy without a stable, secure place in which to live. Among the many good reasons to "do something" about homelessness is that homelessness makes people ill.

Infectious and Communicable Disorders: Homelessness and Public Health

The health consequences of being homeless are borne primarily but not exclusively by homeless people themselves. Unlike most sick people, sick homeless people are not usually isolated from the healthy; rather, they tend to remain in the shelters or in the streets, making frequent contact with others. To the extent that the homeless are more prone to infectious and communicable diseases than the domiciled population, their illnesses threaten not only their own well-being but possibly the health of the larger public as well.

Table 2.4 reports the rates of various infectious and communicable disorders among the HCH adult client base. These disorders range from the trivial to the profound; all of them are characterized by some degree of direct communicability to the otherwise healthy. The last row of the table shows a composite index made up of all the other specific disorders shown and also includes serious respiratory infections (pneumonia, influenza) as well as communicable skin diseases and lice. At any given time about one HCH client in five is afflicted with some infectious or communicable condition, a rate five or six times that observed among NAMCS patients.

The more serious illnesses shown in the table are, of course, AIDS,[44–47] tuberculosis[48–50] (see Chapters 14 and 15), and the various sexually transmitted venereal diseases.

1. *Aids:* We have documented evidence of active AIDS infections in 103 clients; HIV positivity is known in 66 additional clients. Among clients seen more than once, the corresponding numbers are 77 and 58. Taking the latter figures as the more indicative and converting to customary epidemiological rates, we estimate the rate of AIDS infection among homeless adults to be 77/33682, or 230 cases per 100,000. Likewise, the estimated rate of HIV positivity among homeless adults is 58/33682, or 170 cases per 100,000.

2. *Tuberculosis:* Table 2.4 notes 376 documented cases of active tuberculosis (TB) among all HCH adult clients and 326 among adult clients seen more than once. Again taking the latter as the most indicative, we estimate the rate of TB infection as 326/33682, or 968 cases per 100,000 homeless adults. In contrast, the rate of TB infection in the national population at large is about 9 per 100,000, and among the urban population, about 19 per 100,000.*

* Data on the national rate of TB infection are taken from the reference in Note 47. The 1985 NAMCS data for urban adults show 32 cases of active TB among 49,903 patients, about 64 cases per 100,000 adult ambulatory patients, or about three times the observed rate for urban residents in general but only about 7 percent of the observed rate among HCH adults.

3. *Sexually Transmitted Diseases:* One fairly common but inaccurate stereotype about the homeless is that they are relatively old. In fact, they are surprisingly young, with an average age in the middle thirties in most studies. They would therefore be expected to be sexually active, a point that nonetheless surprises many people. Indeed, two pieces of evidence, both indirect, suggest that the rate of sexual activity among the homeless is about the same as in the population generally. The first is the rate of pregnancy among homeless women (about a tenth of all women seen); the second is the rate of sexually transmitted venereal diseases (STDs).

Overall, STDs are observed in 2.9 percent of the adult clients seen more than once, in 1.9 percent of the men and in 5.4 percent of the women. These infections are moderately more prevalent among nonwhites than whites and definitely more prevalent among the young than among the middle-aged and old. The rate of STD infection among the homeless is about twice that of the ambulatory population in general. Analysis of the rates of STD by age and gender combined shows that these infections are more common among women than men at all ages and more common among the young than among the old regardless of gender.

In sum, approximately one HCH adult client in five has an infectious or communicable disorder that poses some potential risk to the public health. The bulk of these disorders are relatively minor—lice infestations, other skin diseases, and the like. Still, serious respiratory infections are observed among nearly 4 percent; sexually transmitted venereal infections among about 3 percent; and active TB infections in about 1 percent.

The principal "population at risk" from these and related disorders is undoubtedly other homeless people. The shelter system itself may well abet the transmission of infectious and communicable diseases.[51] Sleeping arrangements vary from rooms for six to ten persons, to many rows of closely spaced cots set up wherever there is room to do so, to large dormitories housing hundreds. Bathroom and eating facilities are usually communal. Consequently, infectious and infestational skin diseases such as impetigo, tinea, pediculosis, and scabies are easily transmitted. Staphylococcal and streptococcal bacteria will pass easily from one open wound to another. Respiratory diseases transmitted by droplet inhalation, such as TB, and viral and bacterial respiratory infections find abundant receptors, most of all among a population that tends in any case to be malnourished and debilitated. Most of the people who are made ill by contact with ill homeless people will thus be other homeless people. (The staff of facilities serving the homeless represents a second population at some direct risk.)

Homeless people, however, are not quarantined inside the shelters. Many of the facilities serving homeless people are intentionally closed for all or part of the day, thus forcing the homeless to circulate among the larger population. The condition of homelessness itself is also not a static one; there is, rather, considerable "migration" into and out of the homeless condition over any reasonable time period.[52,53] The population at risk from infectious and communicable disease borne by the urban homeless, in short, is *not* coterminous with the urban homeless population itself.

This is not to suggest that homeless people should be isolated from the rest of the population in order to protect the healthy. The point, rather, is to emphasize the urgent need for thorough, aggressive screening of homeless people for communicable disorders and adequate medical treatment for those found to be afflicted; in the long run, of course, the solution to the health risks posed by the condition of homelessness is to eradicate the condition itself.

A Note on Health Problems of Homeless Children

The presentation to this point has focused exclusively on health problems of homeless adults, but about a tenth of all clients ever seen in HCH were children under the age of sixteen. Detailed analysis of our data on homeless children is given elsewhere.[43,54] In general, the configuration of illness among homeless children is different from that of homeless adults; specifically, acute disorders are more common and chronic disorders less common in the children. By far the most common disorders observed among the children are minor upper respiratory infections, followed by minor skin ailments; then ear disorders, gastrointestinal problems, and trauma, eye disorders, and lice infestations. In all cases, differences between homeless boys and girls are minor. See Chapter 8.

Health and Homelessness: Summary

In general, the homeless are exposed to and exhibit the diseases and disorders of the general population, albeit at what appear to be elevated (and in many cases, dramatically elevated) rates. Most of their health problems are acute disorders, but the rate of chronic physical illness clearly exceeds that of the national ambulatory care patient population. Epidemiological patterns characteristic of the general population also tend to characterize the HCH data, with the exception that gender differences appear to be lessened.

The leading health problem of the homeless is probably alcohol abuse, followed by mental disorders of various sorts. Alcohol abuse in particular has many associated health consequences, and the high rate of alcohol abuse among the HCH population certainly accounts for some, but by no means all, of the elevated incidences observed for many disorders. At the same time the rate of most disorders among non-alcohol-abusing HCH clients is still higher than that observed in the NAMCS survey, so while alcohol abuse is certainly an important part of the story, it is not the whole story. Most of the patterns discussed here are the direct result of homelessness itself, not of correlated behavioral and demographic factors.

Research reported here and elsewhere leaves little doubt that homelessness is the cause of a great deal of physical suffering. Tentative conclusions advanced in 1985[4] have subsequently been confirmed in study after study. Indeed, the essential factual finding—that homelessness causes much ill health—is not disputed by anyone. Not that this is a surprising result. No one in his or her right mind would think that being homeless is actually good for one's health.

Knowing the deleterious consequences of homelessness for health, what can or should we do about them? What do the scientific findings tell us about where or how to intervene?

Recent efforts to deal with the lead poisoning of ghetto children provide a useful analogue for this discussion. In view of the largely indisputable scientific findings that lead poisoning was widespread among poor children, two alternative strategies of intervention might be imagined. One could accept the poisoning as inevitable and call for the development of better screening programs and more effective therapies. Alternatively, one could push the scientific findings back to their more basic cause—in this case, the presence of lead in the ghetto environment—and demand that we get rid of the lead altogether. The latter was chosen as a matter of national health policy. It was decided, in short, that lead poisoning of ghetto children was *not* inevitable and that it was within our means and technical know-how to be rid of the lead and in the process to be rid of the health problems that lead caused.

So with the now unequivocal effects of homelessness on health. Now that we know of these effects, do we treat the symptoms of the problem by intervening with more, better, and more accessible health care for homeless people (the strategy being pursued under the auspices of the McKinney Act)? Or do we also push *these* findings back to their more basic causes and attempt to do away with homelessness altogether? Knowing that homelessness causes a great deal of pain and suffering, do we attempt to soften the pain or rid ourselves of its origins? Knowing that a man beats his wife, do we suggest that he beat her less often or perhaps more gently? Or would we prefer that he not beat her at all?

It has recently been argued that "only a comprehensive long-term strategy for eliminating homelessness will permanently improve the health status of homeless persons."[55] This should not be misinterpreted as just a *political* statement; it is, rather, a *scientific* statement that correctly sorts out causes and effects and recommends accordingly. It is an assertion that whatever else we might do in the way of amelioration, people simply cannot be healthy if they do not have a stable place to live; there is now a great deal of scientific evidence to sustain this point of view. All that remains to be learned is whether we have the means, technical know-how, and especially the political will to do it.*

*This research was supported by a grant from the Robert Wood Johnson Foundation. I am grateful for the capable assistance of my many colleagues at the University of Massachusetts, especially Dee Weber, and also Harry Crumpler for assistance in the statistical analysis.

JOHN N. LOZIER

MANDY JOHNSON

JOAN HAYNES

3

Overcoming Troubled Relationships Between Programs and the Community

Introduction

Homelessness reveals unresolved political, economic, and social questions that are often painful to face. Programs that seriously address homelessness push for resolution of important concerns of our times and are involved in controversy with others in the community almost by definition. Major issues are raised in the course of responsible advocacy, but they surface as well in the day-to-day business of getting along with partners in the work.

HCHP projects have also encountered major controversies with those who take a "not in my backyard" attitude. Local persons often express fears for their personal safety and economic well-being when obviously destitute individuals are present in their neighborhoods or business environments. Service agencies are often the most immediately available targets of blame for the presence of the homeless and the very real problems often associated with their presence.

This discussion considers these matters through the experiences of program in three cities: Venice (a Los Angeles beachfront suburb), Seattle, and Nashville.

Venice: Violent Opposition and Successful Mediation
Background

HOMELESS STRAIN TIES THAT BIND was the headline of a front-page article in the Westside Section of the *Los Angeles Times* in October 1987. For months the local newspapers were filled with accounts of citizens whose tempers were frayed because local beaches, parks, and streets had become home for hundreds of people. Stores and restaurants along the beachfront felt the impact on their businesses; citizens were afraid for their personal safety. There was anger about the increased numbers of the homeless, many with antisocial behavior, now so visible in their neighborhood. Residents, business groups, and civic organizations became vehemently vocal and organized against homeless persons, the social service agencies providing services to them, and the city councilwoman and other concerned citizens who were attempting to develop alternatives to living on the beaches.

One meal program in particular, run by the St. Joseph Center in Venice, became the scapegoat in the community battle between property rights and human rights. The lunch line and its move to an indoor location (after two years of operation in a public parking lot) became the focal point of community frustration. A concentrated opposition campaign threatened the nonprofit center by anonymous flyers against the program, angry phone calls by its neighbors, and political pressure. A carefully planned mediation process eventually led to a peaceful resolution. Here we describe the historical events that led to the mediation table as well as the strategies employed during the mediation and the lessons learned.

Community opposition to programs serving the homeless in Los Angeles has its roots in the macro picture: gentrification, the Pacific Rim economic boom that continues to bring a thousand people per day into L.A., and availability of great amounts of capital for new financial ventures; the destruction of older housing rather than its renovation to meet current seismic standards; and the lack of an effective housing policy to provide for low-income members of the community. Additionally, Los Angeles has a dual system of government. The city and the county share responsibility for public services. The city of Los Angeles provides police, sanitation, housing, and transportation. Los Angeles County (which includes the city of Los Angeles along with other cities and municipalities) is responsible for health, mental health, drug and alcohol services as well as administration of the public welfare programs. This division creates an environment fraught with discord between the two governmental bodies in regard to responsibility for an estimated thirty-five to fifty thousand people living in the streets, parks, cars, SRO hotels, and shelters and on the beaches.

Both the city and the county concentrate much of their attention and funding on the skid row area, where an estimated fifteen thousand live in the streets, hotels, and missions. Outlying areas have had to fight to obtain public funding for social services. The county has contracted for voucher hotels primarily in the downtown area. This forces individuals applying for general relief, the entitlement program for able-bodied adults, to choose between housing downtown or a safer but unhoused environment in one of the outlying areas of L.A. Since an address is a prerequisite for general relief, refusing a voucher hotel means that general relief cannot be obtained. Emergency shelter or drop-in center addresses may be used only for three months, after which the person must have obtained a permanent address.

On the local level, Venice (part of L.A. city proper) and Santa Monica (an adjacent incorporated city) had become a community battleground over the homeless issue. Frequent newspaper articles and editorials documented the ongoing community meetings. Organized pressure on both the government and nonprofit agencies escalated to violence. The people who lived on the streets and beaches were equally desperate. The environment of hostility led one mentally ill homeless woman to drive a van through the front window of a restaurant. The owner was an outspoken opponent of the homeless and services for them. That tragic event followed the shooting of a homeless man in the back while he was digging through an alley Dumpster.

The west side of Los Angeles has been gentrified during the last thirty years. SRO hotels, low-income housing, and missions that provided services to homeless persons have been lost. Construction of very expensive replacement housing has brought to the neighborhoods wealthier residents, people who did not realize that the homeless and the very poor had occupied these beach communities for decades.

By 1987 the need for housing and social services had become acute. Yet the community climate was such that programs bringing large numbers of the homeless together in public places raised a tremendous furor from residents who felt that their property values were being lowered and that public safety was endangered. The Westside Ecumenical Council had organized churches, agencies, and interested individuals into the Westside Shelter Coalition in order to create a forum for public education and a way for social service agencies to network and keep abreast of legislative issues. The local chambers of commerce had a variety of responses, but their basic stance was that homelessness was bad for business.

Politics in Venice

The political climate also contributed to volatility. Nineteen eighty-seven was a big election year in Venice. Pat Russell, the incumbent city council member of many years, was unseated by Ruth Galanter in an upset. Galanter, a Venice resident and a city planner by profession, won on a slow-growth ticket. This immediately put her at odds with developers who wanted to continue the development begun under Russell.

Developers in Venice had been trying to improve their image through an organization called the Venice Action Committee (VAC), committed to beautification. VAC had organized to plant trees, paint out graffiti, and press government to provide public sanitation and street improvements. VAC's goals also included exertion of its political influence on the small nonprofit organizations. VAC invited agencies to participate at meetings at which homelessness was discussed.

Just at this time a small nonprofit organization, the St. Joseph Center, sponsored by the Sisters of St. Joseph of Carondolet, was attempting to find a permanent home for its lunch program. Ten years earlier, when it was founded, the center had developed a food pantry, a thrift store, and an outreach and advocacy program to meet the needs of low-income Hispanic families living in Venice. In 1981 the center had noted an increase of homeless people, primarily single men asking for food and other services. In response, the center had developed a separate drop-in center for the homeless to rest, shower, obtain social services, and get a meal.

This very visible meal program created animosity in the neighbors. The drop-in center was a small (eight hundred square feet) storefront located at a busy corner. The meal program was conducted in the open parking lot behind the building, which fronted on a side street. Neighbors had a daily view of homeless persons sitting, resting, and eating a meal. Additionally, they blamed the increasing numbers of people entering the neighborhood for trash and vandalism. The center's building was torched in the middle of the night.

The center in collaboration with both city and county officials restored its food program by distributing sack lunches on the beachfront in a large municipal parking lot several blocks away. This parking lot was already a center of controversy because large numbers of people resided there in cars or vans. The open-air program was intended to be temporary until the center could find an indoor location.

The issues raised must be understood in the context of the location, one of the busiest beaches in Los Angeles. Venice Beach has long been renowned for its tolerance of eclectic life-styles and for decades has been a hodgepodge of neighborhoods, residents, and special-interest groups. Although local humor referred to Venice as "where the trash meets the surf," businesspeople and developers were dedicated to improving the economic and life-style environment. Consequently, local merchants objected to the program in the parking lot. They were already upset with the many unlicensed vendors who illegally set up along the beachfront. The local business community thought that the food program caused further deterioration of their business environment because of its visibility, the numbers being served, the trash on the beachfront, and the public inebriants who utilized the program. VAC asked the St. Joseph Center to plan for a move off the beachfront and offered to locate an unoccupied restaurant.

The center had been trying to find an indoor site without success and appreciated the friendly overture. The center then actually submitted a proposal to VAC to buy a local vacant restaurant near the drop-in center. After waiting for two months for VAC to respond, the center moved ahead on its own to buy the restaurant.

Impact of the Los Angeles Outdoor Campground

In the meantime, the new Venice city council member, Ruth Galanter, had been elected. Downtown, seventeen miles away, Los Angeles Mayor Tom Bradley began his plan to open an urban campground on the Los Angeles River for two months in order to clean up skid row. This expensive resettlement coincided with a visit from Pope John Paul and came in response to complaints from downtown businesses about the numbers of people living in the streets. This resettlement effort had the unexpected effect of forcing people from downtown to Venice Beach. According to Rhonda Meister, the St. Joseph Center's executive director, "The sanctioning of an outdoor campground by the public sector gave a permission to homeless people on Venice Beach to create their own encampment. Prior to the downtown encampment, Venice homeless packed up their belongings each day. But after the City built and funded its campground, the number of shanties proliferated on the beach."[1] Public furor mounted over the increased numbers and the structures that the homeless built for protection from the weather. Citizens and civic groups became more openly vocal about homelessness.

The county responded by organizing a three-day social service outreach "blitz" to connect homeless people sleeping on the beach to services. There was considerable public discussion about whether the beachfront was an appropriate location for social services. The city-owned Pavilion, a large but little-used amphitheater with community rooms, became the focal point because it contained many of the needed elements to run a program. But the business community overwhelmingly opposed provision of any services on the beach and was very critical of the police for failing to remove campers. This pressure eventually resulted in passage of a No Camping city ordinance.

While the center quietly negotiated its own real estate deal to purchase the empty restaurant, the new city councilwoman began developing her response to the situation and conducted a variety of meetings with organizations and a public hearing. Meanwhile, the pope having come and gone, the city prepared to shut its urban campground, and fear ran high in Venice that its closure would relocate even more people to the beach.

The public hearing, held at the local high school, was designed to be a forum for all sides: social service agencies, local businesspeople, experts, the homeless, the police, and the city attorney's office. More than a thousand attended, and the rowdiness of the audience delayed the opening of the hearing. Homeless people who testified were loudly booed; the police (whose presence grew during the evening) had to escort some rude and uncooperative people from the auditorium.

The news of the restaurant purchase resulted in delight to beachfront businesses and anger among the new neighbors of the vacant restaurant. Additionally, City Councilwoman Galanter proposed to expand services for the homeless at a site on Rose Avenue, near the restaurant. The neighbors began to organize against St. Joseph Center's purchase of the restaurant. Soon flyers reading "No Skid Rose" were distributed in the neighborhood. The realtor handling the sale received threatening phone calls. The center staff was harassed by VAC members and anonymous bomb threats. The executive director was personally attacked verbally at a VAC meeting and had to be escorted out as members lost control and the entire session deteriorated into a shouting match. The board chair's automobile tires were slashed.

Mediation

Emotions ran high on every side of the issue. The St. Joseph Center remained determined to open its restaurant. However, the center staff also recognized the clear danger of negative public sentiment. Violence could continue; raising of private funds to purchase and operate the restaurant could be hampered. The strain of trying to operate social services in such an environment seemed intolerable, and the county's Human Relations Commission and the center began to develop a community mediation process. This started by organizing friends to support the concept and getting a commitment of all the parties to participate. The police met with all concerned, telling them to stop the violence, and the County Human Relations Commission played an active role, facilitating information sharing, clarifying positions, and eliminating rumors, all before the formal sessions started.

Eleven formal mediation sessions were conducted by professional mediators, the Neighborhood Justice Center, which was a nonprofit group funded by the County Bar Association to facilitate nonlitigious solutions to disputes. All the players—city, county, nonprofits, the police, VAC, and the Venice Town Council—were involved as well as three new groups: a religious day school which is a neighbor to the restaurant, a temple located on the beachfront, and Neighbor to Neighbor, a group of local citizens who organized to support local social services. The mediation process set up rules, structured discussion of the issues, and gave assignments to the participants in order to move toward consensus. Sessions were held at secret locations, and participants were sworn to secrecy in order to limit public speculation about the hostile situation.

Mediation proved to be a setting in which people were allowed to say mean-spirited and hateful words openly. The sessions were agonizing for the nonprofit agencies involved. For the St. Joseph Center staff the toll was immeasurable, although the community support that came forward in response was remarkable. After the opponents to services had vented all their negativity and agreement that there was a need in the community for an indoor food program had been reached, the mediators moved on to solutions. The opposition coalition members had nothing to offer. They were neither able to find another location nor to offer credible solutions. Their dearth of ideas and the vacuum of their ability to offer positive leadership resulted in the recognition that the center had every legal right to operate the restaurant. The mediators then brought the St. Joseph Center staff together with their local neighbors to plan the restaurant operation in a way that would be acceptable to both. Local people were concerned primarily about appearances: the number of persons walking through the neighborhood, lines in front of the building, signs, and crime. The center was prepared to work collaboratively on these issues.

The leader of the neighborhood opposition group continued to meet biweekly with center staff. He ultimately joined a board committee, and his wife volunteered to design the landscaping for the restaurant.

Seattle

Race and Access to Care

In 1984, when the RWJF's Request for Proposals (RFP) was put forth, the question of minority populations' access to social and health services was a hot issue in Seattle. Seattle has four major minority population groups: black, Asian, Native American, and Hispanic. The demography of Seattle's population (1980) was as follows:

White	79.5%
Black	9.5%
Native American	1.3%
Asian	7.4%
Hispanic	2.6%

The total minority population in Seattle was 20.8 percent, yet it was estimated at that time that over 50 percent of the homeless were minority persons. A special effort was needed to address their needs.

The Minority Executive Directors Coalition was a powerful group within the Coalition for Survival Services (the sponsoring coalition for the RWJF grant) and advocated that a team focused on minority access to social and health services be included in the grant. The three other teams included in the grant were based upon geographic boundaries. Thus the demographic rather than the geographical basis for the minority access team did not fit the overall concept of service provision.

Access of minority persons to health and social services was, and is, a valid concern. However, the design of the service delivery system was not well thought out, and the team, as implemented, did not provide the same range of services as the geographically based teams.

Implementation and Restructuring

The minority access team, as implemented:

- Did *not* provide health services
- Did *not* target homeless persons specifically but rather attempted to serve a wider population of those at risk of becoming homeless
- Could *not* adequately coordinate health care for clients because case managers were not part of the health care system

The minority access team was not really a team at all. Instead, caseworkers were hired by social service agencies to assist agency clients in getting necessary services. On any of the three geographically based teams a client could receive medical care, mental health and substance-abuse assessment and counseling, and social work services. Through the minority access team clients did not have access to the direct medical care, mental health, or substance abuse services.

At its first foundation site visit to Seattle, members of the site visit team recognized that the minority access team did not meet the basic criteria of the grant. While making special efforts to serve minority homeless individuals was seen to be appropriate, until the program was redesigned to meet the program guidelines, the foundation would not approve that portion of the budget. The HCHP Governing Council also had been concerned with the manner in which the minority access team had been implemented. The threat of disappearing grant funds demanded action.

The council, which had responsibility for the overall program, now set guidelines for restructuring the minority access team. The guidelines were based upon foundation criteria, comments from the site team, and legal requirements, such as backup supervision and patient confidentiality. Representatives from the community participated in the program guidelines.

An ad hoc task force was responsible for adhering to the council's guidelines for restructuring the team. The task force was composed of representatives from the minority communities as well as council members. If the program were to survive, the community must continue to have ownership.

It was agreed that the current casework services should not be disrupted. The council negotiated with the foundation for three months' funding of current services while the program was restructured.

Many meetings of the task force were held. The first few served almost solely for venting of emotions. The task force had infinite patience, and members repeatedly made the point that all the concerned groups needed to work together to design a program that met foundation guidelines so that minority clients would be served. Representatives from the community health centers which targeted the various minority populations as well as the social service agencies were invited to all the meetings.

Once the task force had agreed that the focus for this particular grant had to be on health services, an RFP to select a lead health agency for the minority access activity was distributed to the community health centers. Reaching this agreement was a major step since it meant that the social service agencies had agreed that health care should be provided by health care organizations.

There was only one response to the RFP, a letter from the Seattle Indian Health Board (SIHB) which stated:

. . . after careful review of the RFP and the entire HCHP, . . . minority clients could be best served by distributing funds to existing teams for the purpose of hiring minority health/ outreach workers to ensure access to minorities. . . . Under this proposed plan, minority populations would have access to medical, alcoholism, mental health and other needed care through existing teams. Services and access to minorities would be greatly enhanced and less cumbersome through this plan.

This plan was the community-designed solution for which the task force had hoped. The SIHB is a well-respected agency in the minority community, and its plan was discussed by the task force and then recommended for approval to the Governing Council. The new plan was implemented four months after the restructuring process had begun.

Nashville: Battles over a Site

The Nashville, Tennessee, HCHP project encountered determined, sophisticated, and vehement opposition from the operators of businesses near its proposed site for a multiservice center for the homeless. Because the HCHP project had become part of the Health Department in the local government, it was particularly vulnerable to repeated attacks in the local legislative body, the Metropolitan Council. The fierce struggle over the Downtown Service Center illustrates important issues and principles for those who encounter community opposition in their attempts to serve the homeless.

The plan for a service center originated with advocates who recognized a need for additional daytime shelter and services, including employment, counseling, and personal hygiene. The new program was to expand upon the professional offerings of the HCHP project, provide a site for outreach efforts of other agencies, and promote greater coordination among them.

The Nashville Coalition for the Homeless, developer of the HCHP project and the service center concept from the beginning, had important allies. Both local daily newspapers provided strong editorial support for the project, the result of a constant flow of information about the need and the developing proposal. The coalition worked closely with Councilman Ludye Wallace, chairman of the Special Committee on Homelessness, which passed a resolution in August 1986 identifying "a Homeless Service Center as a priority." After the local housing authority's Task Force on Homelessness acknowledged a need for laundry and shower facilities for the homeless, Mayor Richard Fulton identified $200,000 in bond revenues for the purpose. In April 1987 the Metropolitan Council appropriated $30,000 for planning and development of the service center and designated the Health Department as its operator. The remaining $170,000 went to the housing authority for site acquisition, with a provision that the council must approve the final location.

A suitable vacant building was available for purchase just two blocks from the Downtown Clinic primary care site and close to the Nashville Union Rescue Mission and the Salvation Army. Warehouses, a gas station and garage, a blood bank, a security firm, and religious publishing houses lined the major thoroughfare on which the proposed service center building was located. The housing authority signed a contract to purchase the building, contingent upon council approval of the site, and a July 21, 1987, date was set for the council vote. Neighbors of the site learned of the proposal and imminent vote from a newspaper reporter on July 17. Their predictable concern (neighbor Ed Loftis: "This would just further identify this as an area for street people"[2]) was intensified because they had not been notified by public officials about the plans. Early, official notice would have given opponents more opportunity to organize, but it would have been fairer and more appropriate and would have dispelled some of their emotional tension.

News coverage of the imminent vote was intense, and Councilman Wallace deferred the service center site approval vote, calling a public hearing for two weeks later. Advocates and opponents alike tried to organize their constituencies to attend the meeting. Opponents of virtually any proposal, and those who feel their safety or economic interests threatened, have an easier time turning out a crowd than do proponents and people whose motivations are more altruistic. Predictably, the public meeting was packed with agitated service center opponents.

The immediate neighbors of the site had organized other business owners and employees into the South Loop Merchants Association and had published a newsletter devoted entirely to attacks on the service center, which it prominently characterized as a bathhouse. In an era of AIDS hysteria, the bathhouse characterization was a subtle appeal to people's worst fears about the homeless. The South Loop constituents at the hearing described distasteful behaviors of some of the homeless and expressed fear of increased crime and reduced property values. They argued that the facility was poorly planned and not needed. It seemed to proponents, as they tried to describe safeguards for the neighborhood to be built into the service center's operations, that no amount of reassurance could be heard; in such situations, rational approaches have little impact.

Service center proponents at the heated hearing were pressured into a mistake when critics of the proposal asked for utilization projections that had not yet been developed. Pressed for an answer, the HCHP project director estimated that perhaps 75 persons a day would use the facility. When a grant application later analyzed utilization figures of other facilities and projected 115 users per day, the inconsistency was fiercely attacked by project opponents as evidence of bad faith. As it turned out, all projections were far off base, and nearly 200 people per day were registering at the service center shortly after its eventual opening. Estimates, especially those made casually, are dangerous undertakings.

Councilman Wallace, chairing the public hearing, wisely avoided stating a position on the issue, and the matter moved toward a site approval vote by the full council. The full array of resources of both sides of the issue came into play for this site approval vote, which finally occurred in mid-October 1987. Proponents approached the vote like a political campaign, targeting the members of the council as the only decision makers in this situation, seeking members' commitments, and keeping a careful count of votes. Promotional materials were created for the audience of council members, with a lesser emphasis on developing support among the general public. The newspapers remained supportive with strong statements like the Sunday *Tennessean*'s lead editorial on October 16: SERVICE CENTER'S APPROVAL WOULD SHOW COMPASSION.

Service center opponents were aware of their vulnerability to charges of narrow self-interest. Trying to appear more positive, the merchants association proposed an alternative plan that would have homeless people arrested under resurrected vagrancy laws, diagnosed in a "process center," and "rehabilitated" in a "controlled environment" located next to the public hospital, the city morgue, and a vocational rehabilitation office. The chairman of the Coalition for the Homeless, Richard Couto, defined the issue clearly when he wrote in the October 12 *Tennessean:* "The proposal has flaws, in part, because the merchants are clearer on what they don't want than on what Nashville's homeless population needs. The merchants do not want a service center for the homeless in their area."

The service center location was approved in October 1987 by a twenty to fifteen vote, with four abstentions. The merchants immediately sued to block acquisition and development of the site, alleging various deficiencies in procedures. When the merchants' requests for injunctions were denied by the courts, the purchase of the site was completed. Litigation on the issue continued until a Tennessee Supreme Court ruling in August 1989 approved the procedures used to establish the Downtown Service Center, which had by then been open for nine months.

The service center controversy was revived in the spring of 1988, when the Metropolitan Council had the opportunity to accept or reject $391,696 in McKinney Act funding awarded for the project in December 1987. Prominent members of the council publicly criticized the terms of the grant, which required use of the building for at least ten years, again proclaimed the site a poor location, objected to a projection that the center would serve only about one-tenth of the city's homeless, and railed at the supposed inconsistencies in planners' projections of utilization rates. A resolution rescinding site approval was introduced as an alternative to approving the funding.

This second major council battle over the service center was only slightly different from the first. Advocates once again waged a decidedly political campaign targeted at the decision makers; one at-large member of the council was swayed by 250 calls and letters in three days favoring the service center. The opponent's alternative proposal had evolved from a coercive "processing center" into an SRO hotel adjoining a relocated service center. The new mayor, Bill Boner, who did not have "a dog in that fight" during the first round, this time supported the project "simply because I do not see an alternative on the immediate horizon which will give us any additional ability to address the homeless issue."[3] The mayor's support and the very active involvement of a few members of the council helped create a more comfortable margin of victory; the federal funds were accepted on a vote of twenty-six to six, with seven abstentions.

The Downtown Service Center is now open and operating quietly and effectively. The story of its creation, like the stories of Seattle's conflict over race and access to care and of Venice's over a food line, illustrates that more than good intentions, careful planning, appropriate staffing, and adequate funding are required for the successful delivery of services to the homeless. Political acumen, eagerness to work with others in the community, and determination have proved equally important attributes for success.

Lessons Learned: Advice to Health Care for the Homeless Programs

Unstructured public hearings become out-of-control free-for-alls that generate inflammatory press and do not help anyone.

Working with civic and business groups is necessary, but allowing them to dictate leadership on the issues will backfire. Don't continue to participate when you become the target. There will undoubtedly be unsubtle blackmail—hints of support and open threats of eliminating financial backing, in order to force cooperation.

Don't trust the press. Controversy sells newspapers. Do your best to control it. Be prepared to organize your own letters to the editor campaign in order to achieve some balance of ideas printed.

Expect community opposition, and operate your program with a critical eye for how it appears to your neighbors. Avoid lines outside your building; have a code of conduct; prevent people from lying down or sleeping around the building or using drugs and alcohol; keep your whole perimeter immaculate; be a good neighbor. Homelessness has been created in part by gentrification. New neighbors have a low tolerance for social problems that have historically been in the neighborhood.

Go door to door, tell your neighbors who you are, what you do, answer questions, and get feedback. Find out who your supporters are, so that you can call them again. Find out who doesn't support you, and listen closely to complaints.

Have patience. The moral rightness of helping other people and working for community solutions will eventually win out over acrimonious selfishness. Those whose only interest is in preserving property values have no answer for who should feed the hungry.

Use whatever political clout you have to line up your friends, to get support for the politicians who support you.

Take care of yourself and your friends who are involved. The emotional and psychological toll of these battles is enormous. Play tennis, go swimming, or unplug your phone in order to reduce your own personal stress.

During mediation try to articulate and value shared experiences and perceptions—e.g., homeless people can be frightening to the elderly, or public inebriates are a social problem in the community.

Mediation is not easy, but it works. Once the opposition has had the opportunity to express itself and feels that it has been heard, the shared experiences and perceptions can lead to agreement.

Work for a win-win solution.

4

Slouching Toward Chaos: American Health Policy and the Homeless

Introduction

Health care to homeless persons emerged as one of the dominant new themes in United States health policy during the 1980s.[1,2] Intense legislative interest in this issue culminated in the 1987 passage of the Homeless Assistance Act, a sweeping addition to the nation's federally financed health initiatives. Scientific study of the homeless also burgeoned. Virtually every medical and social science journal published major articles describing careful study of all facets of homeless existence.

Why the interest in health care for the homeless? Are their health needs particularly problematic, or does the very existence of their needs demonstrate systemic flaws in an apparently functional system of care? Answers to these questions are not entirely self-evident. The remarkable successes of Health Care for the Homeless Program suggest that with sufficient prodding the health care system can respond. Access to high-quality medical care was accomplished for thousands.[3] However, the extraordinary effort required to achieve this modest goal indicates structural problems with our health care system.

Thomas Kuhn characterizes the scientific paradigm as a shared set of theories and points of view that are sufficiently "open-ended to leave all sorts of problems for the . . . practitioners to resolve."[4] In science, research is undertaken to discover facts that explain and confirm the dominant theory. However, facts that do not fit the theory strain the paradigm until either the fact is found to be in error or the paradigm changes. If the paradigm changes, the scientist embraces a new theory that accounts for more facts and gives him or her a different constellation of problems to study. For example, the discoveries of oxygen and of the benzene ring precipitated paradigm changes. Prior to each discovery, the theories of combustion and organic chemistry, respectively, were increasingly unable to account for numerous facts revealed through scientific experiments. The paradigm changes—that is, the sweeping changes in scientific theory—explained most of the scientific facts.

The United States health care system may be described as a paradigm characterized by the widespread view that a pluralistic network of independent practitioners—doctors, hospitals, clinics, and other medical suppliers—can provide the highest quality and most accessible health care for the population. A corollary proposition within this paradigm is that the health practitioners who dominate this network are the most qualified to ascertain the health care needs of the individual patient and of society. Imperfect and incomplete as this view may be, virtually all policy initiatives derive from it. Thus, the practitioners often acting in the role of health policy experts have an ample array of problems to solve, including access for the uninsured, the health of minorities, prenatal care, and health care for the homeless.

If the theories and explanations about health services delivery were substantially correct, the homeless would not have such grossly unmet health care needs. The nationwide efforts to deliver health care to the homeless dramatically underscore and highlight the flaws and inconsistencies that challenge the assumptions from which health policy is derived. These efforts, providing health care to the homeless, present problems that cannot conveniently find resolution within the paradigm. The homeless are more than a uniquely visible subgroup of the poor, whose severely limited access to care was the health care showstopper of the decade. They are the ghosts in the machine,[5] the glitches that defy conventional explanation.

This discussion considers the complexities of the United States health care system and the policies directed toward solving the problems of access to care. It will explore the fact that the proposed solutions are limited by the intellectual and political views of that system. For the homeless, these policy initiatives run the risk of diverting attention from substantive attempts to improve their health status. Proposals for a national health program that risk additional chaos will be discussed. An alternative view of health services delivery that may change the focus of these debates is offered in conclusion.

The Roots of Chaos in the United States Health Care System

During the twentieth century health programs that appealed to special-interest groups substituted for a national health policy. This phenomenon has established the precedent for the incremental changes characteristic of our pluralistic system.[6,7] On the presumption that health care in this country is the best in the world, legislative efforts were directed toward improving the availability of health insurance to certain groups of people while preserving the status quo. Thus, the 1965 Medicare and Medicaid legislation responded to political pressures from the elderly and from southern Democrats, not to a general hue and cry for universal access to care.[8] The absence of a national health care policy together with interest group politics has resulted in a patchwork health care system subject to constant adjusting by elected officials. It is also a system that can reasonably boast the best as well as feel shame for the worst of care.

Levi was a friend to everyone who knew him. I first saw him in the medical clinic more than six years ago for the management of his hypertension and heart failure. In spite of his advanced disease, Levi never complained and continued to work six days a week as a laborer for a small local real estate developer. Although he did not have health insurance, he was able to afford his medicines most of the time.

Two years ago several diagnostic tests were ordered to evaluate Levi's cardiac condition. The total charge was slightly more than $230. I saw him immediately after completion of the tests to discuss the results and to share with him my thoughts about what additional therapies might be available in the months and years ahead. We joked about our families, and I scheduled a return appointment.

Although I saw Levi around the neighborhood many times, it was in the intensive care unit (ICU) that we resumed our doctor-patient relationship. He had suffered a respiratory arrest in his brother's car en route to the hospital. Only in desperation had he even agreed to come to the hospital. Now he was intubated and in a deep coma.

His hospital course was extremely complicated and long. Levi spent thirty days in the ICU learning to breathe again and learning who he was. After a total hospital stay of forty-five days at a cost of tens of thousands of dollars, he was discharged home. He had lost fifty pounds and knew his wife but was intermittently confused about the world around him. He never worked again.

Several months later Levi's mental capabilities had improved significantly. He could care for himself, knew his friends and relatives, and was enjoying our renewed friendship. We talked often about his hospitalization. I impressed upon him the importance of regular clinic visits. When asked for the hundredth time about why he had not come back during the months before his hospitalization, Levi finally said, "Doc, I just didn't have the money for those tests we did. I figured they wouldn't let me in anyway."

Levi died exactly one year after his hospitalization.

Levi's illness, his remarkable survival, and his ultimate disability bear witness to the roots of chaos in the health care system. Piecemeal, incremental policies have constructed something akin to M. C. Escher's graphic *Relativity* (Figure 4.1).[9] At first glance the scene is one of magnificently coordinated stairs and

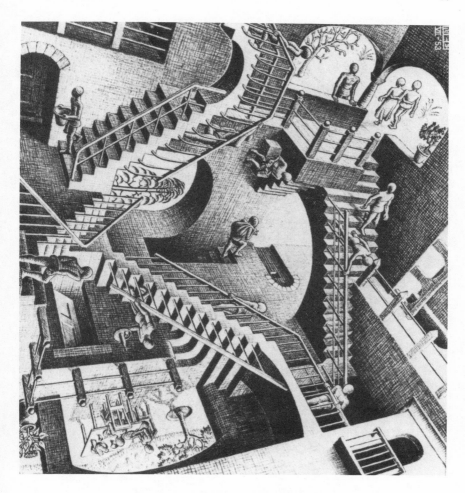

*Figure 4.1 **Relativity** by **M. C. Escher***
© 1990 M. C. ESCHER HEIRS/CORDON ART, BAARN, HOLLAND

passages. On close inspection the scene deteriorates into a collection of isolated structures with connections more an illusion than a reality. The individual parts of our health system may provide excellent care, but there are few connections that ensure access, continuity, or coordination.

Access to health care in the United States is largely dependent upon employer-provided health insurance.[10,11] Prior to 1965, the poor and the elderly were the groups most vulnerable to disease and disability because they generally lacked employer-provided health insurance, while in a response to interest group politics, the passage of the Medicare and Medicaid legislation was seen as a way to begin filling the gaps in health insurance coverage. Although access to care dramatically improved subsequent to implementation, large numbers of individuals remained dependent upon a fragile safety net of hospitals, clinics, and private physicians for their care (Figure 4.2).[10,12]

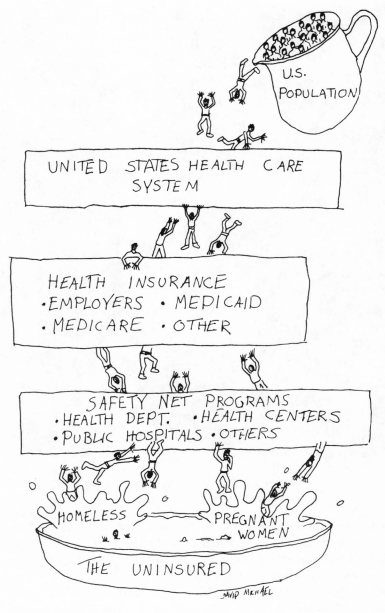

Figure 4.2

For millions of uninsured, including the homeless, hospitals are the primary source of care, usually through the emergency room. Historically, care to the poor in hospitals began with the almshouses for the destitute, the homeless, and the infirm. As medical therapy improved, the almshouse was transformed into the public hospital, which became the repository for the diseases of poverty, segregated from the rest of society. In a parallel development, religious orders built hospitals for the working poor to fulfill their missions of charity.[13]

Hospital-based and health department clinics are another entry point into the system for the uninsured. The birth of the clinic was an outgrowth of the intellectual and scientific blossoming of clinical medicine.[14] From a place to observe and study large numbers of diseased persons, the clinic evolved into a place of care, especially for the poor. Many of the early clinics were housed inside public hospitals. As scientific medicine advanced, the clinic movement expanded to include health departments, community health centers, and other subsidized programs. Taken together, hospitals and clinics are the safety net for people who do not have health insurance.

This hodgepodge of health care services is quite costly.[10,15,16] Spending for medical care has reached more than $500 billion annually, double the amount spent in 1980. The federal government spends about $144 billion annually for Medicare, Medicaid, and other federal programs. Private health insurance contributes $158 billion, and direct patient payments add another $123 billion annually. State and local governments spend more than $62 billion, $24 billion of which represents states' Medicaid contributions. Almost $40 billion is spent to support public hospitals, health department clinics, and other programs for the poor.

The five-hundred-billion-dollar price tag for health care does not include charity care and bad debt, termed uncompensated care. Hospitals assume responsibility for the majority of uncompensated care, in excess of an estimated ten billion dollars in 1989.[17] Most uncompensated care is provided to people who are without any form of health insurance. Because of increasing medical costs, hospital uncompensated care was the focus of much debate and discussion during the 1980s.[18–20]

Uncompensated care costs are important because hospitals have traditionally used a portion of excess revenues to cover the expenses of care to the uninsured through cost shifting. Three pressures have seriously threatened the ability of hospitals to continue care to the poor. First, the cost of medical care has doubled during the past decade.[16] Second, employers and the federal government alike have adopted a number of strategies to control costs, strategies that limit the revenues available to care for the uninsured. Third, the number of people without health insurance has increased by one million a year since 1980, placing an additional strain on hospitals.[21,22] Because they are the institutions of last resort, public hospitals have borne the brunt of these fiscal pressures.

Charity care in the doctor's office is more difficult to identify.[10,23] Although more than 75 percent of physicians claim to provide some form of charity care, the magnitude is poorly documented.[10] Physicians tend to have greater control over who has access to their offices than do hospitals, especially with the 1987 Medicare provision that prohibits the transfer of a medically unstable patient or of a woman in labor to another hospital.

The Stretch for the Uninsured

The fiscal pressures within the health industry have made it increasingly difficult for those without health insurance to get needed medical care. For many hospitals, clinics, and doctors the limits of accommodation have long since passed.

When the social worker from the Birmingham homeless program found Robert, he was sitting on a park bench, crying. That morning the doctor had told him to go to the county hospital for treatment of his cancer. It was the first he knew of any cancer and didn't have the first idea what the man was talking about.

Robert had lived in the northern part of the state, where he had worked in the fields for almost fifty years, since he was fourteen. He never married and lived with his only remaining kin, his elderly, sick brother. Last month he saw Dr. N about the painful swelling on his left leg. Dr. N told him the "growth" needed some looking into by a specialist in Birmingham. The specialist did some tests and told him to come back in a week. Rather than try to travel all the way back home, Robert stayed around town until it was time to go back to the doctor.

The social worker quickly discovered that Robert had no place to stay and that the growth on his leg was metatastic. Apparently he would need radiation therapy. Robert was taken to respite care after he had picked up a prescription for pain pills.

During the next several weeks Robert's condition worsened to the point where he could barely care for himself. His admission to the county hospital had confirmed the diagnosis of metatastic cancer of unknown source, and it uncovered a number of other problems that were preventing him from receiving any treatment other than pain medication. Since he was not a county resident, Robert was not eligible for ongoing care, specifically radiation therapy, at the hospital. More important, his Social Security number was lost or incorrect or both, so that the social worker was not able to apply for Medicaid benefits. She was told it would take six to eight weeks to process another Social Security number and a further six to eight weeks to process Medicaid eligibility.

At the social worker's request, the local congressman's office arranged for the Social Security number within three days. After waiting four weeks for his Medicaid card, Robert decided he was too weak to take any treatments and he was tired of staying in respite care with a bunch of people he didn't know. He knew he was dying, but so was his brother who needed his help. The social worker bought Robert the one-way bus ticket he wanted.

Robert's situation illustrates the problems of those without health insurance.[24-26] The 1987 Current Population Survey estimated that 31.1 million people, almost 13 percent of the total U.S. population,[27] are without such coverage. Estimates of the number of people who are inadequately insured range from 8 to 26 percent of the population.[28] For these, medical costs often exceed 10 percent of annual income. The estimates of the number of uninsured and underinsured combine to a staggering fifty to seventy-seven million individuals not adequately protected against the costs of medical care.[10]

The majority of uninsured adults are between ages eighteen and forty-four years, and more than 35 percent earn at least twice the federal poverty level of $1,008 per month for a family of four.[10,28] Almost 80 percent of uninsured adults are white, although 25 percent of blacks, compared to 15 percent of whites, are uninsured. Two-thirds are in the labor force.[29,30]

For the 12.6 million living below the federal poverty level, access to medical care through the Medicaid program is highly variable from state to state. For instance, Alabama's Medicaid covers fewer than 16 percent of those living in poverty while more than 80 percent are covered in California and Utah. Benefits also vary from state to state. For example, inpatient days are limited to twelve per year in Alabama but are unlimited in many other states.[31]

The surveys conducted by the Robert Wood Johnson Foundation in 1976, 1982, and 1986 indicate that as health insurance has become less available, access to medical care has significantly declined.[21,22] Between 1982 and 1986 there was a 65 percent increase in the number of people without a regular source of care and a 70 percent increase in those who did not have an ambulatory visit in the prior twelve months. For the poor there was a 30 percent decline in ambulatory visits while the gap among ethnic groups also widened. Blacks in fair or poor health had an average of 7.6 ambulatory visits in 1982 compared with 8.6 for whites in fair or poor health. By 1986 the gap had widened to 6.8 for blacks, compared with 10.1 for whites, a difference of 32 percent.

More than 16 percent of the U.S. population reported having difficulty obtaining medical care when needed. Of those with chronic diseases or serious illnesses, 18.5 percent went without seeing a doctor during the prior year. And almost 16 percent of pregnant women failed to have a prenatal visit in the first trimester.

The problems of access to health care for minorities are particularly distressing.[21,32] Compared with 16 percent for whites, 20 percent of blacks and 30 percent of Hispanics reported no regular source of care. Blacks were in fair or poor health 44 percent more often than whites. Hispanics were 80 percent more likely to be in fair or poor health than whites.

The health consequences for the medically uninsured are equally tragic.[33] Nicole Lurie and associates studied the effects of a major reduction of benefits in Medi-Cal.[34,35] Before the change in benefits, 75 percent of people with hypertension had diastolic blood pressures less than 90 mm Hg (millimeter of mercury) while there was 64 percent in the comparison group. After the change only 34 percent of the previously covered adults had controlled blood pressures, and 31 percent had diastolic blood pressures greater than 100 mm Hg. Of the comparison group, 78 percent maintained blood pressure control.

Other analyses have documented the adverse effects of being medically uninsured. C. C. Korenbrot's studies of low-income women enrolled in the California OB Access Project indicated an improvement in pregnancy outcomes associated with a savings of $1.70 for every $1 invested in the program.[36] In a review of black patients admitted to Cook County Hospital in Chicago with a diagnosis of myocardial infarction, mortality was 12.7 percent.[37] Mortality for white patients averages approximately 8 percent. Also, in a study of preventive services, uninsured women received fewer such services than their insured counterparts.[38] Data from the National Health Interview Survey showed a "reverse targeting" of four screening tests: blood pressure, Pap smear, clinical breast exam, and glaucoma testing. Women who were poor and uninsured were less likely to have been adequately screened. In the case of cervical cancer 34 percent of women were not adequately screened compared with 26 percent for nonpoor women. As for breast cancer and glaucoma, 45 percent and 42 percent respectively were not screened compared with 38 percent and 30 percent respectively for nonpoor women.

Even in the public sector the lack of health insurance is becoming a barrier to access for necessary care. B. V. Aiken and colleagues studied two hundred consecutive patients without health insurance who came to a public hospital for care, to determine their potential for adverse outcomes.[39] Almost 80 percent of the patients had diseases "for which medical services were judged to have a moderate or curative impact." Furthermore, for 89.5 percent of the patients the lack of services severely compromised community standards for medical care.

While information has accumulated documenting the extent of the lack of medical insurance and the health effects of limited access to medical care, state and local governments have stretched their resources to provide a level of integrity to the safety net of public hospitals, clinics, and health departments.[40] The approaches taken by these governmental units include high-risk insurance pools, indigent care pools, Medicaid expansion, and statewide planning initiatives. Each of these attempts a solution for one small segment of the uninsured population.[41-43]

High-risk insurance pools have been established in more than a dozen states. Those who are uninsurable because of health conditions can purchase health insurance from the insurance pool. However, the costs are between 150 and 400 percent of community ratings. Only a handful of people are able to afford these policies.

Indigent care pools have been established in several states. The Florida Health Care Assistance Act taxes hospital revenues to provide support to hospitals with high uncompensated care costs and to local health department clinics. South Carolina's Medically Indigent Assistance Act taxes hospitals and counties to cover the costs of hospitalization for individuals who apply for assistance. Indigent care pools have also been established in New York, Massachusetts, West Virginia, and Wisconsin. The Massachusetts Health Security Act is the first and most comprehensive legislation enacted by any state.[44] If the state will be able to afford the costs of this program remains to be seen. Washington and Oregon are planning similar statewide pools. Hawaii recently enacted legislation to provide health insurance to all state residents.

Finally, many states have expanded their Medicaid programs as a means of improving access to medical care. A number of recently enacted provisions permit states to include those heretofore excluded from Medicaid, such as intact poor families. Yet despite generous federal matching, state governments have a difficult time identifying the state revenues necessary to meet the federal requirements.

Strategies for Change

The earliest serious proposals for national health insurance came during the crafting of the Social Security system during the 1930s. Because of opposition by the American Medical Association, Congress passed the Social Security Act without health provisions. In the 1950s the Wagner-Murray-Dingell bill for national health insurance received widespread debate but was sidetracked by more modest proposals for health insurance for the elderly. After enactment of Medicare and Medicaid, serious discussion of national health insurance was absent from the national scene until the late 1980s. Growing frustration with the inadequacies of Medicaid, incompletely controlled Medicare costs, and the growth in numbers of the medically uninsured has led to a renewed interest in more comprehensive solutions.[45–60]

The boldest proposal is from the Physicians for a National Health Program.[61] Universal access to medical care would be guaranteed through a federally administered, regionally operated health insurance program. Care would be received through fee-for-service practices, public facilities, or managed care plans. A negotiated fee schedule for physicians would be similar to that used in Canada for controlling physician charges.[62] There would be no controls on utilization. Hospitals would negotiate an annual global budget for operating expenses. Capital costs would be decided separately by a planning agency. The most radical aspect of this proposal is its funding. By abolishing the private health insurance industry, a national health plan would save approximately fifty billion dollars annually. Health insurance for the uninsured would be paid for with these dollars; any additional revenues necessary for this national health program would come from payroll taxes.

Alain Enthoven and Richard Kronick have proposed a universal health insurance plan utilizing a combination of Medicare, Medicaid, and other public programs and competing managed care plans.[63] Their emphasis is on financial protection against health care expenses and the promotion of cost-conscious behaviors by consumers. Employers and individuals would have the opportunity to select from a panel of qualified, competing health care organizations, thereby leading to cost control. Funding for the consumer-choice health plan would come from three sources: first, an 8 percent tax on the first $22,500 of wages of noncovered workers; secondly, a limit on the employer's deduction for health insurance benefits; and thirdly, new state monies. A first-year increase in total health expenditures of $15 billion would be followed by an annual reduction in health care costs of $15 billion.

A third proposal, from the National Leadership Commission on Health, emphasizes the need for a national system of technology assessment as a method for reducing health care costs.[64] Information from clinical studies would be used to establish practice standards, which in turn might ease the problem of medical liability expenses, another costly ingredient in health care. The commission's report, however, does not address the issues of physical compensation, universal access to care, and funding for the uninsured.

Several bills that would establish a national health program have been introduced in Congress but have received little attention. Among these are the USHealth Program Act of Representative Edward Roybal (Dem., N.Y.) and the National Health Service Act of Representative Ron Dellums (Dem., Calif).

Other proposals come from the Health Security Action Council,[65] the Jesse Jackson presidential campaign,[66] and the National Association for Public Health Policy,[67] along with suggestions for the expansion of Medicaid to cover all the poor.[68,69] Each plan would significantly reduce or eliminate the number of people without health insurance.

Chaos, Paradigms, and Medical Care

They had reached the first step by which man becomes the slave of his property.
    —B. Traven, *The Treasure of the Sierra Madre*

The United States health care system and the policies developed to shape its future have been the focus of this discussion. Since much of the policy debate centers on access to care, the health care needs of the homeless are subsumed in this area. Our nation's health care paradigm is dominated by the widely held view that the overall quality of health care is derived from the network of independent practitioners, who at the same time are seen as best qualified to determine quality. The paradigm has become a tautology, with practitioners defining and practicing it. Attempting to design policies that improve access to care, or enhance quality, or improve efficacy is the chaotic process of incremental pressure politics. Each incremental addition is less an improvement than a testimony to the ability of an interest group to influence the decision-making process. The absolute value of each addition to this scheme is irrelevant since it promotes the institutionalization of chaos.

The institutionalization of chaos means that those who are responsible for national health policy—namely, the U.S. Congress, the medical profession, state and local governments, and consulting firms, to name a few—expend enormous amounts of time and energy tinkering with a grossly inadequate system. Each seemingly genuine effort to improve access to care disturbs the health care system elsewhere, requiring additional effort to preserve it and the paradigm. The currently fashionable and necessarily transient interest in health care for the homeless is an example of the consequences of policy initiatives within the existing paradigm.

The solutions proposed for resolving some of the problems with the health care system range from the demonstrably incremental, such as health care for the homeless, to comprehensive, such as proposals for a national health program. None will be easy to accomplish.[45,70–72] Each is constrained within the limitations of our health care paradigm and, therefore, has the realistic potential to be proved inadequate. The problems of access to care have yet to diminish in the face of many creative and often exuberant efforts to improve the availability of health insurance. Each effort is incremental, adding to a fantastically complex and convoluted health care system. The ideas brought forth in each of these proposals may be positive, but each change has a negative perturbation elsewhere. Health care for the homeless programs may be the final fact that brings about a shift of perspective in the paradigm.

Before the eighteenth century, electricity was a frightening, wondrous, and poorly understood phenomenon. Its study was left to basic scientists, who, through careful experimentation, turned speculation and theory into facts and laws. By the mid-nineteenth century electricity was no longer mysterious. Through science and technology it had become a useful and universally available resource.

Within the last twenty-five years the practice of medicine has started to seem very much the way the use of electricity did a hundred years ago. The often mysterious and always wondrous phenomena of the biological sciences have rapidly yielded their secrets to study and experimentation. The medicine practiced in the late twentieth century is substantially based upon facts that are as available and predictable as the results of flipping an electrical switch. The health care provider need not have an intimate knowledge of medical science to make use of these scientific discoveries. Instead, the practitioner understands and uses a number of generally accepted principles that guide medical practice. These principles, in turn, are grounded in a large body of scientific fact.

If a patient presents problems of chest pain or headache, certain questions are asked, exams performed, and tests ordered, and depending upon the results of each of these, a limited range of therapeutic choices becomes evident. The practitioner uses somewhat standard algorithms to obtain predictable results. The algorithm is either learned from experience or taught. In each case it is based upon scientific facts, the origins of which may be incompletely understood by the practitioner. Like the daily use of electricity, intimate knowledge of these facts is not a prerequisite to their appropriate and accomplished use.

Medicine has matured so that much of its practice is predictable. Doctors take for granted much of the theory underpinning care. Like electrical science in the nineteenth century, medical science is at a crossroad where the distinctions between the practical and the complex are clear. Different kinds of knowledge and skill are necessary for the different uses of medical science. The growing interest in practice guidelines reflects an awareness that good-quality medical care is largely predictable and can be practiced using standards of care or guidelines.[73]

Health policy remains fixed in the paradigm where medicine and medical science are synonymous, understood only by its practitioners, who also largely determine its use and even its progress. By changing our view of health care from the extraordinary to the ordinary and everyday, we change the way we decide to create a system of care that provides universal access to health care that is efficient, efficacious, and of good quality.

Medicine is buttressed by enormous catalogs of fact. With facts, the mysterious and frightening aspects of health and illness become the predictable and available remedies and cures we expect from our doctors. Everyday medicine is the use of facts like our everyday use of household electricity. Ignoring the common need for medicine ignores its power and threatens its useful contributions to the well-being of society. The efforts to provide health care to the homeless can provide a blueprint from which we can build new structures out of a limited view of health care as it exists today, a view that is professionally dominated, fragmented, and increasingly unjust.

STEPHEN A. SOMERS
REBECCA W. RIMEL
NADYA SHMAVONIAN
LAURA D. WAXMAN
LILIA M. REYES
STEPHEN L. WOBIDO
PHILIP W. BRICKNER

5

Creation and Evolution of a National Health Care for the Homeless Program

Introduction

On December 12, 1983, in response to the increasingly visible problems faced by homeless persons on the streets of the nation's major cities, RWJF/Pew announced a joint multimillion-dollar grant initiative, HCHP.[1] The announcement embarked the foundations upon a five-year experiment in community coalition building and health care innovation. These were truly uncharted waters for the two foundations and indeed for the nation as a whole. Few in 1983 had begun to reckon seriously with the devastating health and social effects of homelessness or with the health problems that may have contributed to homelessness in the first place.

The news release issued on that day described a program to provide health care and help in arranging social services—e.g., drug and alcohol treatment programs, public assistance, food stamps, Medicaid, and other entitlements—to otherwise unserved homeless people. The origins and features of this program, the major policy issues learned, and the evolution of representative projects within the program are described here.

The Robert Wood Johnson Foundation

The RWJF is among the nation's largest private philanthropies and one of the most focused in its grant making. All of the nearly hundred million dollars it disburses each year is devoted to developing solutions to this country's health care problems.

Since the foundation became a national philanthropy in 1972, it has invested a significant proportion of its resources in major multisite national programs. The rationale underlying these demonstrations has been to design and implement new models, evaluate them properly, and if they are successful, disseminate them for broader replication by the federal government and others in the public sector. Although in today's fiscal environment expecting such a chain of events might seem unreasonable, it did occur when the federal government replicated the HCHP under the McKinney Act in 1987.

The program attained this level of recognition in significant degree through partnership between RWJF and Pew and cosponsorship by the United States Conference of Mayors. The practice of seeking partners and cosponsors has been at the core of the success of many of RWJF's programs, bringing both increased resources and greater visibility and leadership.

The Pew Charitable Trusts

The Pew Charitable Trusts is also one of America's largest general foundations. Its health and human services program expends more than fifty million dollars annually on national, local, and international efforts. A major thrust of the Pew program is improvement of services to groups at risk. The homeless, along with the elderly, children and youth, and the mentally and physically disabled, are focuses of the trusts' grant making. The HCHP is one of several Pew initiatives seeking creative ways to serve better these high-risk groups.

The United States Conference of Mayors' Involvement in Homelessness

In October 1982 the United States Conference of Mayors brought the growing problem of homelessness and hunger to national attention through a fifty-five-city survey. The survey showed that demand for emergency services, including food and shelter, had increased in cities across the nation and that, on average, only 43 percent of the demand for such services was being met. Alarmed by the new findings, the conference convened in November 1982 an Emergency Meeting on Emergency Needs which brought together mayors, other city officials, and representatives of private service agencies to discuss the emergency service problem and to develop recommendations for national and local actions needed to respond to this growing crisis.

At that meeting the mayors drafted a five-point plan for submission to Congress and the Reagan administration "to help avert a disastrous winter for those in need." The mayors' specific recommendations included an emergency congressional appropriation of five hundred million dollars "to help cities provide the food, shelter, heat, medical care and clothing needed by the growing numbers of homeless families, and individuals" that winter. The request for federal emergency help for the homeless was reiterated at a congressional hearing on December 15, 1982—the first hearing held in Congress on homelessness since the Great Depression—in testimony presented by Ted Wilson, then the mayor of Salt Lake City, on behalf of the Conference of Mayors.

In 1987, nearly five years after the mayors first called for federal emergency aid to address the homelessness crisis, Congress passed the McKinney Act, the first major legislation to respond to the special needs of the homeless. The mayors' conference played a key role in providing information to Congress and the public that substantiated the need for such legislation. At numerous congressional hearings prior to enactment of the McKinney Act, members of the conference's Task Force on Hunger and Homelessness testified on homelessness and on federal initiatives needed to address this growing problem. Through numerous reports, the conference documented the causes and magnitudes of the problems of homelessness, hunger, and poverty in cities, how cities were responding to them, and what national responses were required.

Since enactment of the McKinney Act, the conference has worked to ensure effective implementation of the law, including lobbying for, at minimum, full funding of the amounts that have been authorized for the various programs, such as the HCHP. The conference has continued to make available to Congress, other policy makers, and the public current information on the problems of homelessness and the need for increased national commitment to deal with the problem.[2-5]

The conference has also been involved in efforts to assist cities in improving their responses to the problems of homelessness. In 1984 the conference joined RWJF and Pew in cosponsoring the HCHP.

It has been the conference's long-standing policy that to respond adequately to the growth of homelessness, there must be concerted efforts to address the root causes of the problem. These causes include the shortage of housing affordable to low-income people, unemployment and other employment-related problems, inadequate benefit levels in income assistance programs, and inadequate funding for mental health, social services, and other supportive services.

The Origins of the Program

The development of the program itself began at RWJF in July 1982, under the direction of Drew Altman, Ph.D., then a vice-president at the foundation. He, his colleagues, and members of the foundation's board of trustees had followed the development of homelessness as a national policy issue, personally noting the growing number of homeless persons in Philadelphia, Washington, Chicago, and Los Angeles, cities where they lived or visited while working on other health care programs. Because RWJF is a health care philanthropy, homelessness seemed at first to be a problem not suited to an RWJF-style intervention. But because the issue was not being addressed in any serious way and because it was growing, the health care staff at RWJF began to consider more closely the conditions of home-lessness. They saw rampant physical illness, from tuberculosis to leg ulcers. They also recognized that a twenty-year-long policy of deinstitutionalization had left thousands of individuals with severe mental disabilities helplessly wandering the streets in search of food and shelter.

With that recognition, it did not take long to begin designing a national com-petitive grant program. The first questions to be answered—Who are the home-less? Is health care a serious need among them? Are meaningful interventions possible?—led the foundation staff to develop its own profile of the nation's homeless population.

Staffers found both increasing numbers and much more diversity than the common stereotypes of bag ladies and alcoholics. In general, they could identify three distinct subgroups:

- The traditional skid row population of white older males with chronic alcohol and drug abuse problems
- A newer population of former mental patients who had been deinstitution-alized (or never institutionalized) during the 1970's but still lacked commu-nity mental health, housing or job programs
- The newest homeless population of mostly minority young adults and chil-dren

Many of the latter are casualties of shrinking local or regional economies, drastic reductions in social programs, or other economic dislocations. A deeply troubled minority of the homeless family population suffers from complex medi-cal, psychological, and substance abuse problems that essentially render them dysfunctional without social supports. This rudimentary taxonomy of skid row, deinstitutionalized, and families later evolved to include other subgroups like runaway and throwaway children, homeless veterans, the working homeless, and homeless people with AIDS.

The RWJF staff also consulted a wide range of people with recent knowledge and experience in dealing with the problems of homelessness, ranging from health care professionals to urban officials. It became clear that health care was a crucial need among the homeless and could be a stablizing force in their lives. However, except for sporadic visits to emergency rooms, largely in public hospitals, the homeless did not generally receive health services, making them one of the nation's most medically underserved groups. The few operating shelter programs with health service components had found that when health care was made available in an accessible, nonthreatening, and continuous manner, the homeless used the services.

By 1983 a number of cities had begun to set in motion activities directed toward meeting the diverse needs of the homeless. Some already had in place large public shelter systems, as well as publicly and privately supported health and social services for at least a portion of their homeless. Others had disputatious and quarreling advocates and agencies and poor progress. But foundation staff members believed that communitywide coordination was critical to addressing this problem effectively. Therefore, they decided to accept only one grant application per city and to require applicant coalitions to be citywide, include both public and private agencies, and have the support of the mayor.

In keeping with practices in a variety of other national health care programs, the foundations opted not to administer the program directly. Rather, they turned to the Department of Community Medicine at New York's St. Vincent's Hospital and Medical Center. St. Vincent's had operated a variety of health programs for the homeless in the Chelsea and Greenwich Village areas since 1969. Outreach programs in SRO hotels and in some of the city-run shelters had served as one illustration of successful intervention.

The Program's Selection Process

Eligibility for funding was limited to the nation's fifty-one largest cities in the United States and San Juan, Puerto Rico.[1] Each grant applicant had to develop an overall strategy for delivering health and other services to as many homeless persons as possible, with a minimum of fifteen hundred per year to be served. A citywide coalition, including representatives of public, voluntary, and religious groups, would have to design and implement the project. The intent was to create a leadership structure in each city. As such coalitions strengthened, it was hoped that they would become a stable structure for addressing the health and related needs of the homeless beyond the four-year grant period.

The Request for Proposals required each local program to establish locations where care could be given on an ongoing basis to as large a population of homeless people as possible. Core service teams of physicians, nurses, and social workers were suggested, each team with clearly defined service coordinators and with mechanisms for making successful referrals to other providers (e.g., hospitals and mental health centers). Finally, the RFP embodied the foundations' belief that in addition to the need to provide direct health care, local programs must advocate and seek to assure improved access to other needed services and public benefits programs, such as welfare, housing, and job training, on an ongoing basis. The membership of each local coalition, therefore, was to include representatives of welfare and housing agencies.

Because the RWJF/Pew funding was limited to four years, the RFPs required each city to develop a specific plan for continuing the program after the grant ended. A principal outcome of this requirement was to encourage local coalitions to attempt to mainstream the homeless into existing reimbursement programs (e.g., Medicaid) and delivery systems.

In order to help select grantees, the foundations appointed a National Advisory Committee. Included among the committee members were five mayors, including its chair, Mayor Henry Maier of Milwaukee, and health and social services experts. The trustees of the two foundations made the final decisions on the awarding of grants.

In all, more than four hundred inquiries were received from many different, often competing sources, including health professionals and institutions, major voluntary organizations, religious groups dealing with the homeless, mental health, welfare, and housing. In addition, many ineligible cities expressed interest. In order to avoid division and polarization, competing groups within each eligible city were not recognized or offered application kits until they had formed a single coalition, with the mayor's endorsement. This requirement proved successful, and all eligible cities, even those with deeply antagonistic groups, were able to submit acceptable letters of interest.

Forty-five of the eligible cities submitted full grant applications. Some of the smaller cities declined to complete applications because they had small numbers of homeless, which, when coupled with their transiency or a lack of public hospitals, made the requirement of serving fifteen hundred homeless individuals per year seem unfeasible. Thirty-seven reviewers evaluated the applications. To assure an equitable review process, scores were adjusted under a procedure developed by the Educational Testing Service of Princeton, New Jersey.

The evaluations granted points for responses to four areas of concern:

1. Applicant's case for the need and importance of the grant

2. A workable organizational structure that satisfied the eligibility criteria of the program guidelines

3. A clear and convincing project plan for providing hands-on health care and case management services to homeless persons that could also be sustained beyond the four-year project period

4. The compatibility of the applicant's work plan and budget with the project plan and the goals of the city's overall effort

Additional points were granted for the following:

- The potential number of homeless to be served above the fifteen-hundred-per-year minimum
- The ability to provide services in a continuous manner
- The ability to improve access to existing public benefit programs
- The commitment of other, previously unavailable state, local and private funds
- The ability to assure access to additional health and other services
- The active involvement and participation of local and state governments and hospitals

From this process teams of reviewers selected twenty-four cities site visits as the final step in consideration for funding recommendations. This better enabled the reviewers to assess local commitment and the degree to which the goals and objectives of the proposals were realistic and achievable.

Originally, RWJF and Pew together had pledged a total of $19.4 million to be distributed to coalitions in up to fourteen cities. However, the site visits exposed the extent and severity of the problem and prompted the National Advisory Committee to make funding recommendations beyond the fourteen. The foundations responded by increasing the number of awards to nineteen and the total amount of those awards to $25 million.

Following final approval of the nineteen cities by each of the foundations' boards, the nineteen "winners" were announced at a Washington, D.C., press conference on December 19, 1984, almost exactly one year after the program's original announcement.

Early Responses to the Homeless Program

Prior to the HCHP, the nation's largest cities had begun to respond in a variety of ways to the issue of homelessness in general and health care for the homeless in particular. These local responses had been shaped by:

- Local perceptions of the homeless population and special subgroups
- The city's location and climate
- The range and character of existing shelter, health, and social services
- The overall service and advocacy infrastructure

The response to the RWJF/Pew program highlighted these and other local differences, for instance in the types of coalitions, in the types of organizations that received the grants, and in the proposed service patterns. The governing coalitions that developed the proposals and were to oversee the programs in the nineteen grantee cities could be grouped into three types (see Table 5.1):

Table 5.1 GOVERNING COALITIONS IN NINETEEN
GRANTEE CITIES[6]

COALITION TYPE	NUMBER OF CITIES
Preexisting coalition for the homeless	5
New coalition for the homeless	3
New coalition for health care for the homeless	11

- Preexisting coalitions for the homeless: Some cities had already created coalitions to address the broad range of issues affecting the homeless and simply added a health care component or strengthened the coalitions' existing concern for health issues in response to the national program.
- New coalitions for the homeless: Some cities had no formal citywide groups concerned with the homeless population prior to the national program. RWJF/Pew funding provided the impetus for creating such coalitions with health care one concern among many.
- New health care coalitions for the homeless: Most cities had some preexisting coalitions uniting local groups' concerns for the homeless within a citywide structure, often with an extensive history and established priorities. The national program led these cities to create new, specialized coalitions focusing on health care for the homeless.

Most grantee cities had to designate organizations to receive and administer grant funds since the governing coalitions themselves often lacked the necessary legal incorporation and tax exemption. A review of these revealed even more diversity. Seven distinct types of grantee organizations were identifiable (See Table 5.2):

- Charitable trusts: organizations designed to give or receive grants as a nonprofit agency, often serving as a conduit for developing projects and funding them

Table 5.2 DESIGNATED GRANTEE
ORGANIZATIONS IN NINETEEN
GRANTEE CITIES[6]

TYPE OF GRANTEE	NUMBER OF CITIES
Charitable trusts	3
Planning and coordinating agencies	6
Nonsectarian social service agencies	2
Incorporated coalitions	1
Universities and health providers	3
Religious organizations	3
Public agencies	1

- Planning and coordinating agencies/federations: agencies that serve as planning and coordinating agencies and federated charities that have member agencies, such as United Way
- Nonsectarian social service agencies: traditional social service agencies that provide direct services
- Incorporated coalitions: coalitions of organizations concerned with the homeless that are legally incorporated
- Universities/schools: universities, medical and nursing schools, and hospitals
- Religious organizations: either denominational organizations or coalitions of religious organizations
- Public agencies: city agencies as designated grantees.

The service patterns that emerged involved a wide variety of delivery arrangements. Some cities opted for permanent clinics specializing in health services for the homeless. Others created mobile or outreach programs. Some coalitions became directly involved in service delivery while others contracted with existing providers. Depending upon local resources, some chose to target the homeless population in shelters. Others focused on those who lived on the streets and/or frequented soup kitchens and church basements.

In order to illustrate the wide range of local programs that emerged, three grantee cities have been chosen as case studies: Denver, Nashville, and San Antonio. These descriptions are based on original grant applications.

Programs in Their Initial Stage

Denver (Population 506,000)[7]

Governance: Denver had an existing incorporated coalition eligible to be the grantee organization. The Colorado Coalition for the Homeless was established in late 1983 by representatives from more than forty agencies and individuals concerned about the homeless in Denver. This coalition was broad-based, including homeless service providers, public and voluntary agencies, and religious, business, medical, foundation, and academic communities.

The coalition assumed a dual task for itself. Its short-term goal was to plan, coordinate, and advocate for means to meet the immediate needs of homeless persons. The long-term goals were to raise people's consciousness and to reverse the trend toward homelessness and remove its causes.

Homeless Population: The coalition identified seven different groups of home-less persons in Denver:

- Substance abusers.
- Chronically mentally ill.
- The long-term homeless—individuals resigned to a life of homelessness.
- The new poor—those who recently experienced personal or family crises, including domestic violence, broken marriages, unemployment, evictions and benefit cuts. They were generally people who were well motivated to move out of homelessness but who clearly needed support for a period of time.
- The marginalized—those who moved in and out of self-sufficiency. They were employed (often temporarily) and lived in apartments or SROs for a while and then seemed no longer able to sustain that.
- The new homeless—including the new influx of young people. They seemed to be persons who never had many breaks, having been born into unstable situations carried on into their adult lives. They often appeared to be lost, or disenfranchised, or minimally disillusioned in a way that seemed to handicap their ability to stabilize themselves. They lacked adequate job skills and self-discipline.
- Handicapped and older persons—those, often more near homelessness than actually homeless, who lacked any support system, could not work, and frequented the day shelters along with the homeless for the fellowship and inclusion they found there.

Service Pattern: The Denver program included a stationary clinic site and outreach. By operating a stable clinic, the program could schedule homeless persons for visits and not be concerned about where a mobile team was on a given day. The program staff included a project director, a physician's assistant, a registered nurse, a social worker, an outreach/mental health worker, a reception-ist/administrative assistant, a half-time physician, and a very part-time family physician. In addition, volunteers, including physicians, a nurse practitioner, a nurse, a health aide, and a premed student, took part.

Nashville (Population 455,000)[8]

Governance: Nashville used the foundations' program as the impetus to orga-nize a new Coalition for the Homeless. In 1982 various leaders in Nashville had appealed to the Council of Community Services, a local planning and coordinating agency, to study the homeless problem and evaluate what should be done. In 1983, largely in response to the RWJF/Pew announcement, the council established the Nashville Coalition for the Homeless. It included representatives from social service agencies, university personnel, businessmen, and a judge. The mission of this coalition was to review existing programs and establish coordinated services, including health, substance abuse, mental health, employment, and housing. The board of directors of the council appointed a Project Governance Committee to oversee implementation of the Health Care for the Homeless Program.

Homeless Population: The homeless of Nashville were described as long-term residents recently unemployed, the deinstitutionalized, people traveling north to south in search of jobs, young musicians who hoped to make it in "Music City," and victims of domestic violence and family breakdown. It was estimated that on any given night, there might be as many as fourteen hundred individuals who were homeless. Over the course of 1983 the city's two largest shelters housed ten thousand.

Service Pattern: Nashville's Health Care for the Homeless Program established the Downtown Clinic, a primary care facility in the city's skid row district. The clinic was located between the city's two principal shelters, the Union Mission and the Salvation Army. Staff included a project director, a medical director, a physician's assistant, family nurse clinicians, a medical assistant, case managers, and mental health specialists. Referral to the Downtown Clinic was to come primarily through word of mouth and from other service providers. Outreach to a soup kitchen outside downtown Nashville and to a site in North Nashville was planned. Physical examinations were to be provided for residents of a family shelter and recently released prisoners at a temporary shelter. The Downtown Clinic was also to serve as a medical consultant for a runaway youth shelter. It had a subcontract with the Tennessee Department of Mental Health for a mental health specialist. Metropolitan Social Services and the Meharry Community Mental Health Center also deployed staff to the clinic.

San Antonio (Population 819,000)[9]

Governance: San Antonio was a city with limited services for the homeless. It created a broad-based coalition in response to the foundations' announcement of the grants. The designated grantee was the San Antonio Urban Council, a non-profit organization formed by a coalition of local churches.

Homeless Population: The San Antonio application described the local homeless population as diverse, with more women and children, more minorities, and more young persons than seemed typical in other areas. Also included were the mentally ill and the new and temporarily homeless.

Service Pattern: Services were delivered at two existing shelters. One had been run by the Salvation Army for twenty-five years and provided two meals, showers, and shelter for 250 persons a night. Three years earlier the churches themselves had started a winter shelter for up to 250 additional persons a night. This site was being renovated and was to serve men, women, and children, providing meals, showers, laundry, mail pickup, and storage.

Each shelter team staff included a family nurse practitioner and social worker. Those needing more specialized care were referred to either the county hospital or the closest federally funded clinic. Emergency room care was provided by local hospitals. Mentally ill residents were referred to a county mental health program.

Most direct services were subcontracted with health or social service providers. A corps of volunteers from the Christian Assistance Ministry provided additional support to the staff and the homeless.

Conclusion

When RWJF and Pew initiated this effort to address the health problems of the homeless, the two foundations considered it a very high-risk venture in a brand-new area. Although no foundation demonstration program can solve a national problem, the nineteen-city twenty-five-million-dollar HCHP is considered successful. Indeed, it established a whole new field of endeavor for local health care providers and for the federal government. Over four years HCHP clinicians provided primary care services, assessments, and referrals to more than two hundred thousand homeless persons. All nineteen cities found the motivation and financial resources to continue after foundation funding had ceased.

As foundation support drew to a close, RWJF staff began to examine both the successes and the shortcomings of the service systems that had been established under the HCHP. Aside from the inability to deal with the need for housing, principal among the shortcomings was that there was no guarantee that referral services were obtained or even sought by homeless clients.

Most students of homelessness agree that the population can be sorted into a subgroup suffering principally from economic dislocation and another with fundamental disabling problems. The latter group requires more comprehensive and ongoing care than may be available in a shelter-based clinic. Among those most in need of such follow-up care were homeless individuals suffering from disabling mental conditions, substance abuse, and AIDS and homeless families with a single female usually too dysfunctional to secure services for herself and her young children.

Neither housing by itself nor episodic services provided without appropriate shelter can really help families with complex economic, health, and developmental problems. Indeed, the concept of service-enriched housing, in which financing and delivery mechanisms for health-related services are built into the housing in the design stage seems appropriate for this population. The HCHP moved citywide coalitions to address the health and service problems of their most destitute residents. It also moved federal government and the sponsoring foundations to expand their own limits and to bolster and integrate health and social services for the homeless in communities across the nation.

PART II

CLINICAL CONCERNS

BRIAN C. SCANLAN
PHILIP W. BRICKNER

6

Clinical Concerns in the Care of Homeless Persons

What Is Different About Working with the Homeless?

Primary care is the goal of service programs for the homeless. Primary prevention of illness and identification of individuals at risk for disease can be achieved through the medical interview and physical examination, designed to screen for illness and risk factors. These objectives apply to all health care relationships. However, providers who work with homeless persons must first face the tasks of reaching an isolated and often alienated population before attempting to assess the medical needs of their patients.

The tasks facing providers who hope to manage the *chronic* illness and health needs of homeless persons are more formidable. Upon identifying chronic illness, such as diabetes mellitus or hypertension, providers must attempt to institute appropriate therapy when available, modify the behavior of the patient to reduce the risks of complications, promote compliance with therapy and health instruction, and coordinate the intervention of other disciplines as needed. These goals are elusive for providers working with any patient base, let alone a population without stable shelter, economic means, social supports, or basic trust in the individuals or institutions attempting to help.

Although some analysts choose to simplify the taxonomy of homelessness, claiming the vast majority of homeless persons to be drug-dependent, alcoholic, or mentally ill, in fact, a wide spectrum of subgroups of homeless persons has clearly emerged. Women, children, youth, whole families, and older people are entering the ranks of the homeless in many cities, bringing with them a distinct set of health needs which vary dramatically from those of the stereotypic homeless man of skid row or the deinstitutionalized schizophrenic woman. It is incumbent upon health care providers to understand the contribution of various subpopulations to the patient mix in order to lend specificity to the health service systems they devise.

The inability of homeless persons to care adequately for themselves is often attributed solely to the presence of mental illness and substance abuse, but the behavior of homeless persons is only one of several significant influences on the delivery of care. The attitudes of providers, the locus of care, and the design of the delivery system itself all influence the outcome of any patient encounter.

As a group the homeless may be viewed as bizarre, physically unattractive, dirty, and ultimately unworthy of the level of care provided to the "citizen," a term from the hospital lexicon used to denote a respectable patient. In a recent discussion an attending physician in an urban hospital freely admitted his feeling that a differential standard of care should exist for an executive of a large corporation and for a homeless alcoholic based on the patient's "value to society." This statement is remarkable chiefly for its frankness. Few hospitals would offer this position as policy, yet when homeless patients recount visits to hospitals and encounters with physicians, it is evident that the dispassionate approach demanded by medical ethics is often abandoned. Staff attitudes may compromise the quality of care rendered, and there may be little incentive for staff members to correct their attitudes. The complex medical and social problems posed by the homeless often create serious financial burdens to hospitals resulting from protracted lengths of stay and lack of medical insurance.

Homeless persons who seek help rarely have access to primary care. Episodic assessment and treatment obtained in the crisis-oriented setting of an urban emergency room is perhaps the most common mode of care the homeless experience. Aside from staff attitudes, the setting itself may do little to foster compliance with treatment and follow-up. The sheer numbers of patients seen in an emergency room and the prevalence of critical problems may deny attention to the street person who merely has acute bronchitis or bilateral cellulitis of the legs. Neither problem is immediately threatening to life, and each could be relatively easily treated if there existed a modicum of stability in the patient's situation. The facts of life for the homeless patient, however, are not likely to be the focus of an emergency room encounter, and their influence on effective care may not be appreciated.

A nurse at a New York City men's shelter describes aptly the usual outcome of episodic care for her clients, who often arrive at her clinic's doors on a Monday morning with "three slips of paper": a prescription which has not been filled because the patient has no funds; a list of instructions (e.g., bed rest, leg elevation, warm soaks) which cannot be accomplished in a shelter setting; and a slip for a follow-up appointment which cannot be kept because the patient's condition may have progressed by now to warrant return to the emergency room for admission to the hospital.

The prescription may have been written by a good and compassionate physician, and the instructions given by an equally sensitive nurse, but the demands of caring for shelter residents or the unsheltered often exceed the limits of the individual hospital-based provider. Care provided where the homeless congregate, by an interdisciplinary team that has an established and reliable association with a local hospital, has distinct advantages over conventional modes of care.

Ellen Baxter and Kim Hopper in their ground-breaking analysis of homelessness in New York[1] found that contrary to a common stereotype, homeless people at shelters and soup kitchens accepted assistance in whatever form offered, always in numbers greater than could be accommodated. Health care provided to the homeless where they gather is likely to be met with the same degree of enthusiasm, if offered in a nonthreatening, consistent manner by a team of professionals who are flexible enough to adapt their style to the terms of this population.

Interdisciplinary teams of nurses, social workers, and physicians have worked successfully in HCHPs across the country. Serving in a variety of sites, including shelters, drop-in centers, and SRO hotels, teams have offered an alternative to fragmented, episodic health care. Essential to the success of their efforts is the support provided by a strong connection to a hospital with a stated interest in the medically underserved. Hospital-based care, in specialty clinics, the emergency room, or inpatient services, is more easily provided with this collaboration.

Initial contact with patients is most often made on regularly scheduled site visits or in established satellite clinics. A casual but persistent manner is employed by the team members assigned the task of making initial contact during a site visit at a hotel or drop-in center. Adherence to a reliable schedule of visits and enlisting initial contacts to herald the team members' presence can contribute to continued success. Finding cases is the goal of site visits. Clients who need further assessment or therapy can be referred to the hospital-based clinic or emergency room as required.

The hospital's primary care clinic is the model for the on-site clinics. However, satellite units, which can substitute for hospital-based medical outpatient services in many cases, can be established at sites with the space and ancillary staff to accommodate them. It must be recognized that along with a higher level of care provided by satellite clinics a significant increase in work and responsibility may be generated for shelter staff members. The identification of one or two shelter residents with chronic illness may stretch a shelter's or hotel's meager resources. The health care team must be sensitive to the impact its work may have on the equally important agendas of other shelter staff members.

Homeless Women: A Focus on High-Risk Pregnancies

All pregnant homeless women are at high risk. Daily priorities of their lives may interfere with opportunity for medical care. Finding the means to nurture, feed, and protect their other children may take all the energy and attention available, until labor pains start. Support from adults—a loved one, a spouse, siblings, parents—is a rarity for a homeless woman.

These are women in crisis, abused, burned out of their homes, or evicted. Temporarily placed in SROs, motels, or transient units maintained by such voluntary agencies as the Salvation Army, they generally find themselves in alien environments, bereft of friends. They are unfamiliar with local geography, stores, school, the neighborhood clinics. They are frightened, angry, and intimidated. It is a daunting task for a mother to organize life for herself and her children under these conditions. To add the requirement that she seek out a source for prenatal care is hard, even though good health and life are at stake.

The basic requisites of prenatal care are well understood. They include assuring adequate nutrition, control of blood pressure, elimination of gynecologic disease, limitation of weight gain, classes in parenting skills, and familiarity with birthing procedures. The living conditions and social stresses of these women make good prenatal care hard to offer and a challenge to receive.

Good care of homeless pregnant women requires skilled attention by a properly trained professional. An obstetrician would be most appropriate, although a family practitioner or a nurse midwife might be acceptable. Further, the woman should be seen in a comfortable and properly equipped office. Ad hoc arrangements that may be adequate for other forms of basic health care are not acceptable. The pregnant woman must be encouraged by all reasonable means to attend a genuine prenatal clinic. The health care team members must therefore accept the responsibility of making this happen. They should pay much attention to engaging the patient in the process, allowing her the support needed to keep appointments, arranging for temporary care of her other children, obtaining vitamin supplements and other medications prescribed for her, and encouraging her to avoid conduct that may hurt the fetus. Staff should accompany the woman to clinic visits if necessary and spend time informing clinic staff, from receptionist to billing clerk, nurse, and physician, about the circumstances the patient faces. Helping her plan postnatal care, a complex challenge in these circumstances, demands consideration.

The demographics of pregnancy among homeless women have been reviewed by James Wright, Ph.D.[2] His information derives from reports of the nineteen HCHPs funded by RWJF/Pew. Wright notes that the average age of homeless persons in this country is in the early to middle thirties. The assumption that this is a sexually active population is supported by the fact that 11.4 percent of the women seen in the HCHPs more than once were pregnant at their first contact. Rough estimates suggest that the rate of pregnancies among adult women in the HCHPs is about twice the national rate. Limited understanding of contraceptive technique and lack of access to family planning services are probably the chief explanation for this observation. A higher incidence of rape also may play a role.

In Wright's study, the highest pregnancy rate is found among the youngest cohort, sixteen- to nineteen-year-olds. Of this group, 25 percent have been pregnant during their contact with HCHPs. The rate in twenty- to twenty-four-year-olds is 20 percent, falls to slightly more than 10 percent for those aged twenty-five to twenty-nine, and then decreases rapidly. Differences between whites and non-whites are insignificant.

In a survey conducted by the Pediatric Community Medicine staff at St. Vincent's Hospital in New York City, of children up to age eighteen living in one SRO, 50 percent (four out of eight) biologically capable of pregnancy were pregnant. The present situation of homeless families has led in part to an accelerating cycle of children bearing children, a demeaning and self-defeating metaphor of the homeless.

Clinical Disorders of Homeless Persons

HCHPs throughout the country have shown that most chronic and acute medical illnesses afflict homeless persons at significantly higher rates than in the domiciled population. Data from HCHPs throughout the country have been compiled and analyzed by the Social and Demographic Research Institute.[3] This work provides the most comprehensive view of the health concerns of homeless persons to date.

A comparison of the health of a New York City homeless population and a domiciled population was conducted in 1985[4] by studying the health data collected in clinics for homeless persons and the data provided by the National Ambulatory Medical Care Survey conducted by the U.S. Public Health Service in 1979.[5] Data from NAMCS were considered to represent the health status of domiciled persons seeking care at ambulatory sites nationwide. The SADRI study concludes that most medical problems occur at rates two to six times higher among the homeless than among the domiciled. After the study accounted for significant demographic differences between the two samples, most categories of illness were still found to occur at increased rates among homeless persons. See Table 6.1.

Table 6.1

CATEGORY OF DISORDER	TIMES HIGHER THAN NAMCS RATE
Neurological	6
Hepatic	5
Respiratory	4
Nutritional	4
Skin	2–3
Trauma	2–3

The experience of HCHPs to date further suggests that the homeless are sicker than the general population. Data provided by SADRI[3] show that two-thirds of homeless persons who make visits to seek care do so for a range of acute medical problems, the remaining third for chronic illness. Approximately 80 percent of the acute problems seen are comprised of upper respiratory ailments (33 percent), trauma (23 percent), and minor skin ailments (14 percent). Self-limited illness, such as an upper respiratory viral infection, is more likely to be self-treated by a domiciled population able to limit environmental exposure and afford over-the-counter preparations to relieve symptoms.

Trauma is the presenting complaint of about one-quarter of homeless patients with acute disorders. Youth and male sex are risk factors for traumatic events, which include lacerations, sprains, contusions, and fractures. In settings serving a young, predominantly male population, trauma is likely to be the most frequently encountered medical problem. The mortality rate can be high. J. T. Kelly's review of trauma among San Francisco's homeless[6] is illustrative:

Trauma victims included homeless men and women of all ages, but were typically males from 20 to 39 years of age. They suffered a great variety of severe injuries, including stab wounds, head trauma, blunt trauma, multisystem trauma, gun shots, suicide attempts, burns, complex facial fractures, hip fractures, pneumothoraces, and lacerations of the neck, chest, liver, large and small bowel, and tendons of the hands. Stab wounds and fractures predominated and accounted for 65% of the major trauma injuries. . . . A 46-year-old homeless male diabetic suffered multiple rib fractures when a garbage truck emptied into its compactor the dumpster in which he was asleep. A 35-year-old homeless female alcoholic sustained a skull fracture when she was beaten and raped by four men in a deserted building where she was sleeping.

The course of a minor traumatic event may be complicated from the outset by the presence of concurrent substance abuse or mental illness, which can profoundly affect the patient's ability to recognize the need for care or to seek help promptly and appropriately. The ability to follow instructions, fill prescriptions, and monitor progress may be impaired by a variety of psychological, social, and economic factors. Compliance with follow-up appointments given to homeless patients who were initially seen for trauma in Kelly's review was as low as 20 to 30 percent.[6] The complications of wound infection and loss of function thereby occur more frequently to homeless patients.

The most common infectious diseases encountered among the homeless are acute respiratory disorders. The role of dormitory-style living in promoting outbreaks of acute respiratory illness is undeniable. Characteristics of the homeless patient may conspire to complicate the usual brief illness caused by most viral agents. A high prevalence of tobacco use, underlying chronic illness, incomplete immunization, poor nutrition, and poverty contribute to longer and more serious bouts with colds and influenza.

Chronic obstructive pulmonary disease (COPD) and chronic lung infections also occur with increased frequency. COPD occurs at a rate six times as great as that of a domiciled sample (NAMCS), a difference attributable in part to the elevated rate of tobacco use among the homeless. Considering the tenacity of nicotine addiction and the deprivations of homelessness, it is unlikely that primary care providers can hope for much success in trying to modify smoking behavior in homeless patients. Tobacco use is often linked to other addictive behavior (e.g., alcoholism and opiate abuse) and is common among patients with significant mental disorders. The association of tobacco use with other intractable disorders which occur frequently among the homeless makes the cessation of smoking an elusive goal.

Pulmonary tuberculosis is encountered frequently among the homeless. Outcomes of this infection associated with bygone eras—namely, death and spread of the infection beyond the lungs—are also more frequently seen. The decline in the incidence of tuberculosis observed in the United States through most of this century is probably due to improved living standards and the reduction of late progression of the disease accomplished through prompt recognition and effective antibiotic therapy. Homeless persons do not share in the benefits of a generally improved standard of living and certainly are more likely to elude the efforts of public health workers and primary care providers. Consequently, the homeless remain at increased risk for the disease and its complications. Chemoprophylaxis with isoniazid and antibiotic therapy for active disease both require months of consistent treatment and follow-up evaluations. Homeless patients beyond the reach of primary care efforts will remain a reservoir of untreated or inadequately treated disease.

Chronic illness in general is more prevalent among the homeless population. Of the patients seen by HCHPs,[3] 31 percent had at least one chronic disorder, compared with 25 percent in the NAMCS sample of domiciled patients. The prevalence of chronic illness in the HCHP sample increased with age, male sex, and black race. Hypertension, gastrointestinal disorders, and peripheral vascular disease were the most common.

A higher prevalence of hypertension was encountered among homeless patients specifically screened for the disorder by the St. Vincent's Hospital Department of Community Medicine in New York City.[7] Twenty-five percent to one-third of this sample were hypertensive. Male sex, black race, age, and alcohol use were risk factors for hypertension, mirroring the HCHP sample. Alcohol abuse is a recognized contributing factor to hypertension, as well as to a wide variety of neurological disorders and gastrointestinal diseases. Interestingly, the prevalence rates in each of these disease categories for homeless nonusers of alcohol remains higher than that of domiciled abstainers.

Peripheral vascular disease is a common cause of morbidity among the homeless population.[8,9,4] Between 10 and 20 percent of various study populations have had significant vascular disease, usually of the lower extremities. Venous insufficiency, cellulitis, dependent edema, and leg ulcers are commonly encountered, particularly in settings where there is little opportunity for recumbency and leg elevation to counter the influence of gravity on dependent extremities. Of the medical disorders, exclusive of substance abuse, encountered with greater frequency among homeless persons, disorders of the limbs are perhaps the most strongly correlated to the homeless state. The homeless patient is fifteen times more likely than an age-matched domiciled patient to have significant disease of the peripheral circulation.[4]

Kevin McBride and Robert J. Mulcare[10] have provided an excellent review of the pathogenesis and treatment of the stasis ulcer, the most prevalent form of peripheral vascular disease. The objectives of the care plan they outline are, first, the relief of venous hypertension, and, secondly, the consistent daily application of therapy to established ulcers. The difficulty of establishing and maintaining follow-up of homeless patients in traditional outpatient settings is well recognized. The presence of alcoholism, substance abuse, and psychiatric illness can influence the patient's general ability to keep appointments and otherwise comply. Leg elevation and recumbency are the simplest and most effective means of reducing venous pressure in lower extremities, but many shelters either cannot accommodate this simple maneuver or may place strict limits. Support stockings, if the patient can obtain them, are easily stolen during the night, when they should be removed. The availability of abundant clean water, soap, and sterile dressings for daily care may be severely limited. The presence of underlying disease, such as diabetes mellitus, is likely to remain undetected because of the lack of comprehensive care, and appropriate medical management may not be established. Thus, an array of individual and environmental determinants can render a relatively simple medical regimen ineffectual and contribute to the development of life-threatening and costly complications.

Primary diseases of the skin and cutaneous manifestations of chronic illnesses are common presenting complaints of homeless patients. The incidence of dermatologic afflictions, such as psoriasis, impetigo, seborrhea, and nonspecific dermatitis, may be at least three times higher among homeless patients than among a matched sample of domiciled, ambulatory patients.[4] Parasitic skin infestations (scabies and lice) are two common diagnoses in emergency rooms serving the homeless.[11] Although the majority of infestations are neither intractable nor life-threatening, the development of secondary infection can lead to bacteremia; chronic sequelae, including renal failure caused by poststreptococcal glomerulonephritis; and septic shock.

Treatment for scabies and lice is simple and effective. Difficulty, however, often develops soon after the diagnosis has been made in the emergency room. The phobic responses of providers to the infested patient may result in his or her discharge with incomplete treatment and instruction or with no treatment at all. But even the most thorough intervention in this setting is unlikely to prevent reinfestation if close contacts are untreated, if clothing and bed linen cannot be washed or replaced, or if the patient fails to return to monitor the efficacy of the initial treatment.

The incidence of hypothermia and hyperthermia among the homeless is unknown; in fact, estimates of the incidence of thermoregulatory illness in the general population vary widely.[12] Environmental exposure is obviously more likely to occur if a person is without adequate shelter, but exposure alone is by no means the only element increasing the risk of thermoregulatory disorders among the homeless. L. K. Goldfrank[13] has described the elements that augment the risk for both hypothermia and heat stroke. They include many of the most common physical and behavioral disorders encountered among the homeless. Independent risks for both thermoregulatory conditions include chronic debilitating disorders, trauma, the use of psychotropic agents, alcoholism, the use of central nervous system depressants, nutritional deficiency (Wernicke-Korsakoff syndrome), and psychiatric disorders.

Treatment of many chronic disorders, including hypertension, diabetes mellitus, peripheral vascular disease, and heart failure, have well-established and relatively effective treatment regimens. The increased prevalence of chronic disorders and their complications among homeless persons is a direct consequence of living conditions and the failure of the health care system to reach the needy and maintain contact. Until long-term solutions are devised for the underlying causes of homelessness, health care providers can best influence the health of the homeless by providing consistent on-site service, which includes both patient advocacy and medical care.

Diabetes mellitus provides a paradigm for the management of chronically ill homeless persons. Management requires dietary measures aimed at control of body weight, serum glucose, and lipids.[14] Regular administration of oral hypoglycemic drugs or insulin may also be needed, along with careful monitoring of blood glucose levels. However, meals in most shelters, while adequate, will rarely meet the needs of a diabetic client. A clean, accessible, and safe storage place for insulin, medications, and blood glucose monitoring devices will not be available in most shelters. The street value of syringes and alcohol swabs makes these items particularly subject to theft. Shelter life can be viewed as an independent risk for the immediate and long-term complications of diabetes. Even if ketoacidosis and coma are somehow avoided, the vascular and neuropathic complications will occur after ten to twenty years of uncontrolled diabetes, leaving a population at high risk for stroke, blindness, renal failure, myocardial infarction, amputation, and permanent dependency on the state.

Homeless Persons, HIV Infection, and AIDS

Definition

The fateful consequences of infection with the human immunodeficiency virus (HIV) are broadly understood by health care workers. Acquired immune deficiency syndrome (AIDS) and AIDS-related complex (ARC) are illnesses caused by HIV, with definitions strictly defined in their clinical parameters by the Centers for Disease Control (CDC).[15] It is now recognized that the virus causes numerous other conditions that do not meet the precise definitions of AIDS or ARC but lead to severe morbidity and death.

In discussing the prevention of HIV disease and the treatment of patients, we should understand that we are concerned with a range, beginning with persons at risk and asymptomatic carriers and extending to those with AIDS. HIV infection may be clinically silent for seven years or more in the bodies of infected individuals, who are nevertheless capable of infecting contacts despite their own lack of symptoms.

Issues in Care of Homeless Persons with HIV Infection

Information regarding the number of homeless persons in the United States with HIV-related illness is sparse and largely anecdotal. Experience of the Johnson/Pew HCHP reveals:

- AIDS has been diagnosed in all nineteen cities.
- Education of staff and patients regarding HIV disease is needed.
- Many programs have started to give free condoms to homeless persons in shelters, along with advice about safer sex practices.
- A few programs have started to distribute bleach solution with instructions about disinfecting needles and syringes to intravenous drug users (IVDUs).
- There is a consensus that homeless people are eager to have information about AIDS and that many are prepared to try risk reduction.

Proper and effective care of HIV-infected people raises an ethical matter of great practical significance. The rights and needs of the general public versus the right to privacy of each individual are at issue. An example of recent vintage in a major New York City shelter focused on the conflict between several homeless people who told the shelter nurse, requesting absolute confidence, that they had AIDS and the demand made by the shelter operator to the nurse that all such cases be brought to the attention of management. In this instance the patients' confidence was maintained. However, this kind of dilemma will in all likelihood present itself to many homeless health care programs.

The loss of immunity that results from HIV infection causes the development of aggressive infections in patients. Unusual diseases, such as *Pneumocystis carinii* pneumonia, have been recognized as part of the clinical picture from early in the epidemic. It has been understood more recently that more common conditions, such as tuberculosis, bacterial pneumonias, and syphilis, may present in a highly aggressive form in HIV-infected persons. Health care workers should develop a high index of suspicion for HIV-related disease if their patents are ill with any substantial infection, particularly in an aggressive form and especially if the patient is in an HIV risk group.

Precaution for Health Workers

The CDC has produced definitive statements on this subject.[16,17] These documents should be required reading for all health care workers in the United States, including those who work with homeless persons.

Staff members should apply the following universal safeguards on the assumption that all patients under care are infected with HIV:

- **Blood precautions:** Careful handling of any blood, blood components or products, serum, wound drainage, needles and syringes, instruments, and laboratory specimens is essential.
- **Excretory precautions:** Careful handling of stool, vomitus, urine, or semen of patients is required.
- **Secretion/discharge precautions:** Careful handling of any oral, respiratory, nasopharyngeal, or vaginal secretions or of wound drainage is essential.

Appropriate application of these safeguards for health workers requires that:

- Hands must be washed immediately if they become soiled with blood or secretions.
- Gloves must be worn for any direct contact with patient's blood, bodily fluids, or secretions.
- Goggles and masks should be worn during the performance of any procedure which would be likely to cause splashing or aerosolization of blood or blood-tinged bodily fluids into eyes or into mucous membranes.
- All needles, syringes, and disposable and sharp instruments (sharps) must be placed with care into appropriate punctureproof containers. When filled, the containers should be disposed of in a proper fashion, after being sealed.
- Never break off or recap needles.

- All spills of blood or bodily fluids must be immediately cleaned up and the area disinfected with an appropriate disinfectant solution. Dakin's solution (one part bleach to ten parts water) is an example.
- No health care worker with open skin lesions that are exudative or weeping should have contact with blood or bodily secretions from patients.

Mental Health Concerns

Drug dependency, alcoholism, and chronic mental illness are encountered frequently among the homeless. Alcoholism is historically linked with homelessness. The stereotypic male homeless person is the denizen of skid row. Since the early 1960's, however, the face of the down-and-out has changed significantly with the movement to deinstitutionalize the chronically mentally ill and with substance abuse epidemic throughout the country.

Increasing numbers of former patients of state mental institutions have made their way to the streets and shelter system because the attempt to bring humane long-term psychiatric care to the community has failed.[18] Shelters and psychiatric emergency rooms have also seen increasing numbers of "young chronics," low-functioning, socially isolated, dependent men and women who have eluded formal diagnosis and treatment. Their primary psychiatric illness is often complicated by substance abuse. Studies conducted in a variety of settings[19,20] (e.g., psychiatric emergency rooms, drop-in centers, shelters) indicate that the frequency of substance abuse as either a primary or a secondary problem varies widely. The changing demographics of homelessness in many traditional settings, such as the Bowery in New York City, call for providers and service agencies to adjust to new demands.

Substance abusers, including alcoholics, frequently exhibit disordered care-seeking behavior. They may be acutely intoxicated, they may lack insight regarding their illness, they may be manipulative, and they may not accept needed care. Such characteristics reflect their underlying illness, drug dependency. We know very little about drug dependency, certainly very little about how to cure it. Health providers become frustrated when they cannot cure. When therapy is inadequate, as it is often for substance abuse or psychosis, providers must guard against blaming patients for their frustration. Neither the patient nor the provider is responsible for our current lack of understanding or for the unavailability of adequate treatment facilities.

Violent behavior is a common concern of providers, particularly for those caring for the mentally ill or for drug addicts. These patients are generally perceived as violence-prone, while their history of victimization is easily obscured. The stereotypic view of the mentally ill, including the chemical-dependent among them, fuels the resistance to much needed mental health facilities and drug treatment programs in the community and can adversely influence care by promoting an exaggerated expectation of violence.

The capacity for violence in any individual at any given time is impossible to predict with confidence. A history of violent behavior is one indicator which may be helpful, but this information may not be available. Faced with this uncertainty, health workers can minimize the potential for violence by developing a non-threatening, receptive approach, which promotes a sense of patient participation in the care plan and emphasizes the patient's controlling influence on any encounter.

The experience of the HCHPs has been remarkably free of violence. In more than two hundred thousand patient encounters, many with patients who are mentally ill or have substance abuse problems, no extraordinary episodes of violence against staff members stand out. Yet although accounts of violence or threats are anecdotal, they highlight the need for swift and decisive action to protect other clients and staff members when the concern is real.

J was a thirty-five-year-old man who resided in an SRO hotel in Greenwich Village. He was employed in the hotel's kitchen and was first encountered by a nurse-physician team in 1983 during a site visit. He complained of "not feeling well" and was referred to the St. Vincent's Hospital outpatient clinic.

A history of intravenous drug use was obtained, and acute hepatitis was diagnosed. It was recommended that J suspend his work in the kitchen until his health problems were clarified. Upon being told of the team's decision, J confronted the nurse at the hotel and during their conversation smeared saliva on her arm, stating, "You know what I'm doing." Other behavior suggested to the nurse that J was having auditory hallucinations and that he was concerned that he might have AIDS.

Subsequently J avoided the team for about six months, failing to keep follow-up appointments. Another nurse-physician team visiting the hotel reestablished contact with J, who had become more reclusive and had adopted a disheveled "Rambo-esque" appearance. He was now convinced that the original physician and nurse had altered his body with the placement of "a computer chip in my brain" in an attempt to control or harm him. For this they had "to be killed."

The threat was taken seriously, and J was banned from further clinic visits; hospital security and local police were notified. The police believed there was little they could do in the absence of an overt act of violence.

Despite these measures, J arrived at clinic several times, unannounced, asking for the physician by name. On one occasion, after being escorted from the premises by security officers, he attempted to reenter by using another door. By this time the security department had become well aware of J and the threat he posed, and further visits ceased.

The physician was able to relocate his work area within the clinic building and arranged to be accompanied when he arrived and left the building for a number of weeks, until the immediate threat seemed to have passed.

The patient lost contact with the team, which continued to visit the hotel. A pattern of increasing drug use and vandalism eventually led to his eviction.

In this particular case the use of a team approach was helpful in diffusing the focus of the client's rage, perhaps avoiding a serious violent incident.

The service needs of the mentally ill homeless, including drug-dependent persons, are similar to those of the homeless population in general. Contact agencies, such as drop-in centers, soup kitchens, and outreach programs, are vital means of establishing a helping relationship. The application of the multidisciplinary approach can promote the chances of accurately defining needs of individuals and consequently making appropriate and timely referrals. Teams of social workers, nurses, and physicians with linkages to psychiatric service agencies are effective in making initial contact and in case finding.

On-site clinics at shelters equipped to provide psychiatric care or to refer disturbed people to appropriate agencies, in the course of providing general medical care, are essential. Without access to a wide range of services, shelters are in danger of becoming warehouses for the chronically mentally ill, grim replacements for the dismantled state hospital systems.

The need for residential facilities in the community is most pressing for the homeless mentally ill. Living space with on-site psychiatric care, linked to other community-based and hospital-based services, is in short supply. Programs such as the St. Francis residences in New York City serve as models for meeting the long-term needs of the homeless mentally ill. Each St. Francis Residence has a full-time staff that provides assistance in living skills and encourages socialization, while maintaining and monitoring medical and psychiatric treatment with the help of community psychiatrists and physicians.

Health care providers must become advocates for mentally ill patients. Guiding a client through the labyrinth of the medical and social service system is a task which eventually falls to each member of the team. But staff members must also provide voices for their clients when public issues arise that affect care and services. Advocacy might take the form of confronting community resistance to treatment facilities or of calling upon legislators to redirect mental health funds to community-based programs for the mentally ill and drug-dependent.

JAMES T. KENNEDY

JOSEPH PETRONE

ROBERT W. DEISHER

JED EMERSON

PAULINE HESLOP

DEIRDRE BASTIBLE

MARC ARKOVITZ

7

Health Care for Familyless, Runaway Street Kids

In the autumn of 1969 an infant boy, Eduardo, was born to a Hispanic woman incarcerated in the New York State prison system. The boy never knew his father and was reared by relatives of his mother in an impoverished, inner-city household. Eventually he spent some time in foster care and in city-run group homes. Little is known about his early childhood except that he completed only two or three years of grade school and that from the age of seven he was sexually abused by a male relative. By the age of thirteen he had abandoned his chaotic home— "run away" if you will—and taken up residence on "the street." He survived there by stealing, selling marijuana, and selling his body.

When he was fifteen, he arrived at a runaway shelter, complaining of hunger and depression. The staff found him to be an engaging and manipulative youngster, somewhat overweight. He could not read English or Spanish. A medical check revealed a sexually transmitted infection, which was treated. The boy made "friends" among the staff and other residents, but he refused to see the agency's psychiatrist. "I'm not crazy and I'm not gay" was his standard reply to any personal inquiry. He resisted any serious attempts to find him a stable home. He came to the shelter several more times during the next three years but always went AWOL whenever a plan looked promising. With each visit he seemed more distant and resistant to care.

Eventually he stopped using the shelter, and during the last two years of his life only the outreach staff had significant contact with him, always at sites known for male prostitution. They learned that he had been arrested several times, that he had been beaten by an arresting police officer, and that during one incarceration he had hanged himself in his cell. After four months in a psychiatric hospital he was discharged to the streets with a clinic appointment for ongoing care. He never kept appointments of any kind.

Late in 1987 the outreach team, shocked by his appearance, brought him to the shelter's clinic. He reluctantly agreed to a medical exam, but only by a nurse and physician he knew from previous visits. He was nineteen years old then but weighed thirty-five pounds less than when he was fifteen. He had a large dental abscess, oral thrush, and scabies. He was now addicted to crack. His hematocrit was 25 percent, he was HIV positive and he had diffuse patchy infiltrates on his chest X ray. Before he died of cryptococcal meningitis, he had three hospitalizations for treatment of his dental abscess, Pneumocystis carinii pneumonia (PCP), and severe thrombocytopenia. Throughout his illness he was an uncooperative patient, refusing procedures and antagonizing his care givers. He ended each hospital stay except his last by leaving against medical advice. He complained to the shelter staff, "The doctors treat me like dirt." One hospital refused to readmit him. He was twenty years old when he died of AIDS, and his mother was again in prison.

This boy's life defines "runaway youth" in contemporary America. Knowing his story, and the stories of thousands of other homeless adolescents like him, brings perspective and focus to the delivery of health care, indeed, of all care, to this population of troubled youth. A lot more happened to this boy than infection with a series of pathogens. AIDS was not his only cause of early death. Getting to know children like Eduardo is the essential first step to providing successful medical care for their problems. Yet getting to know the names, faces, and lives of alienated youths is not always easy. Each is an individual, but their backgrounds are surprisingly alike. Before we discuss the health concerns of homeless adolescents, it is essential to introduce them as the professionals working with them know them, as "street kids."

Much confusion and controversy has gone into naming, defining, studying, and counting[1-3] runaways.[4] Just in the last decade the group has been called runaways, throwaways, societal rejects, urban nomads, homeless youth, alienated youth, disconnected youth, disenfranchised youth, missing and exploited children, and, most recently in keeping with an evolving global definition, street kids. No individual patient is a street kid. Each patient, however disadvantaged, has a name and the dignity implicit to it, but "street kids" is a handle that seems to fit the large cohort of American adolescents and young adults abandoned to the streets of our nation. So while the term has no place in the day-to-day lexicon of youth specialists, it is used here as a "best fit" descriptor for a remarkable group of American children.

How many street kids are there? The U.S. Department of Health and Human

Services and the National Network of Runaway and Youth Services estimate that as many as a million youths run away from home each year in the United States and that 25 percent of these adolescents become familyless street kids surviving on their own.[5,6] There is no good count of how many adolescents run from institutions or other nonhome settings, nor is it known how many are spun off from homeless families. The homeless population was once made up of mostly single adults, but today families with children make up more than 33 percent of the counted homeless, with estimates in some cities exceeding 50 percent (Portland, Oregon, Philadelphia, Yonkers, and Trenton) and more in New York.[7] A significant number of these homeless families include adolescents; indeed, many are made up of teenage girls with babies. No national tally is made of how many youth "age out" of alternate care programs onto the street. The U.S. Office of Juvenile Justice and Delinquency Prevention finds it impossible to estimate the number of children abducted in the United States each year, whether by strangers or parents, but the National Crime Information Center lists close to sixty thousand youths less than eighteen years old reported missing on any given day.[8] Significant numbers of these children are exploited by deviant adults or organized sex rings. Many never return home and wind up on the street. Across the southern tier of the United States thousands of Latino street kids cross the border looking for economic improvement they rarely find.[9] Like tributaries to a rising stream, each of these sources adds abandoned children to a rising flood of American street kids.

Conservatively speaking, there are about 200,000 such youngsters—a subpopulation of the United States that is not even recognized to exist. They are not even counted among the population of the homeless. By some incredibly strange quirk of United States counting procedures, the homeless are not counted [officially] until they become 21 years of age. . . . What these youngsters have in common is how good they are, and how brave they are, and how much they desperately want to make it back into society off the street. Very few of them actually succeed.[10]

Although uncounted and lacking a precise taxonomic niche, the abandoned, familyless street kids of America exist in numbers sufficient to overwhelm the hundreds of youth services agencies created to serve them. Whatever the definition, most professionals working with troubled youth agree that the numbers of adolescents for whom the street is home is large and growing. The National Network of Runaway and Youth Services has more than seven hundred member or affiliate agencies, including at least one from each of the fifty states. These member agencies provide direct services to runaway or homeless youth,[11] and most of them function beyond their designated capacities. The New York City police runaway unit estimates there are 20,000 street kids in New York City alone. Covenant House, an international agency providing shelter and other services to street kids, took in 8,500 youths in New York City during 1988, 2,700 in Fort Lauderdale, 1,700 in Houston, 2,350 in Toronto, and 511 in New Orleans. On its second day in operation a new program site in Anchorage, Alaska, had 20 residents. Between January 1984 and July 1989 the health services department at the New York shelter had 43,651 patient encounters involving almost 15,000 patients. The Coordinating Council for Homeless Youth Services in Los Angeles reported that in 1987, 3,000 youths under the age of seventeen came into runaway shelters and another 3,500 were turned away for lack of space. The Orion Center in Seattle referred 502 patients visits to the Pike Place and Pioneer Square clinics for street kids during 1988, and at the Larkin Street Youth Center in San Francisco a single nurse practitioner had 150 patient encounters each month during the same period. The Larkin Street program had 8,983 outreach contacts with youth on the street during 1988, and the clinic had 1,727 patient visits involving 946 individual patients. Of those visits, 85 percent were for treatment of a sexually transmitted disease and 11 percent were for problems of pregnancy.

Project Street Beat is an outreach program that sends its van into "the harshest streets of the South Bronx, in decaying neighborhoods rife with drug abuse. . . ."[12] In its first year on the streets this van recorded 2,508 contacts with 597 adolescent prostitutes. A seventeen-year-old told the staff, "I've been here for four years, and sure I'm scared. It's dangerous here, and girls get killed all the time. But I'm on crack, and, no, I don't want to get off."

The "Nineline" (1-800-999-9999), a twenty-four-hour-a-day hot line for runaway youth, received nearly 2 million calls between September 1987 and June 1989. Of those calls, 256,477 came from youths in crisis. Table 7.1 breaks out the reasons for those quarter of a million calls.

It has been the experience of each of these programs that this group of homeless adolescents brings complex problems to the agencies created to help them, and all put health care high on the list of the unmet needs of street kids. There are thousands of abandoned children and adolescents in the United States, and they are patients unserved by the traditional health care delivery system. Creating a health services program that works for street kids is a challenge best begun with an understanding of who street kids really are.

Street kids are not part of the homeless in America as that population is usually understood. An authoritative scientific study designed to count the homeless pop-

Table 7.1 BREAKOUT OF CALLS TO A RUNAWAY HOT
LINE BY PROBLEM LEADING TO THE CALL

Runaway / throwaway problem	72,525	Peer problems: sexuality	4,747
"Want to talk"	21,026	Abusive parent	4,362
Homeless	18,913	Substance abuse by other	3,814
Health / depression	18,297	Emotional abuse	3,582
Threatened runaway	17,045	Parental divorce / separation	3,026
Pregnancy / teenage parenting	11,829	Legal problem	2,736
Substance abuse by self	10,555	Health / death of friend or relative	1,719
Physical abuse	10,237	Health / suicide of friend or relative	1,716
Other	9,027	Prostitution	1,537
Sexual abuse	7,265	Other domestic violence	1,168
Health / suicide threat	6,334	Rape	1,068
Peer problems: boy / girl	6,048	Missing / abducted	956
Peer problems: school	5,958	Health / STD	420
Parenting concern	5,123	Health / AIDS	297
Alcohol abuse by self	4,921	Pornography	226

ulation of Chicago defined homelessness as "a manifestation of extreme poverty among persons *without families* in housing markets with declining stocks of inexpensive dwelling units suitable for single persons."[13] The National Governors Association defined a homeless person as "an undomiciled person who is unable to secure permanent and stable housing without special assistance." The U.S. General Accounting Office defined homeless individuals as those persons who lack resources and community ties necessary to provide for their own adequate shelter. None of these definitions, except for the emphasis-added reference to familylessness, really gets at what makes an adolescent a street kid.

Adults without resources for shelter may have many concomitant emotional and social problems, but they are not passing through an unrepeatable season of life in which essential human development is supposed to take place with the caring guidance of a nurturing family. Street kids are far more familyless than homeless. Familylessness and abandonment are the consequential features of being a street kid. Runaways from healthy, functioning families only rarely become street kids. They go home as soon as the horrors of the street life-style confront them. To understand these truly abandoned youth well, it is useful to examine both what is missing from their lives and what replaces it.

What is a contemporary family?

The major functions assigned to the family by society are as follows: the meeting of survival needs; the protection, care, education, and rearing of children; the creation of a physical, emotional, social, and economic setting which nurtures the development of individual family members; nurturing of affectionate bonds within the family which will help each member become a contributing member of the family and community; and the responsibility for the social control of its individual members. . . . One of the ways children learn how to relate to the outside world is by experiencing relationships within the family. The modeling that goes on within the family constitutes the most powerful experience children have in learning how to deal with society as a whole. It is generally recognized now that the child's peer group and school influence also play a powerful role in helping to socialize the child. However, the child continues to use his family as a frame of reference for understanding what goes on outside the family unit. Intrafamilial behavioral patterns influence, and in many cases reinforce, what the child experiences outside the family.[14]

Survival, protection, education, nurture, development, modeling, control, socialization, and reinforcement all are lost or distorted when an adolescent's family is replaced by the brutal realities of the street as a home. It is a mistake to describe street kids as resourceful. It implies their ability to make mature judgments about how to live their lives. What street kids do is cope—"survive" is what they call it—in an adult world using the resources of a child, and their choices are often wrong and tragic. What replaces the nurturing process of a family is the lifestyle of the street: violence, drugs, sexual exploitation, and crime.[15] The professional literature on runaway youth frequently tips its hat to Samuel Clemens and his indomitable Masters Sawyer and Finn, but a passage describing Tom's influence on his friend Joe Harper seems presciently metaphorical with regard to the choices made by today's street kids. Tom has resolved to "escape from hard usage and lack of sympathy at home by roaming abroad into the great world never to return" and meets up with Joe, whose resolve is the same.

As the two boys walked sorrowing along, they made a new compact to stand by each other and be brothers and never separate till death relieved them of their troubles. Then they began to lay their plans. Joe was for being a hermit, and living on crusts in a remote cave, and dying, some time, of cold and want and grief; but after listening to Tom, he conceded that there were some conspicuous advantages about a life of crime, and so he consented to be a pirate.[16]

"Consented" overstates Joe's freedom to choose. On their first night abroad these kids were eating stolen food and smoking stuff that Huck stuffed into a corncob and sucked through a weed. With adamant certainty street life erodes the physical and emotional health of abandoned children. Abandoned children persevere by their wits and lug along the unfinished business of their adolescent transition to adulthood. They become like peripheral animals in a herd, undefended and uncared for, discarded, and offered up to predators.[17] It is difficult to overstate the negative impact of being familyless throughout adolescence. Twain's happy endings never apply.

The effects are even more exaggerated if the process of becoming familyless has also been cruel. Physical, sexual, and emotional abuse is routinely identified in the assessment of street kids.[18-21] Poverty is a rule, although not a universal one. Parental substance abuse, parental mental illness, and parental criminal activity are also typical background factors in the childhoods of street kids. The common finding of school failure at a young age implicates unrecognized learning disorders within the group,[22,23] and there is good evidence that runaway street kids have a high incidence of chronic emotional and mental disturbances.[24] Many runaways run from out-of-home placements in group homes, foster care, or institutions. For whatever reasons, such placements represent failed surrogate families for the adolescents who flee them. By deliberately deciding to deinstitutionalize status offenders society has abandoned an important point of control over troubled youth[25] and replaced it with few alternatives.[26] Street kids are often turned out of families unable to deal with behaviors considered intolerable. Drug use, pregnancy, and gender identification conflicts are commonly cited by street kids as reasons for having been "thrown out" of their homes. Street kids are not "emancipated minors"; they are abandoned children. On the street they grow old fast, and as they lose the tolerance adult society usually affords its juveniles, they become perceived of as deviant and dangerous. Their self-perception, self-esteem, and self-regard also become confused and distorted,[27,28] and they are left alienated from peers, adults, and social institutions.

The American College of Physicians recently published a position paper entitled "Health Care Needs of the Adolescent."[29] It states, "Providing health care to adolescents presents a dual challenge: the treatment of immediate health problems, and the opportunity, through health promotion, to influence health habits, lifestyle choices, and health status in adulthood, because health behaviors originating in adolescence may well have long-term health consequences." The current president of the Society for Adolescent Medicine, Dr. S. Kenneth Schonberg, has written, "Our quest to affect adolescent morbidity and mortality through health education is a hallmark of adolescent medicine."[30] These statements assume a broader role for health professionals treating any adolescent, and they state an urgent truth for anyone treating familyless, runaway street kids. Effectively influencing the health habits and life-style choices of a street kid is the home run of therapeutics, medical or otherwise.

Physicians and nurses providing health care to homeless teenagers have a professional obligation to focus most of their attention on accurate diagnosis and good-quality medical care, but it is important that they understand the backgrounds of America's runaways if they wish to engage their patients in a successful plan of care. In large measure the physical health problems of this group do not present difficult diagnostic or therapeutic challenges. Even human immunodeficiency virus infection and all its complications can be managed with a rather straightforward series of clinical judgments, but all the correct clinical judgments in the world do not translate into "doing the right thing" for a patient who remains alienated from and distrustful of his care givers. This is not to say that health care professionals should expand their role to include the responsibilities of social service professionals. That would be folly. Physicians and nurses should, however, understand how profoundly the experience of being a familyless adolescent impacts on both the short-term and long-term health of their patient. Beyond the "doctor-patient relationship" they should be prepared to use their status in society as advocates for these neglected children. They should be prepared, too, to team their clinical efforts with professionals in other fields to work toward complete healing of their patients. "Networking" and "team approach" are now hackneyed jargon in the realm of child care, but there is simply no other "right way" to do it. Homeless children have no homes; familyless adolescents have no families. There are no pills or shots that will cure these problems, and applying only such interventions is merely palliation.[31] Societal interventions, perhaps like the National Youth Academy proposed by the Reverend Samuel Proctor,[32] hold as much hope for the future health and well-being of America's abandoned adolescents as does a cure for AIDS. There were street kids before the AIDS epidemic; there will be streets kids after the AIDS epidemic. AIDS put street kids on television,[33] but so far it hasn't gotten many of them off the street.

Remember Eduardo. He was abandoned by many, abused by most, and failed by all. Had a cure for AIDS been available to him, the cure by itself would have had little impact on the course of his life. That is the lesson that all who work to bring "right thing" health care to street kids should keep in mind. Gain that perspective, and the medical problems of familyless street kids come clearly into diagnostic focus.

Health Services Research on Street Kids

There is little documentation of the health status or health needs of runaway youth and even less information on what health care delivery system best meets their needs.[34,35] Much has been studied and written about health care needs and the provision of health services to the entire population of American adolescents,[36] but most of this work focuses on the topic of teenage pregnancy.[37] A study of disadvantaged adolescents entering the Job Corps program identified significantly increased medical morbidity.[38] Recently there has been more attention paid to young children who are homeless,[39–43] but these children are not adolescents and are usually living in a shelter with at least one parent or guardian.

One interesting study demonstrates how a particular cohort of adolescents can have distinct health needs.

. . . the health care needs of 80 Indochinese refugee teenagers, evaluated during a 4-year period, were determined. The Centers for Disease Control's suggested screening measures were used, and it was found that 52% had positive purified protein derivative skin tests, 38% lacked immunizations, 35% had stool specimens positive for parasites (prevalence and number of parasites greatest among Cambodians), 14% had blood tests positive for hepatitis B surface antigen, and 10% were anemic. Additional evaluations showed that 19% had hemoglobinopathies, 14% were in or below the fifth percentile for height and weight, 12% had goiters, 12% had skin disorders, . . . 5% had visual defects, 5% had hearing loss, 5% had psychosomatic illness, and 4% had idiopathic scoliosis. Although suggested Centers for Disease Control screening measures may be adequate for younger Indochinese children, these data suggest that additional studies are necessary for teenagers. For the sexually active adolescent, identification of and counseling for hepatitis antigene-mia and hemoglobinopathies are crucial. In addition, early identification of emotional and physical problems during screening may enhance assimilation into a new society and facilitate completion of the psychosocial tasks of adolescence.[44]

A similar study of familyless street kids, especially a national one, would be of great value. There is one report comparing runaway with nonrunaway youth seeking health services at an adolescent health clinic in Los Angeles. Of 765 initial health assessments done in 1985, 110 (14 percent) were on runaway youth. Comparison of the runaway and nonrunaway groups revealed that street youths are at greater risk for a wide variety of medical problems and of health-compromising behaviors, including suicide, depression, prostitution, and drug use. Runaways accounted for only 14 percent of the population but suffered 23 percent of the recorded morbidities. Of the runaways, 84 percent were substance abusers, with 34 percent of them using intravenous drugs. Also, 19 percent of the runaway group reported sexual activity prior to their tenth birthdays, and 26 percent were involved in prostitution (compared with 2 percent of the nonrunaway group).[45] In 1984 David Shaffer and Carol Caton conducted a census, including inquiries relating to emotional status and social background, of homeless youth at several shelters in New York City. They interviewed 118 new shelter residents and found that 45 percent of the males and 37 percent of the females were both depressed and antisocial. One-third of each group had attempted suicide. Aside from health care this study reported that 37 percent of the males and 19 percent of the females had been charged with a crime, and 75 percent of the males and 50 percent of the females had been expelled or suspended from school.[24]

Despite the paucity of published studies, many health care providers work in many ways with homeless adolescents and street kids. The experiences of these professionals is that as a group street kids have more health problems and more serious medical morbidities than school-based patient groups and that street kids have almost no access to existing health care providers. A uniform health assessment tool for this patient population would be an important step forward in documenting and meeting their needs. If more resources become available, larger studies can be done to focus health care service strategies for this group of adolescents, but it is already certain knowledge that their medical problems transcend the care available to them now.

Clinical Issues

"Street medicine" is hardly a recognized medical specialty, but the term is used by health professionals treating homeless youth for lack of anything more certified. Street medicine is different because its patient mix presents a concentration of pathologies not unknown but far less common in more conventional practices. Roughly in order of frequency those pathologies are: violent and traumatic injury, substance abuse, sexually transmitted diseases (including hepatitis and AIDS), psychiatric disturbances, skin infestations, ignored pregnancies, "unwell" babies, and the "neglected pathologies"—i.e., common chronic illnesses exacerbated and complicated by lack of simple care. Some of these clinical problems deserve a closer look.

Violence and Trauma

The high incidence of gunshot and knife wound scars noted on the physical examinations of street kids is supportive evidence for all the studies that identify homicide as a leading cause of death among young Americans. If so many casualties survive to grow scars, how many must have died? In 1986, 5,552 homicide victims were fifteen to twenty-four years old.[46] Only motor vehicle accidents claimed more lives in that age group. Essentially all street kids coming into shelters have been assaulted and robbed of whatever possessions they had. If they have resulting abrasions and lacerations, they are generally dirty and secondarily infected. Stitches put in at emergency rooms never come out on time and only rarely survive the wear and tear of street life. Of all age-groups, adolescents sixteen to nineteen have the highest rate of victimization by nonlethal violent crimes. From 1982 through 1984, 1.8 million violent crimes against twelve- to nineteen-year-olds were reported.[46] Street kids rarely report crimes, especially those they commit. As homeless adolescents spend more time on the street, they are as likely to inflict as to be victims of violence. Many reports have linked the background factors of familyless youth with an increased propensity toward violent behavior and delinquency.[47,48]

When he died, Reggie "Gizmo" Brown got a much larger obituary than most street kids, and in The New York Times *at that: "His gift for survival ran out on the streets of Harlem when, three months shy of his 22nd birthday, he was fatally shot in the back. Those who knew him said he seemed doomed by his past and his homelessness, and they were saddened, but not at all that surprised, to learn that he had been killed."[49] Gizmo was a diabetic from the age of six and lived with his mother and three siblings until he was thirteen. Even by street kid standards he left home and entered foster care in an unusual way, defenestration. When he arrived at a group home in a body cast, he told his social worker that a friend of his mother, in a fit of drug-induced rage, had thrown him out a second-story window. The fall cracked his spine and broke some bones, but he escaped paralysis.*

Soon after he "aged out" of foster care five years later, he began coming to the New York Covenant House shelter. He never stayed long. He lived more often in the nearby bus terminal. Reggie met an attorney who included him as a plaintiff in a class-action lawsuit against the city's foster care system. That suit got press notice and eventually succeeded in expanding the responsibilities of the child welfare system to prepare youths in foster care for the transition to independent living. Gizmo's wit and charm made him a media celebrity for this brief period and secured him his obituary when his death came. Although he wouldn't stay in shelters, he made more than fifty visits to the clinic between 1984 and 1987, always to "test my diabetes." Every blood sugar level was far too high except for those that were far too low. Nevertheless, it amazed the staff that someone with his life-style did as well as he did. Clearly, he was a motivated patient. Reggie got involved in drugs and in crime. He hurt some people and did some time. When he was shot, he was peddling street Valium for fifty cents a capsule. It is hard to say what disease killed him.

Gizmo lived a violent life not because he was a violent person—he wasn't—but because he lived his life on the street. Street violence is a brutal reality expressed in many ways. For girls and young women on the street, violent rape is so common that many don't even comment on it. Despite the street rapes that don't get counted, still half of all reported rape victims are adolescents,[50,51] and a growing number of them are young boys.[52] Physical violence is an integral part of the behavior modification practiced by pimps, and in crack dens nothing is done by mutual consent. For girls or boys who have been sexually abused at home, exploitive sex and rape on the street are just more of the same.

Dealing with the abrasions, lacerations, and sprains associated with accidental trauma and deliberate assaults requires no specialized protocols, but the evaluation and early management of rape victims should be performed by experienced professionals. Proper examination, specimen collection, record keeping, and medical and psychological treatment are essential.

Sexually Transmitted Diseases

The prevalence of sexually transmitted diseases among male and female homeless youths is not known with accuracy. One expert estimates that in the average high school class of 500 boys and girls, 40 of the girls are likely to be carriers of an STD.[53] The lack of an estimate for the boys reflects not sex bias but a scarcity of data on screening of asymptomatic adolescent males for STDs. In a 1984 study of 115 pregnant inner-city girls age thirteen to seventeen, 10 percent had gonorrhea, 37 percent had chlamydia (a coexisting infection in most cases of culture-positive gonorrhea), and 34 percent had trichomoniasis.[54] On the basis of the known incidence of STDs among all sexually active thirteen- to twenty-four-year-olds and the clinical consensus of physicians treating runaway youth it is certain that the prevalence of these infections among this group is even higher and rising. The connection to epidemic crack use is apparent. In New York City an epidemic of congenital syphilis has followed on the heels of the epidemics of crack and AIDS. In 1988, 357 cases of congenital syphilis were reported to the city's Department of Health, more than a 1,000 percent increase since the early years of the decade. Mothers younger than twenty accounted for 13 percent of the cases, and women using cocaine accounted for 33 percent of the cases.[55] In 1987 the health services department at Covenant House, New York, treated 16 patients with positive syphilis serologies. The number rose to 104 in 1988 and to 135 for just the first nine months of 1989.[56] At the Larkin Street Youth Center in San Francisco the number of positive syphilis serologies jumped from 3 in 1987 to 60 in 1988. This upsurge of syphilis infections among street kids is mirrored by similar increases in the incidence of all STDs. Of all the patients seen at the Larkin Street clinic in 1988, 56 percent were treated for an STD.

It is the exception to diagnose a single sexually transmitted disease in a symptomatic street kid. Multiple infections are the rule.

Candy came to the Larkin Street Youth Center clinic in San Francisco because her boyfriend told her he had gonorrhea. She was seventeen years old, and her partner was sixteen. She told the staff that she had been treated for venereal infections several times since she was thirteen years old, that she used intravenous drugs on occasion, and that she was involved in prostitution. She figured she had had two hundred different sex partners during the previous three months and had used protection "sometimes." She was unwilling to discuss her family background but did reveal that she had been in foster care and group homes since she was thirteen after being sexually abused by her father. She had attempted suicide twice and had run from most of the social service placements made for her. She considered her home "the street." Candy was treated for gonorrhea and chlamydia,[57] she was referred to a case manager, and as for all street kids her clinic visit became an AIDS education and counseling session as well. She was given condoms, bleach, and a follow-up appointment. When she returned for that visit, she was also treated for syphilis since a routine blood test for that infection was also positive. Despite the intensity of her encounter with the agency staff, she remains on the street and engages in sexual and drug use activities that threaten her life.

In addition to the dramatic increase in the incidence of syphilis and the development of a pattern of multiple infections, there is great concern that many cases of gonorrhea among street kids are resistant to the antibiotics most often used to treat that infection (penicillinase-producing *Neisseria gonorrhoeae* [PPNG]).[58,59] Besides the health problem this trend represents, it has had the practical impact of raising the cost of treatment for a case of gonorrhea by 400 percent, a significant burden for many of the clinics serving street kids.[60] The interplay of HIV infection and STDs, particularly syphilis, has also had a resource impact. Syphilis seems to be a different disease when it infects patients who have HIV infection. It may soon be necessary to do spinal taps on all such patients if they are to get appropriate medical care.[61,62] Professionals in "street medicine" are asking themselves who will perform these expensive and technically demanding tests.

An American Medical Association "White Paper on Adolescent Health" estimated that nearly a million adolescents, one-third of them boys, are involved in prostitution and that their average age is fifteen.[63] Street kids, especially "missing" children, make up a large part of this group, and they play an important role in the increasing spread of sexually transmitted diseases. However, it is important to note that adolescent prostitution is quite different from "adult commercial sex," especially in its motivating forces and in the fact that essentially all male prostitutes are young boys.[64] This interaction between adult homosexual pedophiles and familyless street kids involved in prostitution has certainly played a large role in the spread of STDs and human immunodeficiency virus infection among runaway youth. In addition, many sexual encounters among and with street kids do not get classified as prostitution, and it is this "survival sex," exchanging sex for food, drugs, shelter, or companionship, that contributes prominently to the high incidence of sexually transmitted diseases within the group. Street kids have had their first sexual intercourse at an early age[65,66] and universally have had many sex partners.[67] The full impact of these behaviors on the incidence of sexually transmitted diseases, including human immunodeficiency virus infection, is still forthcoming.

Health professionals treating street kids should have the knowledge and the tools necessary to diagnose and manage cases of syphilis, gonorrhea, chlamydial infections, genital mycoplasmas, genital herpes simplex, genital warts and molluscum contagiosum, trichomoniasis, vaginitis, pelvic inflammatory disease, chancroid and granuloma inguinale, and human immunodeficiency virus infection. Furthermore, they should be prepared to encounter the less traditional organisms transmitted by sexual activities: *Salmonella, Shigella, Campylobacter, Entamoeba histolytica, Giardia lamblia, Cryptosporidium, Isospora belli, Sarcoptes scabiei, and Phthirus pubis.* Also important, physicians and nurses treating street kids should understand that hepatitis is one of the most frequent sexually transmitted infections in the group.[68] Both heterosexual and homosexual behaviors transmit hepatitis A, hepatitis B, and non-A, non-B hepatitis (NANB).[69] Hepatitis B is the only sexually transmitted disease for which there is a safe and effective vaccine. A strong case can be made for routine testing for hepatitis B surface antibody and administration of this vaccine (recombinant DNA hepatitis B vaccine) to all nonimmune street kids. Testing for hepatitis B is also essential for all pregnant girls since the virus is transmitted to newborns at delivery, and vaccination of these infants is effective prevention of chronic hepatitis B infection.[70]

It is often stated that familyless, runaway adolescents are an ignored and neglected group. Really, they are abandoned. It is sadly ironic that street kids' impact on the incidence of sexually transmitted diseases, including AIDS, may prove to be the ultimate "attention-getting device" that forces society to take notice and end their abandonment.

Human Immunodeficiency Virus Infection

American adolescents as a group are known to do all the things that transmit HIV infection: They have sex with many partners, they use drugs, and they have babies. Yet as of September 1989 the Centers for Disease Control had received only 411 reports of AIDS in the thirteen- to nineteen-year-old age-group.[71] Most of these AIDS cases were in males, and most were acquired through the administration of blood products, something most adolescents do not experience.[72] What does this variance from the usual rules of epidemiology mean? It means that AIDS surveillance is misleading and inappropriate for the adolescent age-group. Street kids are already infected with HIV in large numbers, and their behaviors continue to transmit the infection within and beyond their group. Simple addition and subtraction explain why AIDS surveillance fails to reveal this truth. As of September 1989 there have been 105,990 reported cases of AIDS in the United States. For both men and women the thirty- to thirty-four-year-old age-group has the largest representation, 24 percent of men and 26 percent of women with AIDS. If the mean latency period between HIV infection and the clinical manifestations of AIDS is seven years, a representative person from this group alive today would have been infected in 1983, when he or she was between twenty-three and twenty-seven years old. A representative from the adolescent group would have been between six and twelve years old and unlikely to be engaged in "at-risk" behaviors. If we use the same math, we find it certain that a large number of the 22,000 AIDS cases reported in the twenty- to thirty-year-old age-group through August 1989 represents infections contracted during adolescence.

The CDC definition of AIDS served its most useful functions when it identified a new disease, isolated its modes of transmission, and provided a defined patient population for testing diagnostic and therapeutic advances. HIV seroprevalence surveillance is a far better tool for tracking the course of the epidemic and managing its public health consequences. This is especially true for the adolescent population for which AIDS surveillance is really irrelevant.

The threat of AIDS to the general population of American adolescents is very real and has already compelled many health professionals to action. In March 1988 a national conference on "AIDS and Adolescents—Exploring the Challenge" included work groups on most of the important issues facing practitioners treating adolescents. The recommendations of this conference and Dr. Karen Hein's comprehensive analysis of the impact of the AIDS epidemic on adolescent medicine have been published.[73] Significant testimony was given to the Presidential Commission on the Human Immunodeficiency Virus Epidemic regarding the threat of AIDS to American youth[74] and to special subgroups of disenfranchised adolescents.[75] By the time that commission issued its report[76] there was still little evidence that large numbers of adolescents were infected, but among health care professionals working with the subgroup of street kids there was serious reason for concern that among these patients the epidemic was more advanced than public health officials suspected.[77]

Covenant House in New York has a health services department at its shelter for street kids. There are an average of 40 visits each day in the clinic, and about one-third of the program's new residential admissions are seen in the clinic for a complete health assessment. Between October 1987 and July 1989 the clinic staff performed anonymous HIV antibody tests, in accordance with the New York State Health Code regulations on AIDS testing, on 155 patients. The majority of these adolescents were tested because they had histories of significant at risk behaviors and clinical symptoms or signs suggestive of advancing HIV infection. Of these tested patients, 55 (35.3 percent) were positive for antibodies to HIV. The average age at the time of testing was 18.9 years (no infants or toddlers were tested). Infected were 50 of the 125 males (40 percent) and 5 of the 34 females (14.7 percent) tested. Only 32 (20 percent) of the whole group and 11 (20 percent) of the infected patients had ever used needles to inject drugs.[78]

Alarmed by this clinical experience, Covenant House recruited the New York State Department of Health to initiate a blinded seroprevalence study of runaway street kids. Using discarded serum drawn for syphilis serologies at the initial health assessments of all new patients, an HIV antibody test (ELISA and Western Blot to define positives) was performed. Early results of this study were presented at the 1988 annual meeting of the American Public Health Association in Boston[79] and are summarized in Tables 7.2 through 7.10.

Since that preliminary report the study has continued, and 1,840 other street kids were tested through June 1989. Overall, 6 percent of the group are HIV-seropositive. Also, 76 of 1,158 (6.3 percent) males and 34 of 682 (5.1 percent) females have tested positive. The prevalence of infection rises steadily with age (see figure 7.1). Of this larger group, 7.4 percent of the Hispanics, 6.1 percent of the whites, and 5.1 percent of the blacks are seropositive.

Comparison of these results with other seroprevalence studies (U.S. military

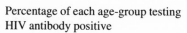

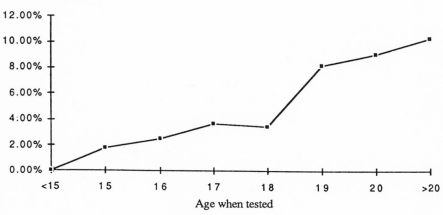

Figure 7.1 **Seroprevalence of HIV antibody seropositivity (October 1987–June 1989) charted by patient's age. Total number tested 1,840.**

Table 7.2 DISTRIBUTION OF HIV ANTIBODY
TEST RESULTS BY THE MONTH COLLECTED

MONTH TESTED	NUMBER POSITIVE	NUMBER TESTED	PERCENT POSITIVE
Oct. 87	4	70	5.71
Nov. 87	8	101	7.92
Dec. 87	11	109	10.09
Jan. 88	5	98	5.10
Feb. 88	8	106	7.55
Mar. 88	5	118	4.24
Apr. 88	4	96	4.17
May 88	5	68	7.35
Jun. 88	7	95	7.37
Jul. 88	11	114	9.65
Aug. 88	6	121	4.96
Totals	74	1096	6.75

Table 7.3 DISTRIBUTION OF HIV ANTIBODY
TEST RESULTS BY PATIENTS' SEX

SEX	NUMBER POSITIVE	NUMBER TESTED	PERCENT POSITIVE	PERCENT OF POSITIVES	PERCENT OF GROUP
Male	52	701	7.42	70.27	63.27
Female	22	407	5.41	29.73	36.73
Totals	74	1108	6.68	100.00	100.00

Table 7.4 DISTRIBUTION OF HIV ANTIBODY
TEST RESULTS BY PATIENTS' RACIAL AND
ETHNIC BACKGROUND

R/E GROUP	NUMBER POSITIVE	NUMBER TESTED	PERCENT POSITIVE
White NH	15	190	7.89
Black NH	32	598	5.35
Hispanic	27	298	9.06
Other/missing	0	25	0.00
Totals	74	1111	6.66

Table 7.5 DISTRIBUTION OF HIV ANTIBODY TEST
RESULTS BY PATIENTS' RACIAL AND ETHNIC
BACKGROUND AND PATIENTS' SEX*

	FEMALES			MALES		
R/E GROUP	NUMBER POSITIVE	NUMBER TESTED	PERCENT POSITIVE	NUMBER POSITIVE	NUMBER TESTED	PERCENT POSITIVE
White NH	2	62	3.23	13	128	10.16
Black NH	16	250	6.40	16	347	4.61
Hispanic	4	85	4.71	23	212	10.85
Totals†	22	397	5.54	52	687	7.57

*There are 25 specimens with unknown R/E status.

† Total (female and male) positive = 74. Total (female and male) tested = 1084.

Table 7.6 DISTRIBUTION OF HIV ANTIBODY TEST
RESULTS COMPARING WHITE AND MINORITY
PATIENTS BY PATIENTS' SEX*

	FEMALES			MALES		
R/E GROUP	NUMBER POSITIVE	NUMBER TESTED	PERCENT POSITIVE	NUMBER POSITIVE	NUMBER TESTED	PERCENT POSITIVE
White	2	62	3.23	13	128	10.16
Minority	20	335	5.97	39	559	6.98
Totals†	22	397	5.54	52	687	7.57

*There are 25 specimens with unknown R/E status.

† Total (female and male) positive = 74 (overall white seropositivity = 7.89 percent, overall minority seropositivity = 6.60 percent). Total tested = 1084.

Table 7.7 DISTRIBUTION OF HIV ANTIBODY TEST RESULTS
COMPARING THE NUMBER OF POSITIVES BY PATIENT GROUP
TO THE GROUP'S REPRESENTATION IN THE ENTIRE STUDY
POPULATION NOT SEPARATED BY SEX

	FEMALES		MALES		MALES AND FEMALES	
R/E GROUP	PERCENT OF ALL POSITIVES	PERCENT OF TOTAL STUDY GROUP	PERCENT OF ALL POSITIVES	PERCENT OF TOTAL STUDY GROUP	PERCENT OF ALL POSITIVES	PERCENT OF TOTAL STUDY GROUP
White	2.70	5.72	17.57	11.81	20.27	17.53
Minority	27.03	30.90	52.70	51.57	79.73	82.47
Totals	29.73	36.62	70.27	63.38	100.00	100.00

Table 7.8 DISTRIBUTION OF HIV ANTIBODY TEST RESULTS
COMPARING THE NUMBER OF POSITIVES BY PATIENT GROUP
TO THE GROUP'S REPRESENTATION IN THE ENTIRE STUDY
POPULATION SEPARATED BY SEX

	FEMALES		MALES	
R/E GROUP	PERCENT OF FEMALE POSITIVES	PERCENT OF FEMALES TESTED	PERCENT OF MALE POSITIVES	PERCENT OF MALES TESTED
White	9.09	15.62	25.00	18.63
Minority	90.91	84.38	75.00	81.37
Total	100.00	100.00	100.00	100.00

Table 7.9 DISTRIBUTION OF HIV ANTIBODY TEST
RESULTS BY PATIENTS' AGE AND SEX*

	FEMALES			MALES		
AGE	NUMBER POSITIVE	NUMBER TESTED	PERCENT POSITIVE	NUMBER POSITIVE	NUMBER TESTED	PERCENT POSITIVE
16	2	39	5.13	2	51	3.92
17	4	70	5.71	3	72	4.17
18	3	92	3.26	4	149	2.68
19	6	94	6.38	19	217	8.76
20	6	78	7.69	22	190	11.58
Totals†	21	373		50	679	

*There are 55 specimens outside the 16–20 age range:
   Age <16 number tested = 36; percent positive = 2.78.
   Age >20 number tested = 19; percent positive = 10.53.
   16> percent positive >20; percent positive = 5.45.
†Total positive = 71. Total tested = 1052. Percent positive = 6.75.

Table 7.10 DISTRIBUTION OF HIV ANTIBODY TEST
RESULTS BY PATIENTS' RACIAL AND ETHNIC
BACKGROUND AND AGE*

	WHITE, NON-HISPANIC			BLACK, NON-HISPANIC			HISPANIC		
AGE	NUMBER POSITIVE	NUMBER TESTED	PERCENT POSITIVE	NUMBER POSITIVE	NUMBER TESTED	PERCENT POSITIVE	NUMBER POSITIVE	NUMBER TESTED	PERCENT POSITIVE
16	2	17	11.76	1	49	2.04	1	21	4.76
17	2	35	5.71	4	64	6.25	1	40	2.50
18	2	44	4.55	1	125	0.80	4	67	5.97
19	4	46	8.70	13	174	7.47	8	85	9.41
20	3	42	7.14	12	148	8.11	13	77	16.88
Totals†	13	184	7.07	31	560	5.54	27	290	9.31

*There are 55 specimens outside the 16–20 age range and 25 specimens with unknown R/E status.
†Total positive = 71. Total tested = 1034. Percent positive = 6.87.

recruits, American college students, prisoners, Job Corps recruits, blood donors, newborns, patients from STD clinics) [80–85] demonstrates that the cohort of familyless street kids in New York City represents an alarming reservoir of HIV infection. New York has been an epicenter of the AIDS epidemic and reported 24,070 of the first 105,990 cases (23 percent) in the United States. Compared with other New York City cohorts at risk for HIV infection (gay men and intravenous drug users), an overall prevalence of 7 percent or even the 16.8 percent prevalence among twenty-year-old Hispanics may not seem disturbing. However, no more than 7 percent of the males seen at this clinic identify as gay, and the number using needles to inject drugs is less than 2 percent. Certainly most of these patients were infected with the human immunodeficiency virus during sexual activity, and in view of the essentially one-to-one ratio of females to males among those testing seropositive, it may be assumed that much of the transmission took place during heterosexual encounters. There are some early data from other Covenant House sites now involved in the blinded seroprevalence study that extend the grave import of the New York findings to a truly national concern. As of July 1989, in New Orleans 7 of 242 specimens (2.9 percent) have been seropositive, in Houston 9 of 549 (1.6 percent), and in Fort Lauderdale 16 of 629 (2.5 percent). The Larkin Street Youth Center clinic in San Francisco began HIV antibody testing in 1989, and 10 percent of their tests are positive.[86] There is no doubt that America's abandoned, familyless street kids are already "players" in the future of the AIDS epidemic, and to date no program in place has a design of proved effectiveness in helping individual youth infected or protecting the public health at large.

Reviewing the case records of those youths known to be infected with HIV gives compelling evidence that the AIDS epidemic is well advanced among familyless street kids, and not surprisingly it documents that the more street time and street activities an adolescent has had the more likely he or she is to be infected. The blinded seroprevalence data support this conclusion with a male:female seroprevalence ratio of 1.2 to 1 and no overrepresentation of any racial or ethnic group among the seropositives. On the street it doesn't matter whether kids have heterosexual or homosexual sex or whether they are white, black, or Hispanic. The survival life-style of the street transmits HIV infection. "Crack gave me AIDS" may not make scientific sense, but it makes street sense.

The case summaries that follow serve to highlight the complexity of treating street kids with any serious medical problem. HIV infection is simply a paradigm. Again and again the same obstacles that frustrate efforts to get these youths off the street obstruct the delivery of sensible medical care.

In June 1988 a social worker from New York City's child welfare service contacted Covenant House to arrange intake referral for Derrick, a fourteen-year-old boy who was being discharged from a psychiatric hospital after three weeks of treatment for depression and a suicide attempt. The only other placement the social worker could find would be a series of overnight stays in city offices, so despite the fact that Covenant House is a short-term crisis intervention program, she felt it was a better choice. This boy had been reared by his mother and had been sexually abused from the age of six by several older male family members.

"It wasn't sexual abuse because I'm gay," he told the nurse. He had been involved in street prostitution from time to time and was treated for syphilis when he was thirteen. He claimed that his mother finally threw him out because she "couldn't deal with my homosexuality." Around the same time he was told at another clinic that his HIV antibody test was positive. Shortly thereafter he took "a bunch of pills to kill myself" and was admitted to the hospital.

Terry was nineteen when he came to the shelter. He had been brought up by both parents until he was nine years old. When they divorced, he lived with his grandmother for five years until she died of cancer. For the last five months he had been staying with his father, who was homeless following an apartment fire and was heavily addicted to cocaine and alcohol. Terry smoked crack every day he was on the street with his father and came to the shelter to get away from his father and drugs. In the previous year he had survived a car wreck in which his cousin was killed—"we were real high"—and he had been incarcerated for thirty days on a drug offense. These events depressed him, and he drank a bottle of gin and a bottle of Comtrex, "to kill myself." His health assessment in the clinic revealed that he was bisexual and that since the age of thirteen he had had serially monogamous relations with ten women and three men. He also had generalized adenopathy and a large, firm parotid mass. He tested positive for HIV infection. A biopsy of the mass was scheduled, and intake arranged at a drug treatment program, but he was arrested and lost to follow-up.

Linda came to the shelter "because this crack and prostitution are getting to me, and I'm afraid of AIDS." She told the clinic psychiatrist that she left her home in Detroit at age sixteen because "there were too many of us, no money, no food, and too many beatings." She was quickly involved in prostitution and had traveled to Chicago and Houston before coming to New York. At a physical done in preparation for going to the Job Corps she was found to have venereal warts, trichomoniasis, and a chlamydial infection. Her rapid plasma reagin (RPR) test for syphilis was positive. Because of her life-style and multiple STDs and wish to go to the Job Corps, where HIV testing is mandatory, she was counseled to have the test before applying. The result was positive. Her STDs were treated, but after several counseling sessions she left New York.

Scott is a nineteen-year-old white male who came to the clinic on the outreach van, requesting medical care for a sore throat, cough, chills, vomiting, and diarrhea. He stated he had been living on the street since he was twelve years old and had supported himself that entire time by hustling. He had lived in New York, Fort Lauderdale, Washington, D.C., Philadelphia, and Newark and had worked the strips in all those places. He claimed to be heterosexual, but he arrived with his current male lover (also a street hustler) and couldn't remember his last sexual encounter with a woman. He stated, "I guess I'm turning gay." He used IV drugs "two or three times" when he was fifteen years old but claimed that he never had since. He had been using crack daily for about two months. Physical examination revealed a very inflamed pharynx and expiratory wheezes. Laboratory tests were *normal, and a throat culture was negative; but a chest X ray showed patchy basilar infiltrates consistent with "crack lung." He was treated with erythromycin and inhaled albuterol. His plan included HIV testing and long-term drug treatment. His HIV antibody test was positive, but despite intensive counseling, he decided he "couldn't make it in drug treatment" and returned to the streets.*

Serrita arrived at Covenant House in August 1987 after living on the street for more than a year. She never knew her father and considered her relationship with her mother to be "real bad." She had left school in the tenth grade because of "problems" and drug use. She had worked briefly at a fast-food restaurant. When she was eighteen, her mother, a health care worker, told her to leave home. She began living in the boiler room of her apartment building and soon had a boyfriend staying there with her, "because he could get me crack." After one month the boyfriend left, and she took in another man, also a local drug supplier. She claimed that these two men were her only sex partners up to that time. She continued daily crack use, and in March 1987 she came to the clinic with a vaginal discharge. She was told she had gonorrhea and was treated. She did not keep her follow-up appointment. In April 1987 she was arrested for attempted murder and was sent to jail. She was released by July 1987 and was living on the street. She denied involvement in prostitution and alleged she was raped by a stranger in July 1987. She denied any IV drug use but continued to use crack daily. Serrita came to the clinic in mid-August 1987 and complained of a human bite on her finger. She had lost forty pounds since leaving home. Her physical examination revealed a sixty-two-inch-tall 124-pound adolescent. She had an infection of her right thumb. Laboratory investigation revealed an elevated serum globulin—3.9 (grams per deciliter), a positive vaginal KOH (potassium hydroxide) prep, and positive rapid plasma reagin and fluorescent treponemal antibody (FTA) tests for syphilis. She was treated with ceftriaxone, benzathine penicillin, and clotrimazole suppositories. She was counseled about the risks of her life-style, and when offered an HIV test, she consented to be tested. The HIV antibody test was positive. Her initial reaction to the result was chaotic, but after counseling and talking with her mother she made significant changes in her life-style. "Crack gave me AIDS" was her comment. She remains drug-free and asymptomatic.

Chantal first arrived at Covenant House in 1982 at age sixteen, when she ran away from an abusive father. When she was seven years old, her mother died of a head injury received in a fight. Her father frequently beat her. At age fifteen she was raped and became depressed. She attempted suicide several times. The psychologist who saw her in 1982 concluded: "She would make an excellent adjustment to a residential treatment center and has the potential to vastly expand her intellectual and creative potential with the aid of therapy and a therapeutic environment." She left Covenant House without permission and returned two years later. She was pregnant and had gonorrhea. She again left the program without a successful placement. She returned in December 1986, stating she had nowhere to stay because her boyfriend had died of "pneumonia and TB." An HIV antibody test was positive. In March 1987 she again became pregnant. She intended to keep the child. Her EDC (estimated date of confinement) was February 1988. When she turned twenty-two, she "aged out" of the program and left to "make it on my own."

Donny was sixteen when he first came to Covenant House in December 1985. He said that he had "problems" with his mother and that he had left home five times previously. He said that his mother was an alcoholic and that she often threw objects at him. Most recently she had beaten him with a shoe, and he wanted to file an abuse complaint against her. He denied substance abuse but admitted to being bisexual. At that time he was sixty-six inches tall (tenth percentile) and weighed 107 pounds (less than fifth percentile). All his laboratory values were normal, including a negative RPR. He left Covenant House before a complete physical exam could be completed. He returned in January 1988 and came to the clinic, stating that he needed medication for asthma. He said he was anxious and depressed because of the way "all those boys" talked about his sexual preference. He said he had a monogamous partner for the previous seventeen months and that they used condoms regularly. He admitted that in 1982 and 1983, when he was thirteen years old, he had been a male prostitute in New York City. Until recently he was able to obtain medication for his asthma with his Medicaid card. He lost his Medicaid eligibility when he failed to appear for a face-to-face interview. His physical examination revealed his weight to be 120 pounds (still less than fifth percentile), two- and three-centimeter lymphadenopathy in his neck, axilla, and submental groups. He was sad, withdrawn, and frightened. Since he planned to go to the Job Corps, he was referred for HIV counseling. The counselor put him in touch with his mother, and it was agreed that he should be tested. His mother told him she would take care of him "no matter what," and indeed, he decided to go home to her despite his knowledge that she was still an untreated alcoholic and that her home was often chaotic. He was discharged from Covenant House to the care of his mother for the first time in seven years. He returned to the Covenant House clinic in early February 1988 to learn that his HIV antibody test was positive. He "expected that" and has joined several support groups and volunteered to work with a PWA (People with AIDS) support group.

Trudy came to the Covenant House clinic in May 1987. Covenant House was the discharge plan resource for her release from a large university-based hospital following treatment for pelvic inflammatory disease. Before her admission to the hospital she had been living with friends. Her mother had died of alcoholic cirrhosis when she was thirteen. Her father had died of alcoholic cirrhosis when she was seventeen. She knew she had twenty-five-year-old twin sisters but was not in contact with either. Whenever she was questioned about her parents, she cried and withdrew. She had been admitted to the hospital complaining of abdominal pain. She had been sexually active since the age of thirteen and currently had a thirty-year-old boyfriend of long standing. He was being treated for nonpulmonary tuberculosis. She did not know where he lived. She had completed ninth grade and had once worked at McDonald's. Her plan for the future was to get a job "working with kids." At Covenant House she complained of bleeding gums, night sweats, and painful intercourse. Her physical examination revealed a fifty-seven-inch-tall eighty-five-pound black adolescent, appearing younger than her stated age. Physical examination revealed large axillary, cervical, occipital, pre- and postauricular, and inguino-femoral lymphadenopathy. Since she had just left the hospital, the only lab test done was an HIV antibody test. It was positive. On June 30 her boyfriend arrived at Covenant House, and she left with him. Neither the Covenant House staff nor the physician who took an interest in her at the medical center has been able to find her.

Jose came to Covenant House in New York in December 1987 after living in the Port Authority bus terminal for six months. His parents separated when he was six years old. At fifteen years of age he was raped by a neighbor. He used intravenous cocaine for several years (seventy-five to one hundred dollars per day), spent the summer of 1986 hustling to support his drug use, considered himself gay, and has had two lovers (twenty-nine and forty). He didn't finish the eleventh grade. He has worked as a home health attendant, but most of his work has been drug dealing. He presented with a persistent cough and a stuffy head. His medical history was significant for a hospitalization in August 1986 for pulmonary tuberculosis, moderately advanced. He was treated and responded. At Covenant House he was found to have chronic hepatitis (both hepatitis-A- and hepatitis-B-antibody-positive) and was treated for phthiriasis. He was tested for HIV antibody and was positive. When informed of the result, he called his mother and told her he had some "bad news." She replied, "If you got AIDS, go cure yourself. Don't come here." Then she hung up. Since December 1987 he seems to be drug-free, and there is no evidence of recurrent tuberculosis. He has applied to a therapeutic community for drug treatment.

Madeline arrived at Covenant House in November 1987 following the death of her mother from a crack-induced stroke. She spent three months on the street before coming to Covenant House. Her father had been in jail for the last two years. She did not complete the eighth grade because of a pregnancy and marijuana use. She had never had a job. She used crack daily for eight months before coming to Covenant House. She was in her third pregnancy, due to deliver in May 1988. Her first child has AIDS and is still in a hospital; her second pregnancy ended with a miscarriage in the fourth month. She commented, "I was so drugged up nobody could have a baby like that!" She had had a total of three male sex partners. The father of her first child was neither an intravenous drug addict (IVDA) nor gay. He did have two other girl friends who were IVDAs. The father of her second child (and this pregnancy) denied IV drug use and homosexuality, but he was raped at the age of eight (with anal penetration) by a male baby-sitter. Madeline has been treated for gonorrhea, syphilis, venereal warts, and phthiriasis. She's been arrested and is on probation for "child abandonment." She told the nurse who interviewed her that she felt good about herself and was looking forward to being an executive secretary. Physical examination revealed a sixty-six-inch-tall 117-pound black female. She had generalized lymphadenopathy, and there was a purulent cervical discharge. Laboratory investigation revealed anemia, a positive *syphilis serology, and trichomoniasis. She and her boyfriend tested HIV-anti-body-positive. She lost custody of the baby when it tested positive for cocaine. The baby stayed in the hospital, and she was discharged to the street, where she lived until 1989 when she again came to the shelter. She had chlamydial cervicitis and was pregnant for the fourth time. She had made three firm decisions: She would stop using crack, she would have an abortion, and she would not tell her current boyfriend she was infected by the AIDS virus. She stuck to all three. Her two surviving children have AIDS and remain in the custody of child welfare agencies. She is well. In the summer of 1989 she met with the president of the United States and the first lady and told them about her life, her ambitions, and her desire to regain custody of her children.*

These patients were tested in the course of their routine medical care and do not represent a controlled study, but it is striking that the infected patients all share chaotic family backgrounds and all have been involved in the street life-style. Eighteen of the infected patients (33 percent) gave a history of physical abuse at home, and fifteen (27 percent) reported they had been sexually abused. Twenty-four (44 percent) had been involved in prostitution, and fifteen (27 percent) had made serious attempts at suicide.

The HIV-infected patients also shared other medical diagnoses. Of the fifty-five HIV-infected patients, eighteen (33 percent) also had syphilis, forth-three (78 percent) had been treated for some other STD, twenty-four (44 percent) had hepatitis B markers, and eight (14 percent) had both syphilis and hepatitis B. Thirty-three (60 percent) had abused drugs, and twenty-eight (51 percent) had been steady users of crack. Another interesting observation is that twenty-two (40 percent) of those testing positive had an elevated serum globulin on a routine chemscreen, while only six (6 percent) of those testing negative had the same finding. Serum globulin testing may be an unregulated "poor man's" HIV infection screen for adolescents. A medical history that includes at-risk behavior is an indication for HIV antibody testing, especially if any of these additional factors are noted on routine evaluation.

Twenty-eight of the HIV-infected patients chose to enter a long-term residential program which included comprehensive medical evaluations. Half these patients had clinical or laboratory findings that qualified them for treatment with azidothymidine (AZT) and aerosolized pentamidine. At the time AZT cost $250 per 100 capsules, and two weeks' treatment required either 168 or 70 capsules depending on the dose prescribed. The cost for monthly pentamidine treatment, the drug and disposable equipment, was $140. Supplying these important treatments, even for the "short" time it takes to secure Medicaid eligibility for patients, represents a serious budgetary problem.

Every clinic for familyless street kids should have, or have access to, as many AIDS educators and counselors as it takes to keep the majority of those patients who are still uninfected from becoming so. Every medical visit must also be an AIDS education session, stressing personal worth and personal control and attempting to influence life-style choices and behaviors that are dangerous. It is well known that knowledge and attitude are more easily changed than behavior, but to their great credit, today's adolescent AIDS educators are "inventing" behavior-changing techniques on the run. They should have the full support of the other medical professionals on their team.

One final statistic says everything about the ongoing tragedy of the spread of human immunodeficiency virus infection among familyless street kids. Of the 155 patients tested at Covenant House, 9 who originally tested negative were retested at a later date, and 3 (33 percent) had converted to seropositive. Each of them had spent the time between visits to the clinic living the life-style of America's familyless street kids.

The availability of antiretroviral drugs like AZT, the ability to diagnose and treat opportunistic infections or malignancies in their early stages on the basis of subtle clinical and laboratory clues, the proved efficacy of primary prophylaxis for *Pneumocystis carinii* pneumonia, the transmission of the virus from mother to newborn during childbirth, and the possibility that AZT may actually reduce the transmission rate (chemical prophylaxis) among patients who have not changed their drug and sex behaviors are important reasons to identify all patients with human immunodeficiency virus infection as well as their sex and drug partners.[87,88] This is especially true for America's street kids. Not to do so because of a perception that resources for counseling or medical care are not available is simply another way to abandon these children. Put the resources in place, test those at risk, treat the infected patients, and protect the patients who are still uninfected. Medical progress on the treatment of HIV infection is progressing rapidly. Within the next few years HIV infection will finally be perceived as a medical problem with social and political implications, rather than a social and political problem with medical implications. That will be a good development for the health of street kids and society at large.

In view of what is known about the life-style of street kids, the prevalence of HIV in the cohort, and their incidence of sexually transmitted infections, it is fair to describe street kids as a population in which some of contemporary America's most serious diseases (syphilis, AIDS, gonorrhea, and stimulant addiction) are now co-endemic. The epidemiologic denouement of this development has implications for American society so profound as to justify any effort to interrupt its natural progression.

Psychiatric Disorders and Emotional Disturbances

Psychoemotional disturbances seem so pervasive among familyless street kids that it is hard to describe any of them as mentally healthy. Indeed, to this day "runaway reaction" remains an American Psychiatric Association diagnosis, and the term can be searched as such on the National Library of Medicine's MEDLINE data base. When we examine the psychopathology of the street kid population, we must consider antecedence.[89] It is obvious to professionals working with familyless adolescents that many were emotionally and developmentally intact before their abandonment commenced, but it is difficult to quantify what part of the entire group they represent. Also, there are psychotic youth, separated from healthy families, living distorted lives on the street, but again a count is elusive. Child care specialists making assessments of individual street kids face the same etiologic dilemma that Police Officer Krupke did in *West Side Story* ("Hey, I'm depraved on accounta I'm deprived"),[90] and it can be just as hard to decide whether a judge, social worker, or psychiatrist should be first in line to deal with their problems. Fortunately, even the most etiologically complex case usually lends itself to interventional simplicity. In other words, for an individual street kid all roads lead to where he stands, most of what is in his past cannot be changed, and his tomorrow begins today if the right amount of nonjudgmental, value-based supportive therapy is applied. For this reason, mental health professionals should play a large role in the design and execution of any program treating runaway youth.

For the group at large, however, the need for early identification of which children are at risk of becoming street kids requires that more rigorous attention should be given to the distinctions between what is antecedent and what is consequent in the overall mental health of adolescents who end up familyless, homeless, and "runaway."

The Institute of Medicine has reported that 12 percent of the 63 million children under the age of eighteen in the United States suffer from a mental disorder. Most of this pathology is concentrated among the poor with as many as 20 percent of that group estimated to have emotional disturbance or mental illness. The institute also reported that in 1985 only 2.5 million of these children were treated, leaving 5 million without care. Although this analysis did not look at runaway youth as a separate group, it did conclude that many of the background factors common to familyless street kids contribute to poor mental health. The problems identified included: developmental impairments which limit a child's ability to think and learn, to form social attachments, or to communicate effectively with others; emotional disturbances characterized by crippling states of anxiety or depression or both; and behavioral problems that lead to disruptive and antisocial acts. "In addition to identifying traditionally accepted causes of mental disorders in children, like having parents who are mentally ill, the report was notable for also identifying as causes things like poverty, homelessness, and growing up in 'crowded, inner-city neighborhoods.' It said that such conditions created 'persistent psychosocial adversity' for children."[91] Ellen Bassuk and Lenore Rubin previously described the common findings of developmental delays, severe depression and anxiety, and learning difficulties among the children of homeless families.[22] A study of children of mentally ill parents demonstrated the fact that these children's risk for behavioral problems is much greater when certain cofactors are present in their environment.

A child's risk status and subsequent behavioral outcomes are a function of the relative balance between personal coping skills and net environmental stressors and protectors. When the at-risk child's coping skills are stronger than the net environmental stress, the child is likely to be invincible—free of significant behavior problems. Conversely, when net environmental stress exceeds the available coping skills, the child is likely to fall victim—manifesting severe behavioral problems.[92]

The environmental stressors of abandonment and street life-style are immeasurable, and only a truly invincible child could escape the psychological wounds noted so frequently in street kids coming into shelters. Among runaways new to a shelter "invincibles," like Tom and Huck, are rare; "victims," like Eduardo and Reggie, are common. With street kids it is difficult to separate the emotional disturbance associated with the acute crisis of familylessness from any underlying psychiatric disorder. Nevertheless, when Shaffer and Caton studied a population of runaway shelter residents, they thought that the high incidence of previous psychiatric treatment, the frequency of school problems, the many criminal justice problems identified, and the high incidence of suicidal behavior among the group all supported the conclusion that for most runaways psychiatric disturbance was present at least prior to the current runaway episode.[24]

Initial assessments of street kids in shelters identify feelings of rejection, isolation, and hopelessness. The importance of severe chronic stresses such as family violence, parental substance abuse, neglect and lack of supervision, placements out of the home, and abandonment frequently surface as the youths discuss their problems. Adjustment disorders and transient symptoms of depression are commonly identified in new shelter residents, and for many the shelter milieu is the major factor resulting in symptom improvement.

Tara was nineteen years old when she came to the shelter. Her mother had died when Tara was two years old. She lived with her grandmother for thirteen years. When her grandmother died, she went to live with her great-grandmother, but she didn't get along with her and started staying away from home. At that time her long-absent father appeared and became increasingly abusive, escalating to facial punching. Tara ran away and after a short time on the street came to the shelter. She was depressed and frightened. She commented, "How can someone hate me so much who has never even known me?" The shelter staff offered encouragement and immediately involved Tara in a "plan of action." She soon returned to school, made plans for college, and did quite well.

For many youths, however, long-standing psychiatric difficulties underlie any recent turmoil, and these individuals require referral to a mental health professional. Having psychiatric and psychological services on-site should be a major goal for any program working with street kids. "Immediacy" cannot be overstressed.

The shelter residents referred for psychiatric evaluation benefit from supportive psychotherapy, an opportunity to ventilate feelings, to discuss issues that he or she might not be comfortable discussing with the child care staff, and in some cases to obtain medications that reduce symptoms. When the adolescent's premorbid level of functioning has been good, there is often an excellent response to even a few sessions of supportive psychotherapy. However, good baseline functioning is the exception rather than the rule for street kids. Many have markers of chronic psychopathology: multiple psychiatric hospitalizations, prior suicide attempts, and previous treatment with psychiatric medications.

For the street kids seen in psychiatric consultation the most common diagnoses are:

- Depression, often with suicidal thoughts
- Conduct disorders
- Drug and alcohol abuse
  "Dual diagnosis"
  "Sexual compulsion"
- Schizophrenia and drug-related psychoses
- Various types of cognitive impairments
  Mental retardation
  Borderline intellectual functioning
  Drug-related delirium
  Learning disorders
  Maladaptive personality traits

Suicide deserves special mention because in the midst of an epidemic of adolescent suicide[93] the suicides of street kids may well go unnoticed. The risk factors are all present among the group,[94] but they seem least likely to complete suicides while in shelter care. On the street a dead adolescent is not always investigated as a suicide, especially if he or she is found in the midst of drug deals and prostitution.

On-site psychiatric services should focus on the acute crisis. Psychotic symptoms can be reduced with neuroleptic medications, aggressive behavior can be managed, and suicidal youth can be monitored. Another important benefit of having psychiatric professionals on-site is that they can communicate with the child care staff members who are often overwhelmed by youth with psychiatric symptoms.

Treatment of this group of street kids can be very difficult and frustrating. Often nonmedical problems thwart care, as with patients who lack the social skills to cooperate in their own care, patients who mistrust health professionals, and patients who alienate the staff trying to help them. Failure to keep appointments for follow-up care, failure to stay in treatment once immediate distress has been relieved, and the difficulty of transferring care when a youth is placed or moves to a different neighborhood are other reasons why longitudinal care often fails for this population of patients.

For adolescents with long-standing and severe psychopathology, on-site services are often inadequate, and a large challenge for mental health professionals treating street kids is the involvement of their patients in programs providing specialized ongoing care. For some this means hospitalization, but for most it means integrating drug detoxification programs, day hospitals, day treatment programs working with chronic mental illness, outpatient clinics, Alcoholics Anonymous, Narcotics Anonymous, and vocational rehabilitation programs into the overall care plan for the child. Whenever possible and realistic, strong efforts should be made to reunite and treat the family as a unit.

Left untreated, psychiatric pathology reduces all other efforts to help a street kid simply to "spinning wheels." Mental health professionals belong on the starting team of any program designed to reclaim America's familyless, runaway street kids.

Substance Abuse

"Most scientists agree that in nature the primary role of many alkaloids is protection against animals. Thus, compounds such as nicotine and cocaine represent poisons produced by plants to ward off feeding insects and other animals."[95]

This simple evolutionary survival strategy of the shrub *Erythroxylon coca*, producing the chemical $C_{17}H_{21}NO_4$ (cocaine), is now having a greater impact on contemporary America than the evolution of grain and its distillate, alcohol. Cocaine in its smokable form, crack, has taken an entire generation of inner-city youths prisoner, and for street kids it has essentially pronounced a death sentence. Addiction to this stimulant puts an end to all normal participation in society and inexorably forces the addict into crime. Child care workers dealing with street kids still have to deal with the substance abuse problems that existed in 1984, before crack made its way from the Bahamas to the streets of America's cities. Alcohol, heroin, hallucinogens, marijuana, and sedatives are still formidable problems, but they pale in comparison with the dominant impact of crack on familyless street kids. Forty percent of all Americans between the ages of twenty-five and thirty have tried cocaine at least once.[96] The incidence of steady use by street kids is certainly higher and involves as many female as male abusers—a new phenomenon with enormous implications considering the compulsive sexuality induced by crack use and the endemicity of STDs and HIV infection in the cohort.

The negative impact of this stimulant on its users is enormous, and in many cases it seems as if the entire litany of problems presented by runaway youth were in some way either antecedent or consequent to this substance abuse. Many studies interrelate adolescent substance abuse with:

- Parental substance abuse[97]
- A history of sexual abuse[98]
- School failure
- Sexually compulsive behavior
- STDs and AIDS
- Psychopathology
- Suicide[99]
- Violence
- Criminal activity[100]
- Prostitution[101]
- Child abuse[102]
- The birth of premature and underdeveloped babies[103]

Beyond the developmental handicaps caused by fetal cocaine exposure, infants born to mothers testing positive for drugs are placed in foster care, and for some that is the beginning of familylessness. Crack smokers suffer cardiovascular and neurologic damage,[104] and binge users develop an unusual pulmonary inflammation known as crack lung.[105]

No treatment modality has yet proved effective in the long-term management of crack addiction,[106,107] yet there may soon be more destructive stimulants appearing on the street. Already crack users are at high risk to abuse other drugs because they need to "treat" the crash that follows the cocaine euphoria.[96] This has led to smoking admixtures of heroine and crack ("speedballs"). Soon "ice," a smokable form of amphetamine moving eastward from Asia with devastating impact, may appear on the streets nationwide.[108] Without doubt prevention of initial use is the most important goal in dealing with stimulant addiction.[109] Once crack is used, memories of the intense euphoria it evoked make repeated use inevitable. Studies have identified a lack of connection to family and school, use of marijuana, and psychopathology as important risk factors for adolescent cocaine abuse,[110,111] but any child exposed to the life-style of the street is severely at risk. Knowing how close so many at-risk adolescents are to becoming street kids is the basis for the strongest argument against the legalization of drugs.

Beyond the release and euphoria associated with stimulant use, the financial incentives to become involved in drug dealing are quite powerful for a street kid with no other marketable skills. In some areas of America's inner cities crack has actually become an alternate currency, traded for goods and sex.

Lisa was eighteen years old when she came to the clinic complaining of chest pain. She'd spent the last few weeks in the bus terminal "doin' blow jobs for crack." She wouldn't accept money for sex because she needed and wanted crack. With money "you gotta go out on the Deuce and buy it. There's pimps out there!" She was treated for her crack lung and entered drug treatment.

The "Deuce" is New York City's Forty-second Street, and Lisa was right: There are pimps out there. Her alternate currency kept her out of their reach, "safe," inside a toilet booth in a bus terminal, "surviving."

These rap lyrics were written by an eleven-year-old who was abandoned by a drug-addicted mother;

> *Hey little dude, Wanna make some bread?*
> *Just run these rocks and do what's said.[112]*

The author of those lyrics found a safe place with another family. Most of America's homeless adolescents (yes, eleven-year-olds are adolescents where street kids come from) are not yet that lucky. Finding a successful treatment for crack addiction and preventing any more children from being destroyed by it must become a crusade for American domestic-policy makers. Although experienced staff members in the drug-free programs that seem to work with alcohol and narcotic addictions are opposed to the idea, some temporizing or adjuvant drug

treatment may be necessary to get control of "crackheads" early in abstinence.[113,114]

If the nation does not get control of this epidemic of stimulant addiction, there
will be terrible consequences: Violent crime will increase, the internecine slaugh-
ter of young drug dealers will escalate, and more social resources will be siphoned
off into the black hole of drugs. More important, if this pervasive abuse of stimulant drugs does not abate, more families will be destroyed, there will be more
familyless street kids, and they will swell the ranks of a sexually promiscuous
group that has a high rate of endemic HIV infection. As a *New England Journal
of Medicine* editorialist who reviewed the Covenant House HIV seroprevalence
data commented, "This is terrifying."[115]

Childbearing Street Kids and "Unwell" Babies

Adolescent sexuality, pregnancy, and childbearing are well-studied and documented problems on the American health care agenda,[36,116–118] and they need
not be reviewed here. However, when familyless street kids have sex, get pregnant, or bear children, these problems assume more worrisome dimensions. Perhaps the most jarring sight on the midnight streets of America's cities is the baby
stroller, and there are thousands of them out there. Infants and toddlers growing
up surrounded by crack deals, prostitution, violence, and crime make a forceful
statement about the tragedy of abandoned youth.

A street kid pregnancy refocuses all the concerns about the negative impacts
of substance abuse, prostitution, syphilis, AIDS, poor nutrition, lack of medical
care, and all the consequences of the street life-style on yet another developing
human being. Fetalescence and adolescence may be the most vulnerable seasons
of human development. A pregnant street kid symbolizes all that can go wrong
with growth and development, twice over.

Street kids account for a significant number of the one million annual teenage
pregnancies in America, but there are some important distinctions to be made
about these pregnancies. Most street kid mothers conceive children deliberately
and hopefully, they have a higher rate of spontaneous abortions and a much lower
rate of induced abortions than the group as a whole, they are far more likely to
have a sexually transmitted disease (including HIV infection and hepatitis), they
are far less likely to get regular prenatal care, they are more likely to have low-
birth-weight babies, and they are also more likely to be having their second or
third teenage childbirth. All the evils and problems of the street intersect these
pregnancies.

HIV infection provides the best example. By the early years of the 1990's HIV
will have orphaned more than ten thousand children in New York City alone.[119]
Many of those orphans will be infant children of street kids, and many will have
HIV infection themselves.[120] The New York State Department of Health has
reported that 1 percent of the nineteen-year-olds giving birth in New York City
are already HIV-infected.[121] Children born premature, drug-addicted, and developmentally retarded represent similar personal tragedies, and the group as a whole

represents billions of dollars in social welfare expenditures that must be committed to their care.[122]

The practical health care problems of pregnant street kids are most pressing during the months leading up to and following the birth. Much has been said about the lack of prenatal care among the group, but it is important to note that infants and toddlers brought to runaway shelters have rarely had "well baby" checkups and are always behind in their immunizations. Exploring the reasons for this "neglect" seldom identifies a "neglectful" mother. Many of these young moms have had little or no counseling around the issues and techniques of parenting, and societal supports for poor, familyless young mothers are simply inadequate. With resources for the homeless population at large so inadequate it is not surprising to find newborns in shelters.

Drug-addicted moms present a sad dilemma. Their children are removed from their care at birth and placed with their families, if anybody will take them, or in foster care. Even if this is the best course for the child, this loss often drives the mother into even more destructive behaviors (heavier drug use and prostitution). New York City has so many pregnant drug addicts that there is a special clinic set up for their care.[123] While it serves women of all ages, the problems seen in that clinic mirror those of pregnant street kid drug users: no prenatal care, malnourishment, epidemic STD infections (40 percent are HIV-infected), a 30 percent incidence of low-birth-weight babies, and an infant mortality rate equal to that of a third world nation.

Street kid moms seldom have the support of their children's fathers. Even during pregnancy they often seek out new male partners, and this behavior certainly contributes to their high rate of infection with sexually transmitted diseases.

In 1990 it is not uncommon to realize, when we do a health assessment of a street kid, that the adolescent patient is actually the child of a street kid. Only fifteen years separate the generations.[124] It is difficult to look at a laughing two-year-old and recognize a street kid, but that's what the children of street kids really are. This short generational interval multiplies the negative impact of abandoned children on society. Perhaps a few "invincibles" will emerge from the group, but without enormous societal intervention the majority is destined for tragedy.

Neglected Pathologies

Nothing about living on the street where violence, drugs, and STDs are endemic prevents street kids from having the "normal" illnesses of adolescence. Many runaways visit clinics for treatment of vision problems, sore throats, dental cavities, acne, conjunctivitis, ear infections, headaches, skin rashes, diarrhea, or bronchitis. Most often, however, these problems have gone untreated much longer than "if Mom had known about them." Delayed treatment of episodic illnesses is a significant problem for street kids, but lack of ongoing care for chronic illnesses is even more serious. Asthma, diabetes mellitus, seizure disorder, and known psychosis are the most commonly seen neglected pathologies in clinics treating homeless youth. Current estimates are that between 10 and 20 percent of all American adolescents have a physical handicap or chronic medical condition.[125,126] The incidence among children abandoned to the street seems higher, and the impact of neglect on the severity of these illnesses is easily measurable.

Dan always had trouble walking. His mother told him he had Perthes's disease. "Most doctors don't even know what that is," he quipped as he was examined in the shelter's clinic. He'd been living in the bus terminal for two months since his sister died. He lived with her after his mother threw him out. "My dad got killed, the mob done him, and she wanted to start over." His sister was killed in an auto accident. The driver, her boyfriend, survived the crash but was convicted of driving while intoxicated. The doctor who saw him knew what Perthes's disease was, was sure Danny didn't have it, and had his judgment verified by consultants who were sure that the boy had cerebral palsy and secondary destructive arthritis of his hip. They recommended a program of rehabilitation and total hip replacement, but Dan didn't show up for the appointment at which he would have learned of his new diagnosis and treatment plan.

Andy came to the clinic for a routine health assessment and was noted to have a purulent green drainage from his left ear. "It's been that way since the operations," he said. Beyond the fact that the operations were performed seven years before, he could offer no information except that "another operation is needed to fix the hearing. My mom couldn't afford that," he said. He tested deaf in that ear and returned to the street and his crack addiction before any further evaluation was achieved.

Treating chronic diseases episodically is a great frustration and challenge for health professionals working with street kids. Aptly, gonorrheal urethritis is the perfect disease for the practitioners of street medicine. It's acute, the diagnosis is straightforward (you can even see the beast through the microscope), and at least for now the treatment is immediate and effective. Sadly, all the enemies on the street do not succumb so easily. The problems of familyless street kids are complex, and there are many familyless street kids; but prioritizing services for those with chronic and neglected illnesses seems a natural "right thing" from a physician's perspective.

Nonclinical Issues

Health Services Strategies and Principles

Health services for familyless, runaway street kids should be centered on strategies of service and principles of practice. The strategies should be "reach out," do it *now!*, and network. The principles should include immediacy and sanctuary.[127]

OUTREACH

Any program for runaways that adds an outreach component is immediately surprised by the number of hard-core street kids who never use any community services.[128] More significantly, these are the most damaged kids. In New York City youths brought into care by outreach vans make up a significant proportion of those infected with HIV. Considering the realities of the street, health care is a low priority for homeless adolescents. Outreach workers should be trained to identify youths with a high probability for having an untreated illness and practiced in the skills that bring those patients into care.

"DO IT NOW!"

"Do it *now!*" recognizes the fact that clinicians may have only this visit for diagnosis and treatment of their patient's medical problem.[129] There is (sadly) nothing magical about the practice of medicine. Practitioners collect facts, organize them, arrive at a synthesis that best relates them, and then exercise experienced judgments to influence their patient's outcome. The only modifications street medicine imposes on this process are the more liberal use of diagnostic testing, a lower threshold for therapeutic intervention, and a "go nuclear" strategy for treatment.

NETWORKING

Primary care is a primary need for all street kids, but often subspecialty backup is called for. Clinics treating homeless adolescents should be staffed by health professionals who can cross some of the established boundaries of medical specialty, but they should also initiate and nurture contacts with hospitals and specialty clinic referral resources. Arranging contact persons, folks at each end of the referral process who know each other, is a simple yet effective program plan. When the reasons for a referral have been clearly explained ahead of time, overworked clinic staffs feel less dumped on. Health care for homeless adolescents can seem like one unmanageable crisis after another, and it is important for program staffs to sense that they are part of a larger net of resources for the problems of their patients.

IMMEDIACY

Immediacy is the principle behind "do it *now!*" It dictates that services should be close to where street kids gather and that the staff, equipment, and therapeutics required to deal with their problems be available. In light of the real impact of the expense of health care relative to other forms of child welfare services, programs should be flexible in their use of staff. Volunteers should be encouraged, arrangements can be made with resident physician-training programs to place these physicians on-site during elective periods, medical students can provide important extra hands, and mid-level practitioners can be made an important part of the staff.[130] If an agency can contract with a medical center to staff its clinic with attending physicians from the appropriate departments, there are many advantages. Highly credentialed staffs with many professional contacts at the backup institutions are a great asset.

The importance of immediacy is best exemplified by the street kid who arrives at the clinic with a crumpled, torn ten-day-old prescription from an emergency room for a pharmaceutical that was urgently needed ten days ago. While we recognize the impact on the program budget, it is essential for health professionals treating familyless youth to stress the importance of being well stocked. "Come back tomorrow" does as much good for a street kid with syphilis as "Have a nice day" does for a patient with depression. If the program can't provide it, have backup that can—right away.

SANCTUARY

Sanctuary really means safety. Nothing bad should happen to a kid because he has come into shelter care. It sounds and should be simple, but it can get complex. Often people, including pimps, abusive parents, and officers of the juvenile justice system, are "looking for" street kids who come into care. Thankfully, health professionals are not immediately involved in the resolution of those sanctuary issues, but the principle of sanctuary is often tested in two areas of medical concern: consent and confidentiality.

CONSENT

The issues involved in obtaining valid consent for the medical treatment of familyless and homeless adolescents are complex in theory but straightforward in reality. For the majority of cases—i.e., those patients eighteen and older, those who themselves are parents, those seeking treatment for drug, alcohol, or mental health problems, those who are in true medical emergencies, and those seeking treatment of sexually transmitted diseases—it is clear that the patient himself may consent to care in almost all of the United States and Canada. Under other circumstances legal exploration of the minor consent issue always involves questions about whether children are the property of their parents under common law, whether the nonconsensual touching of a medical treatment is a technical battery under tort law, and whether persons below the age of legal majority can give consent that is both rational and informed. These are important concepts, but they are topics for conference rooms, not frontline health care clinics. Street kids are usually in health care free fall, and gravity is the only law that applies.

Quite simply, in contemporary America thousands of familyless children have only themselves to consent to health care. Because they were enacted years ago, the laws safeguarding parental rights to control children come at today's problems from the wrong direction and often conflict with newer laws meant to "protect" children from abuse and neglect. Most emancipation cases have revolved around the parents' obligation to support their children, and a ruling that a child is not emancipated serves to protect continued parental support.[131] Such reasoning doesn't apply to health care for street kids. Familyless street kids have been abandoned by their parents and have fallen through all of society's safety nets. If they are the property of anyone, homeless runaways belong to their pimps and other adult exploiters. The issue of minor consent to health care is too often clouded by the notion that an adolescent who has been surviving unassisted on the street for months or years might yet be unable to give rational consent to health care he seriously needs.

There is almost no case law in which physicians have been held accountable for providing urgently needed medical care to minors who have claimed there was no one but themselves to give consent.[132]

Health professionals treating street kids are out in front of the courts and legislatures on this issue, and there is little doubt, in view of the health crisis these patients represent, that out front is where physicians and nurses treating street kids belong. Nevertheless, serious legal principles are involved whenever a minor is treated without parental consent, and physicians should ensure that the consents they obtain from minors are documented to be both informed and written. Although broad legislative and regulatory guidance is needed in this area, currently the issue is dominated by the narrower controversy over informing parents when a minor seeks an abortion.[133–35] However that issue turns, there will remain the need for a legislative delineation of the circumstances under which all familyless adolescents may get appropriate and immediate health care.

CONFIDENTIALITY

The medical records of street kids should be maintained no differently from those kept in any practice or hospital and should be protected from unwarranted intrusion just as carefully. Everything relative to medical care should be recorded in the chart and, especially where different providers see the same patient, should be detailed enough to ensure continuity and follow-through. What takes place between a patient and a physician or nurse during a clinic visit is private, and the record of the encounter really belongs to the patient but is left on loan so the medical staff can manage the patient's care. Street kids have a sense of this and resent the indignity, heaped on top of all the other indignities they have endured, of having details of their personal medical histories shared at large. Even when there is "need to know," individual adolescent patients should authorize the release of their records to nonmedical staff, other facilities, or agencies of the government before the record is abstracted or shared. Whenever a chronic health problem impacts on the overall plan for the patient, the physician or nurse should counsel and advise the adolescent to allow sharing the needed information with those in a position to help, but should the patient refuse, that wish must be respected.

There have always been reasons to provide the abandoned children of America who end up as familyless street kids with specialized health services, but the explosion of morbidity consequent to the epidemics of crack and HIV infection has made such services imperative. Physicians and nurses have a large role to play in the overall healing of this neglected group of children.

The most practical lesson learned by professionals working with street kids is that street damage is directly proportional to "street time." Getting kids off the streets in time makes all the difference. A month on the street is a serious wound; six months on the street are a mortal blow. America monitors and sets goals for its health. An important monitor is YPLL (years of productive life lost to any given pathology). Coronary artery disease, breast cancer, suicide, homicide, and now AIDS are high-scoring morbidities in this tabulation. Goals are generally counts and percent reductions in the incidence or mortality associated with any given disease. Sober reflection on the profound implications of the health status of America's familyless, runaway adolescents should compel the creation of a new monitor, YYLSS (years of youth life spent on the street), and the goal should be absolutely none. No adolescent's transition to adulthood should be guided by the principles of street life. There shouldn't be abandoned children on the streets of America.

MARSHA MCMURRAY-AVILA

Growing up Homeless

I saw her one day, just a face at the shelter
With empty brown eyes that no longer knew tears
She looked up at me and I saw in her emptiness
The future of childhood, the future we fear

Chorus
Growing up homeless, faceless to most of us
Growing up way too fast for her years
Growing up hopeless, she's never known happiness
She's growing up homeless, it's happening here

She stood in the line with her mommy for breakfast
She stood in the line for her lunch at midday
She stood in the line for a bed at the shelter
And never a word did I hear her say

Chorus

Her mommy can't work, 'cause she hasn't got day care
She can't pay the day care until there's a job
Her daddy left home 'cause he thought it was better
So they ended up homeless, just her and her mom

Chorus

She's a child of the streets, she's living our nightmares
She's closing herself off from those who would care
'Cause all she can see is the fear and the hopelessness
And all she can feel is the chilly night air

Chorus

MARY ANN LEE
KAREN HAUGHT
IRWIN REDLENER
ALMETA FANT
ELAINE FOX
STEPHEN A. SOMERS

8

Health Care for Children in Homeless Families

Introduction and Overview

During the past twenty years there has been a substantial change in the homeless population. According to new nationwide surveys of the urban homeless and recent studies of national population trends,[1-4] families have become the most rapidly growing segment.

Nationwide, members of these families now constitute an estimated 34 percent of all the homeless, in New York City 40 to 45 percent, and in Portland, almost 52 percent. The vast majority of homeless families are headed by women with two or three children, most under seven years of age. The proportion of two-parent families varies between regions. In the western United States there are more intact homeless families than in the East. Two-parent families appear to be more common in rural areas than urban areas (18 percent vs. 6.7 percent).[3] Their ethnic status tends to mirror the demographic composition of the area where they live, with blacks and Hispanics overrepresented in the cities and whites in suburban and rural areas.

Table 8.1 FROM THE UNITED STATES CONFERENCE
OF MAYORS 1988 REPORT

CITY	PERCENT INCREASE IN REQUESTS FOR EMERGENCY SHELTER	PERCENT INCREASE IN REQUESTS BY FAMILIES FOR EMERGENCY SHELTER	PERCENT COMPOSITION OF HOMELESS POPULATION THAT ARE FAMILIES
Boston	16	10	26
Charleston	40	100	15
Chicago	13	13	40
Cleveland	20	20+	36
Denver	0	0	27
Detroit	17	35	55
Hartford	NA	NA	NA
Kansas City	14	22	44*
Los Angeles	23	NA	35
Louisville	2	9	NA
Minneapolis	9	−15	18
Nashville	23	NA	24
New Orleans	16	13	15
New York City	1	0.4	62.2
Norfolk	16	16	80
Philadelphia	15	15	33
Phoenix	5	60	20
Portland	7–10	12	52*
Providence	NA	NA	30
St. Paul	NA	8.5	16
Salt Lake City	NA	NA	30
San Antonio	10	3.4	33
San Diego	5	10	25
San Francisco	10	−25	15
San Juan	20	40	15
Seattle	−11	16.1	37.3*
Trenton	35	30	54

*In Kansas City an additional 6 percent are childless couples. In Portland an additional 4 percent are childless couples. In Seattle an additional 2.2 percent are childless couples.

Why Has Family Homelessness Increased So Dramatically?

It is generally accepted that prominent factors in family homelessness include:

- Poverty. The worsening plight of the poor can be documented from the United States Bureau of Census reports and others.[4-6] In March 1989 the House Ways and Means Committee reported that from 1979 to 1987 the standard of living for the poorest fifth of the population fell by 9 percent.

- Lack of affordable or subsidized housing.
- Domestic violence and abuse.
- Substance abuse.
- Personal crises coupled with loss of marginal resources or support network and relationships—e.g., eviction by primary tenant in doubled-up situations, estrangement from family members, overwhelmed informal community support networks.
- Unemployment, underemployment, and lack of marketable skills.

A study[8] in New York City revealed the precipitating causes of family homelessness to be:

- 52 percent from doubling up
- 27 percent from eviction by landlord
- 14 percent because of unsafe building conditions
- 7 percent other

How Do Homeless Families Differ from Other Low-Income Families?

Urban homeless mothers typically are quite isolated and have few supportive relationships.[9–11] Such relationships are defined as attachments among individuals, or between individuals and groups or institutions, that serve to improve adaptive competence in dealing with short-term crises and life transitions, as well as long-term challenges and stresses. Traditionally the network of such relationships includes families, friends, neighbors, religious denominations, and mutual self-help organizations.[12] A substantial portion of homeless families using the shelter system suffers from a complex of difficulties, including chronic psychosocial, economic, educational, vocational, and substance abuse problems. They typically seek assistance from agencies when a crisis occurs but cease contact when the crisis abates.[9] E. L. Bassuk has reported that 45 percent of the women interviewed in a Massachusetts family shelter had histories of abusive relationships with spouses or mates.[10,11] When asked to name three persons on whom they could depend during times of stress, 43 percent of the mothers were unable to name anyone or could name only one person. Almost a quarter named their minor children as principal source of emotional support. Currently 22 percent of homeless mothers were involved in an investigation or follow-up of child neglect or abuse.

In addition, urban homeless families are often displaced from their original neighborhoods, where they shopped, where the children attended day care or school, and where the families received health care. This further alienates and isolates the families. The noxious effect relates both to loss or separation and to the absence of a familiar social and physical environment.

In contrast, low-income, nonhomeless families are more likely to have community and family support systems and histories of residential stability. They are familiar with neighborhood churches, schools, and social and health service providers. They are more likely to have ongoing relationships with community agencies for support in times of stress. A study showed that 23.3 percent of homeless families reported not having a regular source of health care as opposed to 13.7 percent of low-income domiciled families.[13]

In summary, homeless families are characterized by:

- Poverty
- Unstable domicile
- Decreased access to support systems
- Increased risk for mental, physical, and developmental problems associated with temporary housing or shelter arrangements

Barriers to Care

Homeless families face a combination of financial, systemic, and informational barriers to health care.

Financial Barriers

Health services for homeless families in the United States are fragmented, variable, and in some areas nonexistent.[14] Most major cities lack a coordinated comprehensive system that provides health care for homeless families and children. In 65 percent of the surveyed cities, families had to meet certain eligibility requirements in order to receive any public services. Certain states do not extend Medicaid eligibility to intact two-parent families and set eligibility levels for single mothers at a fraction of the federal poverty level.

Homeless families in poor and remote rural communities are even harder hit.[3] Provider availability is at issue. The poor financial status of many rural hospitals severely limits their ability to give uncompensated care. Rural areas attract fewer health care workers and thus have fewer services available. David Kindig has reported that the level of physician availability for counties with populations of less than ten thousand is one-third the national average.[15]

Homeless mothers may have difficulty in following recommended therapy regimens for themselves or their children, especially in purchasing medications and supplies not covered under Medicaid eligibility guidelines, and those that require prolonged bed rest, supplemental nutrition, or special diets.

Even if free prenatal or "well child" care is available, obtaining such care is not first on the homeless family's priority list. The few available dollars are not spent on transportation. In rural areas the ride to the local health clinic costs ten to twenty dollars, equivalent to one week's' food budget for the family. Time spent traveling to obtain care is also equivalent to a half or full day's minimum wage. Homeless families in urban areas with cheaper accessible mass transit systems are more fortunate. However, families with several children still have great difficulty in traveling unassisted. The New York Children's Health Project found that its referral and follow-up compliance rate improved from 30 to 63 percent when escort and transportation services were provided for families.[16]

*Systemic Barriers: Nature and Quality of Providers—Patient
and Provider Interaction*

Hospitals and clinics where the poor traditionally obtain health services are often overcrowded, with complex registration processes and long waits. Emergency rooms (ERs), where a significant portion of homeless families obtain care for acute illness or exacerbations of chronic illness, can provide only episodic crisis care.[17] Neither setting encourages compliance with treatment, follow-up, or preventive medical care. Interactions frequently end in frustration and anger for staff and patients.

Providers who serve a largely middle-class population may actively discourage use of services by the indigent homeless, who may be impatient, poorly clothed, and malodorous.

Aside from staff attitudes, the sheer numbers of patients seen and the prevalence of critical problems in ERs may, for instance, make doing a hearing test on a child with a diagnosis of recurrent otitis media and speech delay of low priority. Acute minor illnesses often go untreated in these children. Consequently, they are not seen until serious complications ensue. This results in increased rates of hospitalization, cost, and morbidity.[18,19]

MR is a nine-month-old black female infant brought to a metropolitan ER with complaints of lethargy, fever, and intermittent vomiting of one-week duration. She was referred by a public health nurse visiting the family living in an SRO hotel. Her eighteen-year-old mother was aware that MR had been crying and pulling her ears for the past week. She had been medicating the child with irregular doses of acetaminophen because she was "too busy" to register the child in the clinic. Her previous experience with the ER, a three-hour wait, had discouraged her. MR was diagnosed with otitis media, mastoiditis, meningitis, and shock. She spent many weeks in the hospital. After her discharge she was found to have significant hearing loss and developmental delay requiring rehabilitation services.

Her two-year-old sibling was treated prophylactically for meningitis exposure and remained well, although he was found to have delayed immunization and iron-deficiency anemia.

It is well established that poor children are more likely to be hospitalized and stay in the hospital longer than middle-class children.[20] They are also more likely than other children to suffer adverse consequences from illness and to die. Garth Alperstein and colleagues reported in 1988 that the rate of admission to the hospital for homeless children was one and a half times that of a comparison group (11.6 per 1,000 vs. 7.5 per 1,000).[18] Karen Haught's review of the records of 101 homeless children showed that 3 were hospitalized in a six-month period. One child required six hospitalizations for asthma. In a socioeconomic comparable group of domiciled children, 1 of 72 was hospitalized once during the same period of time.[19]

Treatment of chronic illness among homeless children presents a great challenge. James Wright has shown that of nineteen hundred homeless children considered, 16 percent suffered from chronic illness.[21-23]

In an unpublished survey by the New York City Department of Health, 17 percent of nineteen hundred children living in welfare hotels were found to have chronic medical problems.[24]

To ensure best outcomes, chronically ill children should receive comprehensive, coordinated care from a stable multidisciplinary team that can also give psychosocial support. Children with unstable domiciles often fail to receive such care.

JR is a two-year-old boy with history of recurrent otitis media, speech delay, and asthma. He has been living at various shelters and SRO hotels since birth with his twenty-eight-year-old mother and two siblings, ages seven and five years. JR had been receiving care from four different ERs irregularly, usually for acute symptoms. His mother was aware that he needed evaluation of his pulmonary status and hearing, with possible surgical treatment for recurrent ear infections and rehabilitative services for his speech delay. However, she was never domiciled long enough at any one site for her son to be connected to one health care provider for recommended follow-up and treatment at the various subspecialty clinics. Because of his multiple episodes of illness, mostly otitis media and upper respiratory infection or asthma, JR has delayed immunizations. He was also receiving subtherapeutic doses of medication for his asthma because different physicians were prescribing different regimens. His mother was unable to keep track of each drug and when and how much of each she should give. Only after he was placed, with his family, in a transitional housing unit was he able to receive all his care at one institution. With the aid of nursing and social services support, his mother was then able to bring JR for the necessary evaluations and therapy, comply with his medications, and keep him symptom-free. JR subsequently was enrolled in day care. His siblings were also able to attend school regularly. Mother is no longer so preoccupied with caring for JR that she cannot devote some attention to the two older children.

Informational Barriers

Most homeless families are headed by single women with minimal employment skills. Many are poorly educated. They may not be aware of preventive health services available or how to apply for entitlements.[17] Some are essentially illiterate and cannot follow medical regimens without supervision.

CW is a fifteen-year-old with a three-month-old infant. She has been homeless since she left her mother's house after an argument shortly after the baby's birth.

She was placed in a shelter for teenagers with children after spending two weeks on the streets. On initial admission examination at the shelter the infant, JW, was noted to have thrush and monilial diaper rash. He also failed to gain weight. Mother was instructed to give medications every eight hours and to feed JW at least three ounces every three hours with ready-to-feed formula.

She was also instructed to keep a record of his feeding and medication times. When seen for follow-up three days later, JW showed no improvement. On further investigation, it was found that CW was too embarrassed to acknowledge that she could not tell time or count. She was actually feeding JW every five rather than every three hours. She was giving his oral medications only once a day, when she remembered.

Only after several weeks of intensive supervision and teaching did she manage to learn basic infant care.

Continuity of Care

Giving continuity of care is a major concern of those serving homeless families, both while the family is homeless and after the family is domiciled.

It is well documented that lack of one consistent care giver fosters patient noncompliance with medical regimens and adequate follow-up.[25,26]

Difficulty in obtaining records and poor communication between various institutions result in the loss of accurate medical information. Absence of vital documents often causes failure to obtain needed nutritional, day care, and other social services, such as Supplemental Security Income (SSI), Medicaid, and counseling. This can lead to poor or delayed treatment and to the duplication of diagnostic procedures.

HL is an eighteen-month-old boy who was seen with his eighteen-year-old pregnant mother, GR, at a shelter-based clinic for initial evaluation. They were admitted to the shelter the night before, after police found them wandering in a subway station. HL was examined and received immunizations and anemia and lead poisoning screenings. His mother received her first prenatal visit. She was noted to have a history of drug use and was five months pregnant. Routine prenatal Pap smears, vaginal cultures for sexually transmitted infection, and screening blood tests were completed.

Both patients missed their follow-up appointments the following week. Further investigation showed that the mother left the shelter with the child two days after the clinic visit after being caught using drugs at the shelter. Multiple inquiries were made to locate them, utilizing all available resources, because both had abnormal test results. HL was found to have lead exposure. His mother had an abnormal Pap smear, had a positive culture for gonorrhea infection, and was a hepatitis carrier. All attempts failed.

Three months later the clinic received an inquiry from the neonatal intensive care unit of a major metropolitan hospital. GR had delivered a thirty-three week-premature infant in the ER. She had given the shelter as her address and primary care provider. Essential medical information, including the abnormal test results, was given verbally to the hospital with the agreement that the complete records would be sent upon receiving the mother's consent letter for release of information.

JW is a five-month-old infant who was supposed to be receiving infant formula from the women-infant-children (WIC) program since birth. However, his mother had four WIC forms filled out at three different institutions and lost them each time prior to the interview date because of theft or multiple shelter moves. Each time JW had to have an examination before another WIC form could be done. JW eventually received WIC after a concerned shelter social worker kept all the documents until the interview date arrived.

MW is the four-year-old sibling of JW. She had three health exams, three blood tests for anemia and lead, three vision screens, three hearing tests, and two extra doses of immunization during a six-month period at three different institutions because her mother had twice lost her immunization card and day-care center forms. She was eventually enrolled in a day-care center after an eight-month delay.

When a homeless family is domiciled at a permanent site, it is vital that the pertinent health history while the family was homeless be transferred to an appropriate neighborhood health provider where the family will receive care. Equally important is an introduction for the family to local services, including school, church, day-care center, counseling, and social agencies, to minimize the delay in receiving needed help.

Patient Confidentiality vs. Public Health

It is the right of all individuals to maintain the confidentiality of their social and medical records. Maintaining privacy is particularly difficult when someone lives in an open shelter, especially if medical problems require treatment. Health care staff may need to notify shelter workers so that patients can obtain needed attention (e.g., appropriate food, bed rest, and separate rooms for infectious disease isolation purposes).

The shelter staff also needs to be notified about exposure to infectious diseases, such as tuberculosis, meningitis, lice, scabies, hepatitis, measles, and chicken pox, so that appropriate public health measures can be taken. This may lead to ostracism, discrimination, and resentment by fellow shelter families. It may also lead to eviction of the family by the shelter. As a result, many homeless families are reluctant to seek medical attention. This may lead to delayed diagnoses, inappropriate treatment, and inadequate prophylaxis of contacts.

EL is a thirteen-year-old Hispanic boy diagnosed in the emergency room as having active hepatitis B after being ill for two weeks. In the course of the investigation of his possible exposure to at-risk individuals, EL was found to be living at a welfare hotel with his sixty-five-year-old grandmother. He had been working as a male prostitute in and out of the hotel under the direction of another hotel resident, a twenty-eight-year-old woman who seduced him and induced him to work as a prostitute by offering crack in exchange. When the hotel management got wind of the investigation, despite assurances that the staff and other residents were not at risk for hepatitis B from EL, he and his grandmother were evicted.

Social workers at shelters may be questioned by health providers when children are seen for possible neglect or abuse. Even though it is recognized that the right of the child to be protected supersedes parental rights to confidentiality, the sense of humiliation, the burden of shame, and the feeling of persecution that families experience during the investigation have to be recognized.

Mental and Physical Health Status

Homeless families have health problems similar to those of poor families. However, homeless children experience some illnesses more frequently and more severely than poor children with homes. Their health problems are exacerbated by difficult living environments. For some, their health is compromised even before birth. In a study by Wendy Chavkin and others in 1987, homeless women living in New York City welfare hotels were compared with women living in low-income housing projects. Pregnant homeless women were less likely to receive prenatal care. They were more likely to have babies of low birth weight (18 vs. 8.5 percent) and have higher infant mortality rates.[27]

Mental Health

The adults and children in urban homeless families live in an unpredictable and insecure world of SRO hotels, shelters, abandoned buildings, and the streets. Parents feel that they can exercise little control over essential elements of their own life settings and those of their children. This leads to feelings of alienation, disorientation, fear, apathy, depression, poor impulse control, and autistic withdrawal. Parenting is most likely to be upset as a consequence of the blow to the adult's self-respect and loss of control. There is increased risk of child abuse or neglect. A powerful message is also conveyed to these children: We live in a world so unstable and insecure that there is no guarantee of a safe future. Long-term goals cannot be envisioned and valued. There is no motivation to master the demands of immediate impulse gratification. Substance abuse (25 to 30 percent in parents) is frequently used as an escape. Antisocial rebellion and risk-taking behavior become the life-style of choice.

Young children are affected by the psychosocial upheavals and insecurity of the family because the parents can no longer function effectively, by giving information about the world, setting consistent limits, assisting in developing problem-solving skills, and offering a safe and positive environment in which their children may develop self-esteem. Day care or schools, which can act as secondary support systems, may also be interrupted because of the unstable domicile. Thus it is not surprising to find that in a study of 395 homeless children by Garth Alperstein and colleagues, 9 percent exhibited behavioral or emotional problems, contrasted with 4 percent in the comparison group.[28] Of 61 families living in an SRO hotel, 66 percent of the mothers reported behavioral and emotional problems in their children that developed while in the hotel. The problems were acting out, fighting, restlessness, moodiness, and feelings of frustration.[29] Emergency room records reveal 8.8 reports of child abuse and neglect per 1,000 homeless children, compared with 2.3 reports per 1,000 domiciled children of similar socioeconomic status living in the same health care districts.[18]

Bassuk showed that in Boston about half of 151 homeless children were found to have developmental lags, anxiety, depression, and learning difficulties.[10] Another significant stress is separation of the family. Karen Benker reported that only 22 percent of women with children interviewed in New York City emergency assistance units were accompanied by all their children.[30] Other children were with friends or family members or in the foster care system.

Physical Health Problems

A clearer picture regarding the health status of children who are homeless is emerging. The HCHP projects in nineteen major cities offer a nationwide overview. Various other agencies that serve homeless families, such as the New York City Health Department, the Children's Aid Society, the New York Hospital Children's Health Project, the St. Vincent's Hospital SRO/Homeless Program, and the Pennsylvania Homeless Family Initiatives, have given additional specific regional information and models. There is wide variation among the projects in approach, configuration, and specific program goals. Although the methodology of data collection and analysis differ too widely for detailed exact comparison between these programs, several conclusions can be drawn:

- Common acute disorders constitute the largest portion of health problems seen in homeless children, often exacerbated by environmental factors and delay in seeking treatment.[17,22,31,32] Minor upper respiratory infection is most common (41 percent), followed by minor skin infections (20 percent), ear infections (18 percent), gastrointestinal complaints (15 percent), trauma (10 percent), and eye problems (8 percent).[22] There is little difference between sexes. When compared with the illnesses of the NAMCS housed children, certain diseases have a significant increase in occurrence rates among the homeless.[33] In NAMCS children, 0.2 percent are found to have lice infestations, compared with 7 percent of homeless children with scabies or lice. Upper respiratory infections are twice, gastrointestinal disorders four times, and ear infections twice as common in homeless children.
- Immunization delays occur in 25 to 52 percent of the children.[17,18,31,32]
- Chronic illnesses, especially anemia, asthma, and recurrent otitis media are often untreated or undertreated.
- Unrecognized disorders, congenital and acquired—congenital heart disease,

hernia, genitourinary tract problems, mental retardation, seizures disorders, and short stature—were found in several studies.[31,32,34,35]

- Nutritional status showed very little difference in comparisons of abnormalities of weight (8.7 vs. 6.4 percent) or height (7.7 vs. 7.5 percent) and rates of anemia (14.7 vs. 14 percent) between homeless children and low-income domiciled children.[18] However, these are only gross measures and do not reflect a trend over time. A prospective study looking at growth parameters might well reveal the development of nutritional deficiencies and growth retardation for children in prolonged states of homelessness. When compared with middle-class children, low-income and homeless children are approximately five times as likely to have iron-deficiency anemia (3, 14, and 14.7 percent respectively).[36]

New York Children's Health Project (NYCHP)

The NYCHP started in November 1987 to give pediatric services at specified family shelters and SRO hotels where substantial numbers of homeless children were housed by New York City. The program is an outreach project of the Department of Pediatrics at the New York Hospital-Cornell Medical Center. Pediatricians lead the provider teams, which include nurse practitioners, nurses, registrars, and drivers. Comprehensive primary pediatric care is offered by the health care teams on fully equipped two-examining-room mobile medical units (MMUs) which visit selected sites on a scheduled basis. Complete medical records as well as extensive demographic data are kept on all children. A major outreach and transportation program helps ensure follow-up of continued primary care needs as well as compliance with specialty and referrals.

In addition, the NYCHP provides mental health services, both diagnostic and therapeutic, a substance abuse prevention program, and special services for adolescents.

FINDINGS

From January through December 1988, 3,084 children (ranging in age from one week to twenty-one years) received health services in 6,420 total encounters with project staff. Thirty-three percent of encounters were for "well child" or preventive care. The remainder were illness-related visits.

The NYCHP outreach team coordinated 319 referrals of children seen in the program. Challenges experienced by the outreach staff were substantial in the areas of transportation, communication, and follow-up. Table 8.2 shows the distribution of referrals by service during 1988. Aggressive outreach, use of car services, and active communication with the subspecialty services yielded an overall compliance rate of 63 percent of all referrals kept, canceled, or rescheduled.

Children of homeless families in New York experience definite problems regarding access to primary health care services. This absence of preventive and regular medical care is reflected in a high incidence of incomplete immunizations

Table 8.2 NEW YORK CHILDREN'S HEALTH
PROJECT MEDICAL SUBSPECIALTY
REFERRALS
(*January–December 1988*)

SPECIALTY AREAS	NUMBER OF REFERRALS	PERCENT OF REFERRALS
Emergency room	55	17.2
Ophthalmology	48	15.0
Speech and hearing	33	10.3
Pediatric surgery	33	10.3
Dermatology	22	6.9
ENT	17	5.3
Cardiology	13	4.0
Adolescent/gynecology	12	3.8
Child development/behavior	12	3.8
Neurology	11	3.4
Evaluation	11	3.4
Urology	10	3.1
Psychology	9	2.8
Allergy	8	2.5
Endocrine	6	1.9
Orthopedics	4	1.3
Hematology	3	0.9
Miscellaneous	12	3.8
Total referrals	319	

among patients new to the project. Only 52 percent of children were confirmed as up-to-date in their expected immunizations for age. In addition, many were seen with undertreated chronic and acute illness secondary to poor access to traditional providers.

Medical diagnoses among homeless children seen by the NYCHP rarely include exotic illness. Rather, there is increased incidence of health problems usually seen in domiciled indigent children. Table 8.3 shows the breakdown of health problems noted among NYCHP patients in 1988.

Newark Homeless Health Care Project

The Newark Homeless Health Care Project began in July 1985 with funding from the Robert Wood Johnson Foundation specifically to provide health services for the homeless. The program initially gave health care and social services at seven shelters and two soup kitchens. Services were expanded in 1988 to include two SROs and three family shelter sites.

The teams include a physician, nurse, social worker, psychiatric case worker, substance abuse counselor, and psychologist. Mental health counselors offer individual, family, and group counseling on-site on a rotating basis. The goal of the project is to provide high-quality health care and address the immediate social

Table 8.3 NEW YORK CHILDREN'S HEALTH PROJECT
MEDICAL PROBLEMS—1988

Total illness diagnoses   4,942
Total illness encounters   3,871

DIAGNOSIS	NUMBER OF DIAGNOSES	PERCENT OF TOTAL ENCOUNTERS
Upper respiratory illness	1,059	27.4
Dermatologic conditions	999	25.8
Otitis media	876	22.6
Gastroenteritis	289	7.5
Iron-deficiency anemia	209	5.4
Pharyngitis	178	4.6
Asthma	153	4.0
Conjunctivitis	147	3.8
Bronchitis/bronchiolitis	125	3.2
Thrush	103	2.7
Cerumen impaction	84	2.2
Allergy	70	1.8
Trauma	69	1.8
Strabismus/other ophth.	65	1.7
Caries	60	1.5
Inguinal hernia	45	1.1
Pneumonia	36	0.9
Speech delay	28	0.7
Failure to thrive	25	0.6
Other	322	8.3
Total diagnoses	4,942	

Note • Percentages do not reflect a total of 100 percent because
patients are not limited to a single diagnosis.

needs of the family. In addition, it works to create a network of public and private partnerships to advocate for the homeless.

The majority of the families seen consist of a single head of household, most female, between twenty-four and forty-nine years of age, with an average family size of 2.5 children. Ethnic distribution is 58 percent black, 26 percent white, 13 percent Hispanic, and 3 percent other.

The most common social problems encountered are substance abuse in the parent and child abuse or neglect.

The most common children's physical health problems are anemia (11 percent) and pulmonary disorders (4 percent). In addition, 3 percent of the children were judged to be at risk for HIV exposure because of parental life-styles.

St. Vincent's Hospital (New York) SRO / Homeless Program

In October 1984 the Department of Community Medicine at St. Vincent's Hospital expanded its health services for the homeless to include 160 families (approximately 500 individuals) housed in two SRO hotels in New York City. The program has five major components:

- Outreach team: A team of social worker, nurse, and physician pays regular weekly visits as well as emergency visits to families in the two hotels. The team serves as an information and referral resource. Initial health assessments are made, and treatment is initiated for new families if possible. Informal health education is given.
- Satellite clinic: All the families seen are referred to an established St. Vincent's satellite clinic five minutes' walking distance away for follow-up and regular health care. At least one member of the outreach team is at the clinic when the family is seen, to ensure continuity of care. Every attempt is made to complete all the necessary immunizations, treatment, and age-appropriate preventative screening such as hematocrit, lead, free erythroprotoporphyrin, urine analysis, vision and dental assessment concurrently. Medical regimens are made as simple as possible. Medications are given if the family has no means to fill prescriptions. Every attempt is made to educate the family with regard to their health problems and to how they can help themselves stay well or get well.
- Subspecialty referrals: If subspecialty care is needed, patients are referred to the main site of St. Vincent's Hospital by appointment. The outreach team reminds them of the appointments. Escort and transportation assistance is provided if needed. Missed appointments are rescheduled. The outreach team visits the family to determine why appointments were not kept and whether the family needs assistance to keep future appointments.
- Hospitalization and discharge planning: If patients are hospitalized, involved staff members visit them and serve as advocates, assisting in discharge planning and follow-up.
- Advocacy, networking, and aftercare: The staff maintains close contact with crisis intervention workers, hotel management, local schools, day-care centers, churches, and community counseling agencies that could provide services for these families. Often they function as coordinators and advocates for the families to obtain essential support.

The administrative staff also acts as advocates for the homeless at local, state, and national levels in hopes of influencing policy makers to correct underlying socioeconomic conditions. After the families are domiciled, the staff serves as their informal support during the transitional period while they connect with their new communities.

METHODOLOGY

A total of 173 charts of children seen consecutively at the satellite clinic from June to October 1988 were reviewed. Of these children, 101 were from the two SRO hotels and 72 from the poor working-class families around the neighborhood. The majority of the latter were on Medicaid and lived in high-rise housing projects or run-down apartment buildings close by. Biographical data for each child were counted once. Diagnoses for each clinic or ER visit were tallied for the whole of

1988. The purpose of the review was to learn if there were any significant difference in the health status of homeless children vs. low-income children who are domiciled.

The age structures of the two groups differed (Table 8.4). In the homeless group, 44.5 percent of the children were between ages one and three years vs. 30.5 percent of the domiciled children. The homeless children were predominantly black (63 percent), and the nonhomeless children predominantly Hispanic (65 percent) (Table 8.5). The sex distribution of the homeless children was 55.4 percent male and 44.6 percent female. In the housed children 47 percent were male and 53 percent female.

Table 8.4

	HOMELESS		NONHOMELESS	
AGES	NUMBER	PERCENT OF TOTAL	NUMBER	PERCENT OF TOTAL
0–2 mo newborn	3	3	5	6.9
2–12 mo. infant	8	7.9	3	4.2
1–3 yr. toddler	45	44.5	14	19.4
3–5 yr. preschool	17	16.8	11	15.3
5–11 yr. school age	17	16.8	23	31.9
11–18 yr. teenage	12	11.8	16	22.2
Totals	101		72	

Table 8.5

ETHNIC GROUP	HOMELESS		NONHOMELESS	
	NUMBER	PERCENT OF TOTAL	NUMBER	PERCENT OF TOTAL
Hispanic	30	29.7	47	65
Black	63	62.3	17	23.6
White	6	5.9	7	9.7
Other	1 (Arab)		1 (Asian Indian)	
Totals	100		72	

FAMILY CHARACTERISTICS

In regard to family characteristics (Table 8.6), it is noted that 8.3 percent of the housed children were in the custody of someone other than their natural parents. In homeless families it is notable that 9.9 percent of the families had children not in their own custody at the time of our review. Indices of substance abuse and parent in jail were comparable. Substance abuse was probably underreported because of the hesitancy of parents to divulge such history. Of the homeless children's families seen, 4 percent were involved with Special Services for Chil-

Table 8.6 FAMILY CHARACTERISTICS

	HOMELESS		NONHOMELESS	
	NUMBER	PERCENT OF TOTAL = 10	NUMBER	PERCENT OF TOTAL = 72
Not being reared by natural parent	1	.9	6	8.3
Parent has other children not in her custody	10[1]	9.9	0	0
History of substance abuse in parent	9[2]	8.9	8[3]	11.1
History of substance abuse in parent who is in the home	4	3.9	4	5.5
Parent in jail	6	5.9	3	4.1
Known SSC report during 1988 for parent	3	3	1[4]	1.4
History of being involved with SSC	1	1	2	2.8

1. Of these ten, four involved leaving children in other countries of origin.

2. Of these nine, eight involved drug use and one involved alcohol.

3. Of these eight, six involved alcohol use and two involved drug use.

4. This report was later found to be unsubstantiated by SSC.

dren (SSC), and 5.2 percent of the housed children's families were so involved, currently or previously.

IMMUNIZATION STATUS

The immunization status of the groups is considered in Tables 8.7 and 8.8. An immunization delay is defined as the missing of one or more immunizations by two months. In the homeless children initially 23.7 percent of the children were delayed, and 41.7 percent of these (or 9.9 percent of the total number of children) were caught up by the end of the year. In the nonhomeless a total of 12.5 percent

Table 8.7 IMMUNIZATION STATUS IN TOTAL
POPULATION

	HOMELESS		NONHOMELESS	
	NUMBER	PERCENT OF TOTAL	NUMBER	PERCENT OF TOTAL
Up-to-date for age	71	70.3	59	81.9
Delayed	14	13.8	8	11.1
No records available	6	5.9	4	5.5
Initial delay—caught up	10	9.9	1	1.4
Total	101		72	

Table 8.8 IMMUNIZATION STATUS IN POPULATION
UNDER AGE FIVE

	HOMELESS		NONHOMELESS	
	NUMBER	PERCENT OF TOTAL	NUMBER	PERCENT OF TOTAL
Up-to-date	49	67.1	26	78.7
Delayed	12	16.4	6	18.2
No records available	2	2.7	0	0
Initial delay—caught up	10	13.6	1	3
Total	73		33	

Table 8.9 ANEMIA

	HOMELESS		NONHOMELESS	
	NUMBER	PERCENT OF TOTAL TESTED	NUMBER	PERCENT OF TOTAL TESTED
HCT under 34	14	19.9	10	17.5
HCT 34 or greater	56	80	47	82.4
Total	70		57	

of the children were delayed, and 11 percent of these (or 1.4 percent of the total number of children) were caught up at the end of the year. It was probably more pertinent to consider the immunization status of children under five years of age because school-age children are required by law to have completed their immunizations. In the seventy-three homeless children under the age of five, 30 percent were delayed, and 45.4 percent of these (or 13.6 percent of the seventy-three children) were caught up by year-end. In the thirty-three nonhomeless children under the age of five, 21.2 percent were delayed, and one of these (14 percent [or three of the thirty-three children]) was caught up by the end of 1988.

ANEMIA

Anemia was defined as hematocrit under 34 percent. Of the 101 homeless children, 70 had hematocrit (HCT) results available. Of the 70 children tested, 14 (19.9 percent) were anemic. This is similar to results in the domiciled children, in whom 57 of 72 had hematocrit results available. Ten (17.5 percent) were anemic. (See Table 8.9.)

NUTRITIONAL STATUS

When growth parameters, weight and height, were reviewed, 5 of the 101 homeless children were under the fifth percentile weight for age and 5 were significantly overweight. No domiciled children were under the fifth percentile in weight, and 5 were overweight. (See Table 8.10.)

Table 8.10 GROWTH

	HOMELESS		NONHOMELESS	
	NUMBER	PERCENT OF TOTAL N = 101	NUMBER	PERCENT OF TOTAL N = 72
Weight less than 5th %	5	4.9	0	0
Overweight	5	4.9	5	6.9
Total	10		5	

SPEECH DELAY AND LEARNING DISABILITY

As speech delay is usually a diagnosis of preschool children and learning disability a diagnosis of school-age children, the percentages of each diagnosis were based on children under and equal to or over five years of age respectively. Homeless children were approximately twice as likely as housed children to have speech delay and learning disability. (See Table 8.11.)

Table 8.11

	HOMELESS		NONHOMELESS	
	NUMBER	PERCENT OF TOTAL	NUMBER	PERCENT OF TOTAL
Speech delay*	8	7.9	2	2.8
Learning disability†	3	2.9	2	2.7

*Percent of total homeless (73) 5 years or younger = 10.9; percent of total nonhomeless (35) 5 years or younger = 6.0.

† Percent of total homeless (28) 5 years or older = 10.7; percent of total nonhomeless (39) 5 years or older = 5.1.

The diagnoses for each visit to the clinic or the ER during 1988 were reviewed to determine the presenting health problems. Some patients (particularly children from the hotel) were partially underrepresented because they had not lived in the area or attended the clinics during the full year. The diagnoses from only the index period June to October 1988 were also tallied, to control this bias. The diagnoses are represented as episodes rather than persons (i.e., if one child had three different episodes of otitis during the observation period, it was counted as three rather than one). The diagnoses in Tables 8.12 and 8.13 are those that occurred with significant frequency.

EMERGENCY ROOM

Emergency room utilization patterns were derived by counting the number of ER visits during 1988 and from June through October. There was relatively more utilization of the ER by the homeless. (See Table 8.14.)

All children need a safe, permanent dwelling and a supportive and nurturing environment to grow and develop. They also need excellent comprehensive child health care and appropriate educational opportunities. Homelessness is chaos for

Table 8.12 DIAGNOSES DURING 1988

	HOMELESS (TOTAL 101)		NONHOMELESS (TOTAL 72)	
	NUMBER	AVERAGE NUMBER OF EPISODES PER CHILD	NUMBER	AVERAGE NUMBER OF EPISODES PER CHILD
Otitis, sinusitis	74	0.74	40	0.55
Asthma	45	0.44	11	0.15
Gastroenteritis	19	0.18	6	0.08
Trauma (includes lacerations, fractures, soft tissue injuries, burns)	18	0.18	6	0.08
Skin infections (excluding monilial diaper rash)	18	0.18	4	0.05
Pneumonia, bronchiolitis	6	0.06	4	0.05

Table 8.13 DIAGNOSES FOR JUNE TO OCTOBER 1988

	HOMELESS		NONHOMELESS	
	NUMBER	AVERAGE NUMBER OF EPISODES PER CHILD	NUMBER	AVERAGE NUMBER OF EPISODES PER CHILD
Otitis, sinusitis	29	0.287	9	0.125
Asthma	17	0.16	1	0.013
Gastroenteritis	9	0.089	6	0.08
Trauma	10	0.099	2	0.027
Skin Infections	13	0.128	2	0.027
Pneumonia, bronchiolitis	4	0.04	0	0

Table 8.14 VISITS TO EMERGENCY ROOM

	HOMELESS		NONHOMELESS	
	NUMBER	AVERAGE NUMBER PER CHILD	NUMBER	AVERAGE NUMBER PER CHILD
1988	66	0.65	37	0.51
June to October 1988	36	0.35	13	0.18

children, an event of extraordinary stress, increased vulnerability, and unmet needs.

We all recognize the severe negative impact that life in temporary shelters can have on the well-being of a child. Programs that prevent a family from becoming homeless are crucial. If homelessness occurs, however, attempts must be made to minimize the homeless time period. Much can also be done to improve the various temporary living conditions. Families housed in smaller shelters with privacy and supportive services such as hot meals, health services, counseling, and day care fare better than those in large congregate shelters. Their health status can be improved by such preventive measures as immunizations and teaching parenting skills. National guidelines for basic nutrition, health, and safety standards for temporary residences housing families should be developed and enforced.[37] Public, private, and joint efforts with a wide variety of program designs are needed to solve the more complex problems of high rates of child abuse and neglect, substance abuse, low birth weight, infant mortality, and excess hospital admissions.

JENNIFER BURROUGHS
PENTHEA BOUMA
EILEEN O'CONNOR
DONEBY SMITH

9

Health Concerns of Homeless Women

Introduction

Over the past decade increasing numbers of women have joined the ranks of the homeless on our streets and in shelters. These women are at risk for numerous health problems. Acute illness, trauma, and exacerbation of chronic illness are often the only reasons a homeless woman makes contact with a health care provider. Because of the crisis nature of the social situation of homeless women, important health interventions such as screening, education, and family planning are often neglected. This discussion addresses the needs of homeless women and reflects the experience of four primary care providers in Boston, the Bronx in New York City, Washington, D.C., and Philadelphia.

The persistent stereotype of the bag lady does not reflect the diversity of this population.[1,2] Though there are often other issues that contribute, the lives of homeless women share the common threads of poverty and loss. Many are alienated from their families, have few or no friends, and lack long-term partners. Some seek shelter with their adult children. It has been suggested that homeless women are more invisible than men,[3] perhaps because they hide themselves; the shame of being a woman without a home or family in our society is devastating. One study has shown that women more frequently become homeless after eviction or domestic violence, while men cite unemployment, alcohol/drug abuse, or release from jail as causes of their homelessness.[4] Other factors which complicate the lives of these women include alcohol and substance abuse, violence, and chronic mental illness. Each of these factors may cause or be exacerbated by a period of homelessness.

While there are certainly women who have severed emotional and financial ties with their offspring and who navigate through the world as single entities, some of the "single" women seen in shelters, in soup kitchens, and on the street have children living with relatives or in foster care whom they visit and plan to reunite with. Of the four cities discussed here, this seems to be most frequently the case in the Bronx. When mothers seek emergency shelter alone, they are considered single regardless of their possible contact with children and their own self-images as part of a family network. Although they are usually required by courts to have adequate housing in order to regain custody, the programs for housing search that assist homeless families do not include them. Other women have lost custody of children. A discussion of the health concerns of women must take into account the powerful ties that may still exist with family and children.

Prevention and screening, sexuality and family planning, sexually transmitted diseases, violence, and mental illness all will be discussed. Only brief mention will be made of such important topics as HIV, alcohol and drug abuse, and the problems of elderly women because they are covered elsewhere.

Women constitute approximately 25 percent of homeless individuals seen by the projects nationally, though the numbers vary from city to city.[5] In Philadelphia, where the nurses see clients in day programs and shelters, women constituted 28 percent of clients in a one-year period. Similarly, over eight months in 1988 and 1989, the nurse practitioners, physicians, and social workers in the Boston project saw more than twenty-five hundred individuals, 24 percent of whom were women. This figure does not include women with dependent children.

Prevention and Screening

Preventive health care among homeless women requires careful consideration of two flawed assumptions. The first assumption is that because homelessness is a crisis, routine screening and prevention are inappropriate in the health care of these women. Despite frequent crises, routine health problems and chronic illness do not bypass homeless clients. The second assumption is that routine prevention and screening should be the same for homeless women and nonhomeless women. Effective prevention and screening require sensitivity to the woman's situation and consideration of the impact of homelessness on certain health problems.

Special assessments and interventions are required for good screening and prevention among homeless women. A homeless woman's life may be relatively stable if she has been homeless for a long period, is receiving appropriate benefits, and is aware of community resources for food and shelter. She therefore may be in a position to participate in screening and preventive care. However, many homeless women have pressing needs, and health care providers and social workers are in a position to assist with knowledge of entitlements, housing options, and community meal and day programs.

Despite assistance, there are many barriers for homeless women seeking care, and these have been enumerated before.[6] Lack of medical insurance, overcrowded public clinics, the attitude of providers, hospital bureaucracy, substance abuse, and mental illness may be insurmountable obstacles for this population. In Philadelphia a woman with a long history of IV drug use saw the nurse in a soup kitchen about a leg ulcer. She knew that she should seek treatment because it was infected, but she explained that she could not face how the emergency room staff would treat her, a drug addict without health insurance. She let the ulcer fester for a week before she detoxed herself and sought medical care. If she hesitates to seek care with an acute and painful infection, it is unlikely that she will seek care for an annual pelvic screening exam.

Providers can help homeless women overcome these obstacles in a number of ways. Prevention and screening have been done in all of our cities on-site at day programs, at meal programs, and in shelters. While there is often a lack of adequate space and privacy, providers are able to gain the trust of women who have long been alienated from the health care system. Enlisting the help of various staffs at our sites to make announcements about scheduled visits and encouraging staff members to refer clients they are concerned about have allowed us to reach many new clients. Encouraging women to bring friends is also a strategy that has worked at many sites to engage clients who may not use shelters otherwise. When providers spend outreach time in the sites, homeless women have a liaison in the health care system they know and trust. Sometimes one good experience with the health system enables a woman to pursue a second. Knowing that she can receive sensitive care may help her gain the skills for access to the health care system in the future. In Boston the primary care program at Boston City Hospital allows two medical residents each year to spend one night a week at the nurses' clinic at the Pine Street Inn Shelter. This has led to some long-lasting primary care relationships.

Health providers can also use acute care visits to do routine exams, health teaching, and lab work. Emergency room staff can help with preventive care by referring clients for follow-up at primary care sites and provide information about their visits and referrals in writing. While this may sound futile, many homeless women are remarkably organized with their papers (a few women in Boston use their infamous bags for elaborate filing systems). Hospital admission is also an important opportunity for screening and prevention. Despite outreach efforts, there are many women whom our projects have been unable to reach. It is often the sickest and the most desperate who cannot initiate contact on their own.

Individual women should be encouraged to seek primary care when they have attained a degree of stability. A woman who is newly sober or is participating in drug rehabilitation is often in a hopeful frame of mind, and taking care of herself is a new priority. Information about prevention and health care should be made available in day programs, soup kitchens, and shelters.

Prevention and screening for homeless women should include a complete baseline history and physical examination as well as all the recommended annual exams and tests for women. Special attention should be paid to tuberculosis, substance abuse, mental illness, STDs, physical abuse, and HIV transmission and infection. Finally, a note should be made about hygiene. While a number of authors have pointed out that poor hygiene can be an important defense for homeless women,[1] urinary incontinence in a number of middle-aged and elderly homeless women in Boston has been a source of embarrassment and discomfort. The lack of access to bathrooms during the day, and dangerous or filthy bathrooms in the shelters, only make this problem worse. The nurses' clinic at the Pine Street Inn has managed to provide bladder retraining in a few cases and now stocks the pads designed for this problem. New onset incontinence in a mentally ill woman can also be an important sign of decompensation or depression. Though it is often a difficult problem to solve, medical evaluation and treatment when appropriate can improve a woman's sense of self-esteem and quality of life.

Sexuality

Contraception, pregnancy, sexually transmitted diseases, sexuality—these all are delicate topics in any environment. Discussing these intimate issues with homeless women who often have good reason to be suspicious and alienated is particularly difficult. At a seventy-five-bed single women's shelter in Washington, D.C., homeless women rarely mention these topics unless they are experiencing acute symptoms. The experience is similar in the nurses' clinic on the women's side at the Pine Street Inn in Boston. Lack of privacy during interviews must account for some of this reticence, but it may be that the problems of finding clothing, shelter, and food present more pressing concerns. Most shelters do not permit sexual activities or allow the privacy people may seek, but it is certainly absurd to conclude that homeless women do not have sexual relations. Many women have partners who are also homeless and have access to private shelters during the day or occasionally sleep out in order to spend intimate time with their partners. Prostitution is often the only way for a woman in poverty to support a drug habit, but that is difficult information for a client to reveal to providers. Sensitivity toward sexual orientation is important for providers in this population, in which self-esteem is low and women may be quickly alienated.

Few homeless women seek contraception. It is thus important for providers to broach this subject. A complaint that requires a pelvic exam is the ideal opportunity. All the birth control methods hold particular drawbacks for homeless women. Oral contraceptives, diaphragms, sponges, condoms, tubes of jelly, and canisters of foam are a bulky lot subject to theft or loss. The difficulties posed by daily medication for homeless persons has been described elsewhere: lack of routine, loss, memory possibly clouded by alcohol, drugs, and mental illness, and theft.[6,7] The drawbacks of barrier methods for all women (the mess, the inconvenience) are exacerbated by homelessness. Male partners are frequently unwilling to use condoms. However, providers who do outreach or provide care on-site can carry appropriate supplies to offer, unless sites run by religious institutions object.

Although the intrauterine device (IUD) would seem a relatively good option, the medical requirements are rarely met by a sexually active homeless woman: a woman in a monogamous relationship with no history of pelvic inflammatory disease (PID) or STDs, preferably one who has completed most of her childbearing, and one who will seek regular follow-up. In addition, the woman must be attuned to signs of complications and have access to health care because pelvic infections in the presence of an IUD can become fulminant. One woman who was seen in Boston for mid-cycle vaginal bleeding had had an IUD placed sixteen years before and had not had it checked in the ten years she had been using drugs and drinking heavily. The instability inherent in homelessness makes the IUD a poor choice for most women.

Even with the limitations mentioned above, oral contraceptives are the most popular method. Pills are easy, compact, and effective. However, the problem of birth control for homeless women who are mentally ill may be an exception. A young schizophrenic woman who had recently arrived from Europe with plans to settle in Boston sought birth control from a provider in a shelter. Though a heavy smoker, she had taken oral contraceptives in Europe but had had one abortion "because the pills didn't work." She had taken her psychiatric medications regularly for the month the shelter staff had known her and had kept her appointments at the local mental health facility, but because of her smoking, her history of failure with the pill, and her possible transience, it seemed less risky to encourage her to continue to use condoms and foam with her boyfriend. Three weeks later she had left Boston.

It is interesting to note that some providers have found that a significant number of homeless women report they have had unprotected sex for years without pregnancy. Further questioning frequently reveals a history of PID, episodes of abdominal pain that could represent undiagnosed/untreated PID, or irregular menstruation and amenorrhea. While past infections and the poor nutrition associated with drug and alcohol dependence and homelessness may be factors, providers should evaluate these complaints and rule out the many possibilities that are treatable.

Pregnancy

Many shelters that serve homeless women do not allow children on-site, but unborn children are another matter. Although pregnant women are considered "a family" in some cities and thus eligible for placement in shelters designed to serve families, shelters for single adults serve many pregnant women. Among these women, prenatal care is often not a priority or viewed as inaccessible. Data from a New York City study showed that women living in hotels for the homeless reported "significantly less" prenatal care than did women living in low-income housing projects or all other women citywide.[8] Of the "hotel" women, 56.4 percent had three or fewer prenatal visits, compared with 22.5 percent of "project" women and 15 percent of women citywide. From our experiences, it is safe to say that women living on the street receive less prenatal care than women temporarily housed in hotels.

Pregnancy is high-risk if the woman is homeless. In the study cited above, both the "project" women and the "hotel" women had a higher rate of babies with low birth weight than women citywide. However, "hotel" women had babies whose birth weights were decreased twice as frequently as the "project" babies, regardless of adjustments for maternal variables. In addition, infant mortality rates were highest among the "hotel" women.

In the seventy-five-bed single women's shelter in Washington, D.C., pregnant women present most often to the health providers on-site because of vaginal bleeding, decreased fetal movement, pain or unusual discomfort, or the need to make arrangements for the upcoming delivery. Despite a public prenatal clinic within walking distance, few of the women receive regular care.

Meeting increased nutritional requirements can be difficult or impossible for a pregnant homeless woman. The challenge of obtaining a balanced diet for homeless people has been well described.[7,9] WIC supplements are clearly useless if the woman has no space, refrigeration, or access to kitchen facilities. Many shelters require residents to leave during the day, so pregnant women may have to spend the daytime walking the streets. In Boston a young pregnant woman left her estranged family in the South to stay with an elderly aunt, to find that the aunt's housing allowed guests for only two weeks. When she was approached by shelter staff, she had been in the shelters for two months, was in her seventh month of pregnancy, and had lost eight pounds because of the increased walking and change in diet. She had no knowledge of possible benefits or housing options. Providers need to be familiar with these resources to assist pregnant homeless women in their transition to "homeless family" status.

Drug and alcohol abuse puts the fetus at risk for withdrawal and fetal alcohol syndrome and usually interferes further with a woman's fulfillment of her nutritional needs. Few facilities are willing to detox pregnant women, and those that do frequently have waiting lists. Providers should take advantage of any contact a woman is willing to make to educate her about the effects of her addictions on her baby. Also, realistic discussion about her life after the birth of the baby may inspire a woman to seek treatment. Sometimes a new baby seems like the ticket to leaving streets and shelters. Fantasies of reuniting with the baby's father or finding an apartment just in time should be balanced with the reality of the intervention of social services if toxic screen tests are positive at delivery.

Mental illness presents several problems. A woman who requires antipsychotic medication may be unaware of possible teratogenic effects. Psychosis may interfere with the maintenance of a proper diet and ability to seek medical care and may mask physical symptoms. These are problematic for mentally ill women with intact support systems and are clearly much more so for homeless women.

Caring for homeless mentally ill women who are pregnant can prove tremendously frustrating for providers. In Washington, D.C., a pregnant schizophrenic patient planned a trip to Maine for her due date. Despite health provider and shelter staff protests, she somehow came up with the money for her ticket. Her trip was prevented only because her labor began as she boarded the bus. In Boston a schizophrenic woman who had lost custody of three children was clearly pregnant. She avoided most attempts at contact, and when she did talk with a shelter staff member, she stated that she felt no movement and thought the baby was dead. Because she refused to be examined, the providers on-site were unable to assist her. She delivered a healthy baby a few weeks early. The infant was immediately placed in the custody of the Department of Social Services.

Women who are HIV-positive, homeless, and pregnant clearly need priority treatment. Extensive counseling is required, and enlisting trusted shelter staff members or providers to accompany women to prenatal counseling and care may assure attendance. Such a seemingly bleak situation may actually serve to motivate the woman to change her situation. A twenty-nine-year-old woman well known as an IV drug user at Boston's Long Island Shelter had three children in foster care when she learned that she was pregnant again. Despite her positive HIV status, she chose to keep the pregnancy. The nurses at the shelter were able to arrange for the city's maternal-child public health nurses to meet weekly with her (sometimes on street corners). When she delivered a healthy baby boy, she was placed in a hotel for homeless families and was seen once a week by the health care team. She found an apartment with her public housing assistance three months later and continues to be drug-free. The baby has remained healthy so far, though his HIV status will not be determined for a few more months.

When homeless women present early in pregnancy or have just missed a menses, options for termination can be discussed along with shelter options. Urine human chorionic gonadotrophin tests done on-site can be of great service to women who might otherwise wait another cycle rather than pursue a test at a hospital or clinic. For homeless women who opt for abortion, the already difficult and complicated process for women of low income is made almost impossible in some cities. Women who have been healthy and may have existed on the street without Medicaid are suddenly faced with the task of navigating the often complex welfare systems in order to pay for the procedure. Controversy over public funding of abortions has made access difficult or impossible in some places. Hospitals and clinics may require someone to escort the patient from the procedure and to promise that she will not be alone in case of complications. This may not be possible for a homeless woman. Finally, homeless women who do have abortions rarely return for follow-up visits after the procedure.

Sexually Transmitted Diseases

STDs are one of the most common diagnoses made by the providers in the North and Central Bronx. Interestingly, this is not the case in the three other cities considered in this chapter. However, this probably may not accurately reflect incidence in these other cities. For instance, the STD clinic at Boston City Hospital is well known in the community and accessible without appointment, so symptomatic homeless women may be more likely to seek care there than to approach the providers on-site in shelters and day programs, perhaps for fear of a lack of confidentiality. Women more often than men harbor asymptomatic infections. Infectious salpingitis can scar fallopian tubes and lead to ectopic pregnancies. Chlamydia infection has surpassed gonorrhea as the number one cause of female infertility in the United States.[10] Pelvic pain may be a woman's first symptom, and documenting chlamydia or gonorrhea by culture at that stage of infection can be difficult. Diagnosis of STDs in women is often less than straightforward. A history complicated by the haze of vagueness that drugs and alcohol may lend or by the delusions of psychosis may make the diagnosis in some homeless women impossible. Performing diagnostic tests on-site may be ideal but poses challenges for processing lab tests, particularly for fastidious organisms like gonorrhea, chlamydia, and herpes. Negative results in such situations may be of dubious value. When a diagnosis is made, treating the client's partner may be difficult or impossible, but it should not be forgotten, for treatment rendered is worthless if exposure to the infectious organism continues. As with any population, education is an important task. Though infection with condylomata is often painless, if women are aware that it may affect the likelihood of the occurrence of cancer, they may be more willing to pursue treatment. Knowledge of the possible implications for their fertility as a result of their partners' harboring infectious agents may enable them to persuade their partners to seek care.

The problem of HIV warrants separate consideration and is also covered elsewhere in this text. Education regarding sexual transmission is an essential part of any discussion of sexuality with clients. Despite local public health, community, and federal government attempts at education (the surgeon general's education packet was delivered only to Americans with addresses), much confusion remains. The concept of the virus on dirty needles is often more readily grasped than the risk involved in intercourse with males who may not identify themselves as bisexuals despite previous homosexual relations or with male IV drug users. Discussing and encouraging safe sex are an essential part of any appropriate interaction. The provider should not wait for the woman to bring up sexuality. Dispensing condoms may be controversial at some sites but is an important intervention. However, most providers find that condoms are rarely used. Women are often unable even to suggest their use to male partners who may be violent. While some women who prostitute themselves require their use in Boston, others just increase the price of the interaction if no condom is used. In the Bronx the women who prostitute themselves to support drug habits rarely report using condoms.

Many of the women who are infected with HIV seen in the four cities have IV drug use as their risk factor. In Washington, D.C., over a six-month period in 1988, four women at the seventy-five-bed women's shelter died of AIDS. Three were known IV drug users. The fourth had no clear risk factor except a past lover who had spent time in jail. Women who are infected with HIV and who are homeless and drug-addicted often continue to use drugs despite illness. This can make the engagement process and access to health care difficult. A thirty-six-year-old woman in the Bronx had a sixteen-year drug habit. When the team first met her, she had severe thrush and pneumonia. It took four visits to convince her that she needed hospitalization for both her drug habit and her physical condition. She has since been discharged back to the shelter and is enrolled in a methadone program but continues to inject cocaine. Attempts are being made to enroll her for public AIDS benefits and services, but she may not qualify since she does not yet have an AIDS diagnosis. In Boston a forty-two-year-old woman with two children who lives with relatives has a twenty-year drug history with intermittent drug-free periods. When she learned of her positive HIV status, she began to use more heavily and prostituted herself to support her increased habit. After a binge of ten months she was able to limit her use to the methadone and is attending an immunodeficiency clinic every two weeks.

Violence

Homelessness puts women at great risk for all kinds of violence. Trauma has been cited as a leading cause of disability and death among the homeless.[7,11] Women on the street are easy targets for robbery and assault, especially when mental illness and drugs and alcohol increase their vulnerability. Physical and sexual abuse in family and intimate relationships has been identified as a frequent factor both in the process of becoming homeless and in the lives of homeless women.[1,4,12] A significant number of women eventually reveal to a trusted provider that they became overwhelmed, withdrawn, and hopeless after a traumatic event such as rape or assault. Low self-esteem and alienation can only be heightened by such events. When the perpetrator is a lover, friend, or relative, the effects are more devastating and profound. Social isolation has frequently been described as a part of homelessness;[5] homeless women who are victims of violence often lack any source of emotional support.

Although shelters have been described as sanctuary spaces, in the lives of some homeless women,[12] they can also be violent and dangerous places. In general, large public shelters tend to be less safe for women than small private shelters, especially those that serve only women. Some women in Boston and New York prefer to stay in abandoned buildings or in the street because of their fear of the shelters. In shelters that are completely gender-segregated, violence among women occurs occasionally. Overcrowding, tension caused by the diversity of the population, intolerance of mental illness, and the escalation of an argument all can lead to violence. Elderly women are occasionally the victims of humiliation and harassment by younger women.

Unfortunately women who are homeless are as likely as other women to be victims of battering, regardless of the lack of a "domestic" dwelling. Providers who see homeless women who are victims of violence must use the history to reveal battering situations, as they would with other women. Excellent tools for this have been developed.[13,14] Gleaning such information from a history may be difficult if the woman is inebriated or combative. However, providers should operate with a high degree of suspicion when injuries are inconsistent with the history given, when there are lacerations to the face, injuries located on or around genitals, breasts, abdomen, and back, or when there are obvious bite, belt, fist, or hand marks.[13] Head injuries can be difficult to interpret in an alcoholic woman with a history of blackouts or seizures. In Boston a thirty-eight-year-old alcoholic woman who was frequently battered by her boyfriend died of complications from a subdural hematoma. Shelter staff and providers were upset and frustrated by their inability definitively to place blame for her death on her boyfriend because although she had clearly been beaten, there was at least one witnessed fall in the forty-eight-hour period before her hospitalization.

Homeless women should be offered the community resources other victims of intimate violence have access to. In Boston this has presented a problem on at least one occasion, when the only battered women's shelter bed available was in a shelter unwilling to house a homeless woman! In communities where this is true, creative solutions can be explored. Information and hot line phone numbers should be made available in shelters. Detox programs may be the appropriate choice for drug- and alcohol-addicted women and are well known for their commitment to client confidentiality. If possible, a woman can seek shelter in another part of town.

Providers may be susceptible to blaming the victim in situations where a homeless woman returns to a batterer. Because the woman has few or none of the economic or family reasons other women may have for returning to such situations, it is hard to understand. However, at the root of homelessness for many women is estrangement from family and lack of a social network. A study done in Chicago revealed that almost 25 percent of homeless people had no contact with friends or families.[5] A homeless woman who is battered has often lost everything, including her children, and thus has little or nothing to turn to. Despite these obstacles, homeless women do leave batterers. Appropriate intervention and encouragement by providers may be the first and only chance for a homeless woman. However, rescue fantasies will do neither the provider nor the client any service. In Philadelphia the nurse practitioners offer literate clients Ginny NiCarthy's book of interviews with women who left abusive situations, *The Ones Who Got Away*. This is easy to read and may decrease a woman's sense of isolation.[15]

The violent crime of rape probably occurs more frequently to homeless women if only because of their increased public exposure. Women who are alcoholics or drug abusers and are inebriated or high during rape are often met with insensitivity, if not sarcasm or disbelief, by police and emergency room staff. Homeless women who reveal the experience of rape often do so for the first time weeks to months after the event and rarely seek care or justice. A training program is in the works for the staff at the Pine Street Inn Shelter in Boston to increase the sensitivity and timeliness of intervention. A familiar shelter staff member or provider accompanying the victim to the police station and emergency room can make a tremendous difference in the woman's experience. Homeless mentally ill women are in an especially difficult and vulnerable position in the case of rape and other violent crime. Paranoia often seems to be a powerful part of their illness and defense on the street. After such a crime they are not in a position to speak for themselves or even accept assistance. A mentally ill woman living on the streets of Boston was frequently visited by the Pine Street Inn's all-night outreach van at the site of a bank teller machine where she often slept. She was difficult to engage and very paranoid. One night the van arrived in time for the staff to pull a rapist off her. Though the entire event had been recorded by the bank's camera, no case was pursued in court because the woman was unwilling and unable to press charges.

In a recent study researchers were surprised to find a high rate of depressive and anxiety disorders among women who had been sexually assaulted as adults.[16] Crisis intervention strategies stress the importance of emotional support and the understanding of family and friends in the recovery or posttraumatic phase following a rape.[17] Clearly, many homeless women who are victims of sexual assault are at a disadvantage because of social isolation. The role of the provider may thus be unusually important. A team approach may be most effective so as to avoid an overwhelming situation for a single provider. Because of the emotional intensity of such intimate and violent events, providers should consider those of their own values and attitudes that may interfere with their ability to intervene appropriately.[17,18]

Incorporating questions regarding sexual abuse and assault in a routine history will make the subject a safe one for the woman to broach later.[18] When women are examined in a timely fashion after rapes or sexual assaults, it is important for providers to be familiar with evidence collection techniques. The existence of correctly collected evidence may make an important difference in a case where a woman's mental status was impaired by alcohol or drugs or where mental illness makes testimony difficult.

The feelings of low self-esteem, guilt, and self-blame associated with rape and battering are often part of the psychological construct of homeless women who are alcohol and substance abusers. The psychological impact of violence on the lives of these women must be taken seriously.

Mental Illness

Although this topic is covered in detail elsewhere, it is an important health concern for some homeless women. Some studies have suggested that the incidence of mental illness is much higher among homeless women than men;[19] however, this seems to vary from site to site. National data suggest that the incidence of mental illness is higher among homeless women the older they are, compared with men of the same age.[5] In Boston providers have noted that in general, interactions with homeless individual women often take longer than interactions with homeless men for similar complaints. Anxiety and paranoia are frequent obstacles to engagement and intervention among individual women in Boston. Several studies have found a high rate of undiagnosed physical illness and an unexpectedly high rate of mortality from infectious causes and suicide among the mentally ill.[20,21] These findings underlie the importance of outreach efforts and thorough evaluation of mentally ill homeless women who frequently exhibit paranoia and avoidance. In Boston a fifty-eight-year-old woman with a history of schizophrenia requested cough medicine. Because she had never before approached the nurses, the nurse wisely checked her temperature, which was 100° F. She was referred to the nurse practitioner, who found decreased breath sounds throughout her lungs. She refused to go to the emergency room that night but said she would go the following day. She did not, so the day after that the nurse practitioner accompanied her to the hospital and stayed with her through the process of admission. She was found to have an atypical interstitial pneumonia, which had probably progressed over a few weeks before she sought treatment.

Also of interest are a number of cases in which delusions are centered on sexual or reproductive matters. A fifty-eight-year-old woman appeared for a blood pressure check and said that she felt fine except for the pregnancy with Muammar Qaddafi's twins whom she had carried for four years while on pregnancy leave from the White House, where she had been Mrs. Reagan's personal general. Further work-up revealed that this chronic schizophrenic had large, symptomatic uterine fibroids. Although she denied it, there was concern that "Qaddafi" actually represented a rapist or attacker. A twenty-one-year-old woman new to Boston presented to the nurse practitioner in a shelter requesting tubal ligation by "burning" as soon as possible now that she was "of age." She denied a history of sexual relations and denied sexual abuse or rape. However, the disturbing and lurid detail with which she described the procedure she desired compelled the providers to seek consultation from the psychiatric nurse. Unfortunately the young woman refused any intervention and left the city shortly after.

While mental illness is a health concern for homeless men and women, in our experience homeless women with mental illness are more difficult to engage. This may be due to the self-protective nature of paranoia, but it often means that special outreach and flexibility are essential in order to provide health care to these women.

Conclusion

Homeless women have many health concerns. Effective intervention can begin with outreach and provision of direct care on-site in shelters, day programs, and soup kitchens. Despite their homelessness, many of these women are sexually active and need family planning, STD counseling, and HIV education. While it has been recognized that homeless people are at high risk for trauma, women may need support and intervention with violence in intimate relationships. The devastating event of rape can only be more traumatic for those who are socially isolated.

Acute illness, exacerbation of chronic illness, trauma, and the nature of her mental illness may be directly related to a woman's homelessness. Any discussion of the health concerns of homeless women must address the need for permanent housing alternatives. In addition to low-income housing, our communities need long-term substance abuse programs and more supervised and group housing for the mentally ill.

JAMES J. O'CONNELL

JEAN SUMMERFIELD

F. RUSSELL KELLOGG

10

The Homeless Elderly

Introduction

Nowhere is the tragedy of homelessness in America more starkly contrasted than in the excited eyes of children playing in the corridors of welfare hotels and the weathered countenances of the elderly sleeping on park benches. History is a harsh judge, and each government and culture will be remembered for the care given their most vulnerable and helpless citizens. While much attention has been focused on homeless children, a dearth of data has rendered information concerning the homeless elderly largely anecdotal. This discussion considers the demographics and epidemiology of homeless older people and examines their particular health care problems. We describe three model programs that respect the primacy of independence and function for the elderly homeless while giving them access to an array of flexible multidisciplinary services.

Demographics

The 1985 *Statistical Abstract* showed 12 percent of Americans to be age sixty-five and over. A significantly smaller percentage of the homeless population is elderly. The U.S. Department of Housing and Urban Development has estimated 6 percent of the homeless population to be older than sixty.[1] The Ohio Department of Mental Health completed a statewide survey of 979 homeless persons in both rural and urban settings in 1984 and found 6.4 percent to be sixty or older.[2] A study of Baltimore's homeless that same year, funded by the National Institute of

Mental Health, found 2 percent older than sixty-five, in contrast with 18.1 percent of the total population.[3]

The Boston Health Care for the Homeless Program served more than twelve thousand homeless persons from 1985 through 1988. Only 3 percent were age sixty-five or over, a percentage consonant with the cumulative data gathered by the nineteen cities in the national Health Care for the Homeless Program.[4]

There is a process of natural selection, and those older individuals who remain on the streets are indeed the "survivors" who have defied the odds. The risks and hazards of chronic homelessness lead to premature death, long-term hospitalization, or institutionalization, resulting in the low percentage of elderly among the homeless population.

Some evidence suggests that homeless people die relatively early and that those who survive into the sixth and seventh decades have higher mortality rates than their domiciled counterparts. A mortality study of homeless persons in Boston during 1986 found fifty-six who died in hospitals, on the streets, or in shelters. The greatest number of deaths occurred among men in their thirties or fifties. However, fourteen (25 percent) were sixty years or older, while six (11 percent) of those persons were over seventy. The causes of death, noted in Table 10.1,

Table 10.1 CAUSES OF DEATH AMONG THE
ELDERLY HOMELESS*

		NUMBER	PERCENT
Cancer		5	36
Lung	3		
Gastric	1		
Head and neck	1		
Coronary artery disease		4	29
Chronic lung disease		3	21
Chronic liver disease		2	14
Total		14	100

*Statistics based on fourteen deaths in 1986 among homeless persons sixty years or older in Boston.

reflect those of the general population in that age range, with cancer, coronary artery disease, chronic obstructive lung disease, and chronic liver disease most common. Calculations of standard mortality ratios are virtually impossible because the exact number of homeless in Boston is not known. Estimates range broadly from three to more than ten thousand. Nonetheless, mortality is high among the elderly homeless, for in this small study 3 percent of the population accounted for almost 25 percent of the deaths. Existence on the streets for the old is undoubtedly dangerous.[5]

Further characterization of the homeless elderly seems to vary from city to city. Sharon Keigher found a 300 percent increase in the number of elderly clients seen by the Chicago Department of Human Services between January 1986 and August 1987. Among these, the elderly homeless were more likely to have been found lost or wandering, to have been evicted from an apartment or been victims of crime, and to have had substantially more medical and psychological problems than those who were housed.[6] Another study by Keigher found recent homeless-ness to be more common than chronic, in contrast with Boston's elderly (see below). Those living alone without family or social supports appear to be the most vulnerable to homelessness. The immediate precipitant tended to be an eviction for failure to pay rent, usually because of forgetfulness, dementia, substance abuse, or medical and psychiatric problems. The elderly living in congregate housing or SROs fared better, probably because of the established relationships and social interactions common in such living situations.[7]

In November 1986 a prospective assessment of the elderly homeless was undertaken by the Boston Health Care for the Homeless Program.[8] Thirty persons aged seventy or older were identified as active patients in the HCH clinic sites. Ages ranged from seventy to eighty-six, with a mean of seventy-seven and a median of seventy-five. Nineteen (63 percent) were male, and eleven (37 percent) female, in contrast with the overall population served by the program, which has a four-to-one ratio of men to women. Rather interestingly, twenty-eight (93 per-cent) were white, and two (7 percent) black. The ethnicity of Boston's adult homeless population is 60 percent white, 31 percent black, 5 percent Hispanic, and 4 percent Asian or Native American, similar to the general population of the greater Boston area.[9]

Reliable information was obtained on the duration of homelessness for twenty-one of the thirty patients. The range was from three months to more than forty years, and the average was twelve years. Thus, many of Boston's elderly in this small group typify the classic description of the "chronically homeless person." Peter H. Rossi and James D. Wright studied the homeless in Chicago and noted a heterogeneous population, including one-third that had been homeless for less than two months and one-quarter that had been without homes for more than two years.[10] Most of Boston's older homeless people have been living on the streets for years; neither recent loss of housing or income nor acute medical or psychiatric illness is a common cause of their homelessness.

Gerontology and the Homeless Elderly

Escalating numbers of older Americans and the staggering costs of their health care have focused national attention on the field of gerontology. Alan Pifer col-lected several papers, entitled "The Aging Society," which elegantly characterized the graying of America as unique in world history.[11] Modern technology and medicine have lengthened the life-span, and the U.S. Bureau of the Census esti-mates that there will be more than a hundred million Americans fifty-five years or older by the year 2050. Indeed, more than thirty million of those will be older than seventy-five, a group of minor impact in American society until the 1940s.

Increased utilization of health care services has been repeatedly documented in this elderly population, as evidenced by the continual crises in the Medicare program and the paucity of nursing homes and chronic care facilities for the poor elderly.[12]

In addition, an awareness of the unique needs of the elderly has led to the evolution of the subspecialty of geriatric medicine, now recognized by the Amer-ican Board of Internal Medicine and the American Academy of Family Practice with an accredited geriatric training fellowship followed by a certifying examination.[13]

A striking philosophical parallel exists between the young field of gerontology and the national HCHP. The major tenet of gerontology has been the primacy of function and independence. Prevention, assessment, diagnosis, and treatment are oriented less toward cure (e.g., coronary artery disease, hypertension, and Alzheimer's dementia are never "cured" in the traditional sense) than toward maximal function within the limits of each individual's situation. Much of geriatric care requires a multidisciplinary approach by a team of physician, nurse, and social worker, and the availability of a coordinated network of services, such as day-care centers, meal programs, respite and hospice units, foster care, and substance abuse treatment programs. These outreach teams, firmly based in hospitals or neighborhood health centers, must deliver direct care services at sites where the elderly live and congregate in order to assure access of good-quality health care and accurately to assess function within the individual's daily surroundings.

The same combined medical and public health model describes the approach to the health care of homeless persons in general. Unfortunately, the emphasis of gerontology on care and prevention in the home environment distorts the parallel. Home care of the aged is in stark contrast with the violence and extremes of weather experienced by the homeless elderly wandering the streets of our cities without asylum.

Health Care Problems of the Homeless Elderly

The homeless elderly suffer from multiple medical problems. Table 10.2 lists the total number of diagnoses in the cohort of thirty elderly patients whose medical records were reviewed in the Boston study noted above. The average number of major chronic illnesses was four. Every elderly person in this study suffered either from chronic alcohol abuse (alcoholic hepatitis, pancreatitis, withdrawal seizures, or a previous detoxification admission documented in the hospital record) or from major psychiatric illness (DSM-III diagnosis confirmed by a psychiatrist and documented in the chart). Nine persons (30 percent) suffered from both alcoholism and chronic mental illness.

Chronic obstructive pulmonary disease was present in one-third, all of whom had many decades of heavy cigarette smoking. Peripheral vascular disease was noted in seven persons, most of whom suffered from chronic venous stasis and repeated episodes of lower-extremity cellulitis. Hypertension, urinary incontinence, and previous exposure to tuberculosis were common medical problems as well.

Case studies illustrate some of the more common health care problems of the elderly homeless. The complexity of the major medical problems encountered by these persons emphasizes the importance of a multidisciplinary team approach and the necessity of a coordinated network of social services.

A seventy-eight-year-old deaf man, a heavy drinker and a smoker of three packs of cigarettes a day for almost sixty years, has adamantly refused efforts by

Table 10.2 MAJOR MEDICAL PROBLEMS AMONG 30
ELDERLY HOMELESS IN BOSTON

Acute or chronic alcoholism	19	Deep venous thrombosis	2
Major psychiatric illness	18	Lung mass	1
Obstructive lung disease	10	Fecal incontinence	1
Peripheral vascular disease	7	Cardiomegaly (alcohol)	1
PPD positive	6	Heart failure	1
Arrhythmias	6	Frostbite	1
Hypertension	5	Pulmonary tuberculosis	1
Urinary incontinence	5	Peripheral neuropathy	1
Coronary artery disease	4	Diabetes mellitus	1
Cancer	4	Tremor	1
Anemia	4	Chronic renal failure	1
Benign prostatic hypertrophy	3	Esophageal stricture	1
Peptic ulcer disease	3	Syncope	1
Cellulitis	3	Splenomegaly	1
Dementia	3	Urethral stricture	1
Deafness	3	Herpes zoster	1
Seizure disorder	3	Hypothyroidism	1
Pneumonia	3	Rheumatoid arthritis	1
Inguinal hernia	2	Blindness	1
		Upper GI bleed	1

Total number of major medical problems = 132

the Boston senior home care coordinator to find appropriate placement. He had absconded from two nursing homes, was deemed "competent" although "mildly demented" by two psychiatrists, and returned to the streets, where he had dwelled for more than twenty-five years. Very unsteady on his feet, this man walked with a wide-based gait and suffered from a profound peripheral neuropathy secondary to chronic alcoholism.

For the past four years he remained a guest of a large shelter where the nursing and social service staffs worked closely to provide a safe environment for this fiercely independent man. His pattern was to leave the shelter each month or so and drink heavily for several days before returning for rest. After two hospitalizations for pneumonia and lower-extremity cellulitis, each diagnosed early by the shelter clinic staff working with the HCH provider, he suffered a generalized seizure at the shelter and died in the hospital of complications of an aspiration pneumonia.

The Environment: Prevention, Safety, Flexibility

The story of this frail alcoholic aged man reveals important health care issues. Typical of many elderly homeless persons, he had spent much of his life on the streets and valued his independence above all else. Despite the exhaustive efforts of many social workers and health care providers, and in spite of staff exasperation with issues of competency and his reluctance to accept placements, this septuagenarian simply chose to remain in the familiar surroundings of the shelter. After several meetings with staff and providers, all agreed to respect his wishes for independence while attempting to make the shelter a safer environment for him. Given a permanent bed on the first floor, he was allowed to remain indoors during the daytime if he chose. In the evening he was seen by the clinic nurses for a foot soak and examination of the legs. With early infection of any ulceration, a course of oral antibiotics was initiated. Any cough associated with fever or purulent sputum was promptly treated with antibiotics, preventing costly hospital admissions.

Continued binge drinking necessitated a degree of tolerance on the part of the staff, as it was abundantly clear that this man would not accept detoxification or a rehabilitation program. His deafness barred his participation in the weekly AA meetings at the shelter. During and after the binges, care was taken that he received all his meals and did not become dehydrated.

The man died with dignity after a very short hospitalization. His independence was perhaps a defiance of death or indicated a fear of death, while his rugged individualism ultimately drew the respect of the shelter staff. One lesson learned from this man was that rather than force persons into idealized situations, shelters must make available an array of services. In this case, the necessary services included the shelter clinic for nursing care of lower-extremity ulcerations, diagnosis and treatment of early infections, and provision of adequate nutrition.

Alcoholism

Alcohol abuse in the elderly is common.[14] About 10 percent of alcoholic men in the United States are age sixty and over.[15] Most of these began drinking early in life and have managed to survive despite numerous medical and social complications. Social theorists have found that male drinking behavior is defined at an early age and changes very little after thirty.[16] Some evidence suggests that many alcoholics "burn out" with age and stop drinking after twenty to twenty-five years.[17] However, these elderly persons will still suffer the medical complications of chronic alcoholism, especially cirrhosis, peripheral neuropathy, cerebellar degeneration, and organic brain disease. Despite multiple medical problems, detoxification is rarely necessary in elderly alcoholics, as our patient clearly demonstrated.[18]

From the practitioner's point of view, knowledge of the elderly patient's alcohol intake is imperative. As we have seen, the average elderly homeless person in the Boston study suffered from four major medical or psychiatric problems, most of which required one or more medications. Drug interactions are extremely common among elderly alcoholics. Fifty of the one hundred most prescribed drugs, and all of the ten most common, interact with alcohol.[19]

This seventy-five-year-old Russian immigrant and World War II veteran suffers from a major thought disorder as well as chronic alcohol abuse. Homeless for more than five years, he is a graduate of a local university and a former professor of Hebrew. Despite offers to live with his children, one a psychiatrist and the other a nurse, he stubbornly refused to "burden anyone" and chose the shelters. After an admission for hypertension and heart failure, he finally agreed to placement in elderly housing arranged by Senior Home Care. After more than a year he deteriorated and returned to the streets. He was admitted to the hospital with a nodule in the liver but refused diagnostic studies and left against medical advice after the psychiatry service found him to be paranoid but competent. A brisk upper-GI bleed brought him to another hospital within weeks, and he was found to have a fungating gastric carcinoma. Again he refused treatment, and he now avoids the shelters and spends most nights in a drop-in center downtown. His alcoholism seems to have burned out, but his paranoia has progressed to the point where he will no longer speak with health care providers. With death imminent, his resolve to remain independent has solidified despite the pleas of family and workers.

Competency and Guardianship: An Ethical Dilemma

This man's story dramatizes several ethical and moral dilemmas familiar to those caring for the elderly. While the paranoia and thought disorder are indisputable, the issue of competency to make one's own decisions is problematic. Several psychiatrists concurred that this man was indeed competent, while his providers pleaded that his decisions displayed poor judgment and placed him in grave danger on the streets. On the other hand, the gastric carcinoma, with probable metastases to liver, carried a poor prognosis of several months at most, even with surgery and proper nutrition. He has remained on the streets, continues to socialize each day at a soup kitchen and sleep most nights in a chair at the drop-in center. Doctors and nurses from the HCHP are able to monitor his condition at each site.

Chronic Mental Illness

While several studies have found from 20 to 40 percent of homeless populations suffering from chronic mental illness, little has been written on the mental health of the elderly homeless. Leona Bachrach has emphasized the diverse qualities of the homeless, warning that the interpretation of research on the homeless mentally ill must carefully consider the differences within the population.[20] C. I. Cohen and colleagues have studied the mental health of elderly men on the Bowery of New York and found over one-third to suffer from depression (many of whom met the DSM-III criteria for major depression), while another one-quarter were psychotic or had histories of previous psychiatric hospitalization.[21]

Two conclusions are especially worth noting. First, the authors found no difference between psychotic homeless persons and other homeless persons in terms of social, economic, or health parameters. Secondly, the older homeless Bowery men had smaller social networks, far less income, more chronic illness, and more significant depression than a comparison group of domiciled men living in the community.

As with the ex-Hebrew professor, such studies support the importance of extending the social network of the elderly homeless. Day-care centers, meal programs, drop-in centers, on-site health care clinics all assist older homeless persons through interaction and interpersonal contact while respecting the paramount need for independence.[22,23]

Independence vs. the Need for Intimacy

The tension that can be experienced by an older homeless person between the need for independence and the desire for intimacy and community is illustrated by the odyssey of a seventy-seven-year-old woman with chronic mental illness and three decades of sporadic homelessness. Wandering the streets in sub-zero temperatures, she was found to be disorganized and psychotic and was admitted to a Department of Mental Health (DMH) transitional shelter, where she remained for almost a year. An apartment was finally found, although she returned each day to the DMH shelter to eat meals, play cards, and watch the soap operas. After three months she had become so lonely and depressed that she abandoned her housing and returned to live at the DMH shelter.

———————

This eighty-seven-year-old deaf woman, veteran of the Women's Army Corps who served in the Philippines, left her apartment in 1986 because of fears about the home care providers "invading my home." She spent all her life savings on hotel bills, followed by a brief stay in a Boston shelter before taking a bus to Florida. She was found by the local police in Miami and taken to the Salvation Army, where she remained for two months.

She then returned to Boston and was subsequently evicted from a local hotel for nonpayment of her bill. Returning to the same shelter, she refused all efforts at placement. The social service and nursing staffs of the shelter, working with the HCH team and the Senior Home Care representatives, were able to obtain a guardian for this woman, and she was placed in a nursing home.

The legal basis for her nursing home placement was developed at the neuropsychiatric unit at Boston City Hospital, where she underwent an extensive medical and psychiatric evaluation. It was determined that she suffered from multiinfarct dementia. This thorough evaluation provided the unequivocal documentation which facilitated the legal process of obtaining guardianship, after which appropriate placement became easy. She was content at the nursing home and continued to join other shelter guests for lunch on weekends until her death from chronic lung disease at the age of eighty-nine.

Dementia

A demented homeless person offers a particularly challenging responsibility to those giving care. The differential diagnosis of dementia is expansive, covering many pages of the neurology textbooks. Health workers must remain aware that many dementias are treatable.[24] Each elderly homeless demented person is entitled to a full evaluation and assessment by a specialized team.[25,26]

HCH providers across the country have been exasperated by the moral, legal, and ethical issues posed by demented elderly people wandering the streets of our major cities. Only three of the thirty elderly patients followed in the Boston study had documented dementia; most others refused neurological or psychiatric assessment. Many demented persons have been living on the streets for decades, and placement in hospitals or nursing homes often produces the additional problems of acute delirium or depression. Such people have difficulty forming new memories but frequently do well within the structure of a daily routine. It has been established that the elderly who function well in the familiar environment of their own homes have a high risk of acute confusion and delirium when they are hospitalized. Homeless persons whose familiar environment is the streets will also become confused, angry, and depressed when institutionalized or placed in new SROs or apartments. Yet can we as providers feel comfortable allowing such demented souls to suffer the dangers of the street?

A final dilemma in the care and management of a demented homeless individual is the absence of a family to engage. A major tenet in the care of Alzheimer's disease and other dementias is the involvement of family members and others close to the patient. With demented homeless persons, the few familiar contacts are scattered along the route of the daily trek through the inner city, and in many cases they have long been involved in the protection of these people. The insulin of a sixty-five-year-old diabetic man is kept in the refrigerator of a nearby tavern where he has gone for an eye-opener each morning for twenty years. The tavern's owner draws up the daily dose and tests the urine for glucose and ketones. Several attempts by the HCH team and the shelter staff failed to alter this routine because the patient could not remember to come to the newly established morning clinic at the shelter.

An eighty-five-year-old man, a World War II veteran, with innumerable detoxifications for chronic alcoholism, developed smoldering multiple myeloma with increasingly severe pain in several bones as well as a profound anemia requiring transfusions every one to two months. He developed urinary incontinence and was admitted to the VA hospital several times for urinary tract infections and pneumonia. In the fall of 1987, unable to tolerate a chronic care hospital, he insisted on returning to the shelter, where the staff cared for him by bringing meals and allowing him to remain inside during the days. Eventually the requirement for pain medication escalated, and he became cachectic, while a dedicated shelter staff embraced the burden of caring for this dying man. He remained bedridden in the shelter until several days before his death of cardiac and renal failure in April 1988.

Cancer

Cancer is common among the elderly homeless in Boston and is the second leading cause of death among the elderly in America. Unfortunately our experience mirrors the results of two recent studies that demonstrated that older persons are less likely than others to participate in screening programs. Only 6 percent of elderly women over sixty years of age had ever had a mammogram.[27] Our cohort of patients revealed that all the men had received rectal examinations and stool tests for blood, but none of the women had agreed to mammograms or breast or pelvic examinations during the thirty months of follow-up. While the high incidence of mental illness, particularly paranoia, may explain this reluctance, more effective ways of screening for early cancer in this high-risk group must be found.

Death and Dying Without a Home

The situation of the eighty-five-year-old man with multiple myeloma reveals the difficulties of homeless people who suffer from chronic terminal illness. Hospice care is not available in most major cities; the options for the homeless elderly remain chronic care hospitals, nursing homes, or the streets—with most choosing the latter.

For many, the streets and shelters constitute a community that provides material support (food, clothing, shelter) as well as some degree of "intimacy" (shared cigarettes, passed bottles, card games). Another elderly man in the Boston cohort was diagnosed with esophageal cancer and required a gastric feeding tube to bypass the obstructing lesion. He absconded after several days in one of the city's finest nursing homes, stating that he knew he was dying, "but I don't feel old and out to pasture just yet." He pleaded to return to the shelter where he had been sleeping for more than twenty years so that he could die near his friends.

Each death of a guest at Pine Street Inn, a large shelter in Boston, is commemorated with a service. These funerals have been profoundly emotional, attended by scores of homeless friends as well as relatives and staff, and a worthy attestation of the culture and community within the shelters. It is hardly surprising that when faced with the specter of death, fiercely independent individuals, many of whom have thwarted convention for decades, should refuse to die in the confines of a hospital or nursing home.

Nonetheless, care of the ill and dying homeless person can be overwhelming in the shelter setting. On-site health care clinics can facilitate early diagnosis, making as effective as possible the available treatment regimes such as radiation, surgery, or chemotherapy. Continued care requires frequent monitoring, with emphasis on nutrition and prevention of infection. In the case of the man with myeloma, the shelter clinic staff worked collaboratively with the oncology group of the VA hospital to arrange appointments for transfusions and monitor the management of pain medications.

The death of this man was difficult for the staff and guests of the shelter. Despite an understanding of the inevitability of his death, the process of his dying was emotionally exhausting for all who cared for him. Several guests of the shelter were able to articulate their own fears of dying and described an "emptiness" within their own lives. While shelters often can provide respite care, the concept of hospice care within such settings must be cautiously considered, if at all.

Urinary Incontinence

Urinary incontinence is an exceedingly difficult problem in large shelters, where scores of people sleep in close proximity. Many older persons become embarrassed and ashamed and leave the shelters to sleep away from taunting crowds. The problem is further compounded by the paucity of public toilets in the downtown areas of most cities. Urinary incontinence can often be improved or cured.[28,29] Recognition and acknowledgment of the problem are the essential first step, followed by a referral to a urologist for an assessment.[30]

For the man dying of myeloma, no treatable cause for his stress incontinence was found, and he was given absorbent diapers to allow him a greater range of mobility while sparing him much embarrassment. In addition, his bed was moved near the first-floor bathroom, and the staff encouraged him to urinate every two hours during the day whether or not he felt an urge. This simple behavioral change virtually eliminated his daytime incontinence.[31]

Progress and Pitfalls in the Care of the Homeless Elderly

By June 30, 1989, the cohort of thirty elderly homeless persons in Boston had been followed for thirty months. Twenty-two of them (73 percent) were hospitalized during this period, and most had two or more admissions. One man developed active pulmonary tuberculosis and required several months of inpatient care because of a virulent and multiply resistant organism. A woman became progressively disheveled and disorganized and was committed after the shelter staff found her washing in feces and "speaking in tongues." After a prolonged psychiatric hospitalization she is now in a nursing home.

The situations of these elderly homeless after thirty months are depicted in Table 10.3. Despite intense health care and social service intervention by a coordinated network of public and private agencies, only three (10 percent) were in permanent living situations in lodging houses or apartments or with family members. Four (13 percent) in nursing homes, while one man with dementia and a history of chronic mental illness spent six months in an acute-care hospital awaiting placement in an appropriate chronic-care facility or nursing home.

Eight persons (27 percent) had died. Of the twenty-two alive, eleven (50

Table 10.3 DISPOSITIONS OF THE ELDERLY
HOMELESS IN BOSTON AFTER 18 AND
30 MONTHS

	18 MONTHS	30 MONTHS
Shelter / streets	11	11
Deceased	6	8
Nursing home	6	4
Family	2	2
DMH transitional shelter	1	1
Alcohol rehab program	1	1
Acute-care hospital	1	1
Lodging / rooming house	1	1
Apartment	1	0
Medical respite unit	1	0
Unknown	1	1
Totals	30	30

percent) were still living in shelters or on the streets at the thirty-month mark. One person had been lost to follow-up. Remarkably, fifteen (50 percent) persons were placed in nursing homes at some point during the thirty months and subsequently chose to return to the streets.

Despite an array of support systems, including health care and multidisciplinary services, most of the elderly persons in this study had been chronically homeless and adamantly resisted traditional placement opportunities, choosing to remain in the shelters or on the streets. We need to explore the reasons if we want to influence public policy to build new types of group housing and alter existing facilities to accommodate the specialized needs of this population. This section discusses three programs designed to address the specific needs of the homeless elderly.

Chicago: Senior Reach Program

The Chicago Health Care for the Homeless Program was originally designed to service the small overnight shelters and drop-in centers that are widely scattered throughout the city. Mobile teams of health care and social service providers were oriented toward episodic interventions of moderate intensity, although some clients were seen over much longer periods. Within weeks of initiating services, the project staff realized the unique stresses caused by relatively small numbers of elderly homeless persons. Mrs. M's case dramatizes the poignancy of the problem.

Mrs. M is in her eighties and lived for years in a complex for senior citizens subsidized through the Chicago Housing Authority. Convinced that a city "bigwig" had arranged for her to pay less rent, she had made only partial rent payments for more than three years. One night while walking alone in a dangerous section of Uptown, Mrs. M was mugged and sustained a fractured shoulder. During the prolonged hospitalization she was evicted from her apartment for nonpayment of rent.

Mrs. M was brought to a drop-in center by the Department of Human Services soon after discharge. The HCH staff advocated on her behalf, insisting that more appropriate placement be found. Accompanied by an HCH social worker, Mrs. M was taken to the police station, then to a psychiatric unit for evaluation, back to the police station, and finally, at 4:00 A.M., to the overnight shelter that had been deemed inappropriate earlier in the day.

The HCH staff became involved with this unfortunate woman, who remained homeless for eight months in the shelter system. Several failed placements, all in unfamiliar sections of the city, exasperated the Department of Human Services. This frail woman insisted on returning to her familiar apartment in the BHA senior citizen complex, and she would accept nothing else.

The Illinois Guardianship and Advocacy Commission assessed Mrs. M on the recommendation of the HCH staff and found her competent to make her own decisions. Although she was not openly choosing a homeless life-style, her resistance to resettlement alternatives made it a choice by default.

Mrs. M deteriorated considerably and was admitted to Cook County Hospital. After an extended stay she agreed to a nursing home placement.

———————

The Senior Reach Program, a short- and intermediate-term intensive case management and resettlement service for the elderly homeless, became the first specialized component of the Chicago HCHP. Funded by a twenty-five-thousand-dollar emergency shelter counseling contract of the Chicago Department of Aging and Disability, Senior Reach combines flexibility and assertiveness to identify and serve these vulnerable people. Psychiatric and medical evaluations are arranged, often on park benches, while legal and housing services are made accessible in the outreach setting. The program recognizes the tension between respect for individual autonomy and the need to protect when judgment becomes impaired. Senior Reach relies upon the legal procedures surrounding protective interventions such as commitment and guardianship whenever necessary. Fortunately only a small number of clients have required such intervention, since staff members have learned to work for extended periods to arrive at a resettlement plan that meets both the needs and the desires of the client.

In 1986 the Retirement Research Foundation funded a study of the undomiciled elderly conducted by the University of Chicago School of Social Service Administration in collaboration with the Chicago HCHP. Profiles of 157 Senior Reach clients were analyzed. The study group comprised 87 women and 70 men. Ages ranged from fifty-seven to one hundred two, with a mean of seventy-two and a median of seventy-one years. Minorities were significantly underrepresented when compared with the general homeless population of Chicago, similar to findings in Boston.

At the time of initial contact with Senior Reach, 24 percent had been evicted, 13 percent were found wandering or lost, 20 percent showed signs of marked deterioration in behavior, 7 percent had been victimized, 6 percent were without funds, 7 percent mentioned family problems, while 23 percent were unable or unwilling to answer questions and hence no cause of homelessness was ascertained for them. Only 12 percent of the clients were known to have been homeless for a year or more.

Despite few documented histories of chronic mental illness, 45 percent of the women and 31 percent of the men were confused, disoriented, or paranoid. Poor health was reported by three-quarters of the women and two-thirds of the men. Senior Reach staff had significant difficulties arranging medical and psychiatric evaluations, especially in the inpatient setting. Considerable resistance by many medical facilities to the Medicaid and Medicare reimbursement levels was a hindrance to proper assessment.

Senior Reach identified a dearth of specialized shelters for the elderly. The transience and instability of the shelters caused considerable physical strain to these elderly clients and also impeded efforts to assess clients and arrive at resettlement plans.

Resolution of Senior Reach cases required an average of four months, with a range of several days to a full year. Almost half the 157 clients received placements in apartments, in room-and-board facilities, in nursing homes, or with family members. Hospitalization and subsequent placement were recommended for 23 percent of the women and 10 percent of the men. Approximately one-fifth of the group (22 percent of women, 17 percent of men) remained in the same living situations as at the time of intake. More men (29 percent) than women (9 percent) walked away from temporary shelters after intake but before any intervention.

The Senior Reach staff filed fifteen guardianship petitions, eleven of which were for women. Several factors may account for this gender difference, including cultural biases toward the protection of women, the tendency of men to flee before service intervention, and a greater resistance to supportive or protective placements among the women.

The success of Senior Reach, despite these several gaps in the service network, is due to an assertive but flexible case management that recognizes the vicissitudes in the life of each elderly homeless person. This program continues to work creatively for interim solutions, while striving both for a range of affordable housing (such as SRO hotels, congregate living facilities, and rooming houses) and for efficient health care and social services responsive to the immediate needs of this population.

Boston: Cardinal Medeiros Center

The Kit Clark Senior House (KCSH) is a large multiservice center with a mission to serve the forty-two thousand elderly living in the downtown area and the neighborhoods along Boston Harbor. This agency is composed of a nutrition project for one-third of the city of Boston; a home health agency with adult day care; a mental health clinic; an alcoholism unit; a transportation program; in-home services with homemakers, home health aides, and personal care attendants; and a senior center.

The basic needs of Boston's elderly alcoholic street people for food and day shelter, as well as protection from the violence of the streets, were not adequately addressed in 1983.[32] KCSH responded with an age-integrated meal program designed to serve two hundred lunches to the homeless in a downtown site. Intended as a safe haven from the streets and a place to socialize, the program soon became dominated by younger and more vocal guests. Security and crowd control became dominant issues, while the design of a day center with case management and counseling became impractical. Most elderly simply avoided this program, which essentially mirrored the frightening and impersonal model of the larger night shelters.[33] Within the first six months of operation the day program was asked to find another site, and the KCSH was able to consider an alternate plan.

In November 1984 the Cardinal Medeiros Center began in the basement of a church about two blocks from Boston's largest shelter. Open only to those forty-five years of age or older, this program serves a maximum of one hundred lunches each weekday. Each meal is planned to provide at least one-third of the required daily allowance of vitamins and minerals.

The day program is relatively unstructured, and a tour of the facility finds the elderly playing checkers, reading newspapers, conversing with staff and friends, and resting. The atmosphere is safe and secure, with respect and dignity afforded each quest. The current staff of two are streetwise case managers facile in the areas of housing and entitlements as well as mental health and substance abuse.[34]

A Boston HCHP team assisted volunteer nurses from Massachusetts General Hospital in organizing an on-site clinic at the center. Elderly guests are screened for hypertension and treated for episodic illness, with the HCH clinicians providing consultations as well as full access to the hospital clinics.

The site of the Cardinal Medeiros Center is provided by the Boston Catholic archdiocese, while primary funding for the program is available through the Massachusetts Executive Office of Elder Affairs.

New York City: Respite House

The Single Room Supportive Residence, known as Respite House, is a seventy-four-bed congregate housing SRO site developed under the auspices of Educational Alliance, Inc., to provide permanent housing for the homeless or near-homeless elderly. The criteria for entry include: age of fifty-six years or greater, functional independence, absence of active alcoholism or drug abuse, and lack of a major psychiatric disorder. Residents pay a modest monthly rent and receive a variety of medical, ancillary, and social support services. Because this site does not provide personal care services offered by an institution, applicants must be fully independent.

Since Respite House opened in February 1988, St. Vincent's Hospital and Medical Center, through its Department of Community Medicine, has provided on-site medical services for purposes of screening applicants and treating the residents who are ill. The status of the first seventy-two residents seen for medical care or screening at this unusual site is reviewed here.

The average age for this group was sixty-six years, with a range of fifty to eighty-three (Table 10.4). The majority were white (Table 10.5), most were male, and very few were married (Table 10.6). Of those whose educational attainment was known, 41 percent had completed high school, and nearly a quarter had at least some college experience (Table 10.7). Recent occupations for these individuals were largely at the unskilled level, yet a significant minority had professional backgrounds (Table 10.8). Prior to moving into Respite House, 61 percent had resided in private or city shelters, 14 percent in shared housing, 12 percent in apartments, and 12 percent in hotel rooms, while 1 percent had come from an institution. Several were recent immigrants.

Initial history and physical examination revealed that the vast majority of individuals had at least one chronic medical condition, and most had multiple medical problems (Table 10.9). Almost one-third had a history indicative of alcoholism, although in most of these cases it was no longer an active problem. Fifteen percent had a history of psychiatric illness. Of the medical disorders, the most frequent were hypertension, cardiac and pulmonary conditions, peripheral vascular disease, and arthritis.

A review of the status of the initial seventy-two residents, after an average of seven months, found sixty-three still living in Respite House. One person had

Table 10.4 AGE

AGE	PERCENT
50–54	1
55–59	8
60–64	34
65–69	31
70–74	13
75–79	10
80–84	3

Table 10.5 RACE

RACE	PERCENT
White	57
Black	17
Hispanic (Latino)	20
Asian	4
Native American	1

Table 10.6 MARITAL STATUS

STATUS	PERCENT
Married	4
Widowed	26
Single	25
Separated / divorced	31
Unknown	14

Table 10.7 EDUCATION

EDUCATION	PERCENT
Less than high school grad	31
High school graduate only	17
Some or completion of college	20
Professional school	4
Unknown	28

Table 10.8 OCCUPATIONAL HISTORY

WORK HISTORY	PERCENT
Unskilled	54
Clerical / marginal	23
Professional	13
Unknown	11

Table 10.9 COMMON CHRONIC MEDICAL
CONDITIONS

CONDITION	PERCENT
Alcohol abuse (prior or current)	32
Hypertension	44
Cardiac	27
Psychiatric	15
Orthopedic	15
Pulmonary	14
Neurologic	13
Peripheral vascular disease	13
Diabetes mellitus	13

died, one had disappeared, two had been evicted, one had been hospitalized for acute alcoholism and had not returned, and four had moved to private apartments.

Few of the individuals selected to reside at this site were subsequently found to have active alcoholism (four) or major psychiatric problems (six). The majority have adapted well to congregate living, as illustrated by the following case histories.

SR is a sixty-year-old Hispanic single man who has resided at the SRO for five months. Although he had two years of college, he dropped out for economic reasons and never completed his education. He moved from Puerto Rico to New York City and spent many years working as a short-order cook. In 1980 he began to experience angina pectoris, and since 1983 he has been on disability. He lost his apartment eighteen months prior to entry into this residence because he couldn't pay the rent, and he managed to double up with friends for six months before he was forced to rely on the city shelter system. He has no history of alcohol or drug abuse and denies mental illness. He was referred to this residence by the shelter staff and adjusted well to congregate living. He currently receives his medical care at the on-site clinic.

AP is a sixty-six-year-old divorced black man who has lived in the SRO for eight months. Never having completed grammar school, he worked his entire life as an unskilled laborer, with the exception of a brief stint in the military. At the time of his application to the SRO, he admitted to a distant history of heavy drinking but denied active alcohol use in recent years. He had spent the prior six months in a city shelter after he was burned out of his apartment. On his initial screening exam, performed at the on-site clinic, he was found to have evidence of mild emphysema and vascular insufficiency, but there were no peripheral stigmata of alcoholism. However, within two months of entering the residence he began drinking again and was unable to remain at Respite House.

BW is a seventy-four-year-old widowed white woman who emigrated with her husband to this country from Europe after World War II. After their children were grown, she resumed work as a nurse until her retirement in 1980. She was widowed in 1982 and soon fell into financial difficulties, largely because of the costs she incurred to manage and treat her diabetes and hypertension. Twelve months before entering the SRO she lost her apartment because of nonpayment of rent. Although she spent a few months living with one of her daughters in a neighboring state, she left because of her unwillingness to be a burden upon her family. She was referred by the shelter staff to the SRO, where she has done very well, with the on-site clinic staff providing primary care for her medical problems.

Conclusion

The homeless elderly are vulnerable. They are prey to the desperate violence that characterizes much of street life, poorly suited to withstand extremes of temperature and weather, suffering from chronic debilitating disease, yet they are survivors who embody the American Dream gone astray.

The stories told in this chapter are not fiction. One cannot help wondering about fate, how fragile and precarious is the health of our parents, ourselves, and our children, and how easily any of us can become homeless in the twilight of life.

Prevention of homelessness among our nation's elderly is a complex problem bereft of immediate solutions. However, several innovative programs have cared for older persons who have lost or forsaken their homes, often succeeding in addressing idiosyncratic wishes and finding adequate housing to meet those wishes. Their considerable health care needs are inexorably woven into the social pattern of these homeless elderly persons and can be addressed only by multidisciplinary teams with access to an array of flexible services.

The lives of older people change frequently, often dramatically. It is to be expected. Programs that demand rigorous compliance and permanent solutions will fail. Rather, the elderly homeless must have available a spectrum of flexible, interrelated services and placements that can accommodate the movement, change, and unpredictability that characterize them. As John Gunn noted in his 1974 paper on "Prisons, Shelters, and Homeless Men," "Maybe we are much too keen on curing and not keen enough about tolerating."[35]

JANELLE GOETCHEUS
MARY ANN GLEASON
DEBORAH SARSON
TOM BENNETT
PHYLLIS B. WOLFE

11

Convalescence: For Those Without a Home — *Developing Respite Services in Protected Environments*

Introduction

The shelters and streets of this nation harbor people who are very sick. Many are slowly dying. On a daily basis, medical practitioners are faced with trying to treat these people, only to send them back to the streets or the shelters to survive until the next visit. Further, because a majority of shelters are open only at night, many of these individuals must walk the streets throughout the day in all types of weather without adequate rest and nutrition. Creating protected environments in shelters for respite, convalescence, and treatment of illness will help the homeless stay out of hospitals and receive care that most others, with homes and families, receive as a routine measure.

Need for Respite Care

The exigencies of homelessness exacerbate the most minor health problems that often become major simply because they go untreated. Placing health professionals directly in shelters has proved useful in identifying homeless persons who need respite care.

In March 1985, on the opening day of the HCHP in Washington, D.C., the first patient seen at a health station was a forty-seven-year-old man with pulmonary tuberculosis. He had been in a hospital and then discharged back to the shelter. He had large cavitary lesions in both lungs and was malnourished, anemic, short of breath, and very weak—too weak even to walk eleven blocks away to a soup kitchen to eat.

The following vignettes further describe the range and severity of illness among those often found languishing in shelters, subsisting on streets, or discharged from hospitals.

Thomas R is as fifty-two-year-old man with an open, infected ulcer on his painful swollen leg. For most of his life he worked as a day laborer, usually helping empty trash trucks. Over the past five years TR's legs began to swell by the end of each day. Three months ago he noticed drainage from a small sore on one of his legs. He was not sure whether he had hit the leg against something. TR attempted to keep the area clean, but this was difficult because he lived in a shelter that was open only at night and had no showers.

As the weeks passed, the tiny open area grew into a large ulceration. TR went to a hospital ER where he was treated and given a prescription for an antibiotic. He took the prescription to a pharmacy, but the medication cost fifty-six dollars, and he could not afford to buy it. During the ER visit TR also had been told that he should lie down and rest and that if he did not, he could eventually lose his leg.

Frank L, a sixty-four-year-old postsurgical patient with cancer of the colon, was discharged from a hospital with a prescription to buy colostomy bags. He took the prescription to a pharmacy only to find that the cost was more than he could pay.

After hospitalization FL had planned to return to the rooming house where he previously lived. On his arrival at the house, however, he found that it had burned down. He could not find the person who was to have received his subsistence check while he was hospitalized.

FL went to a shelter where he had lived three years earlier. Staff at the shelter suggested that he return to the hospital to see if he could get more bags there. He was given two bags, the most that could be spared at that time. When these had been used, FL decided to use plastic sandwich bags as a substitute. Because of the ill fit and the leakage of stool onto his skin, he now has a painful, inflamed, weeping area around the colostomy site.

John M is a thirty-three-year-old man with a jaw fracture who was found wandering the streets. He was frantically searching for liquid foods, the only nourishment he could ingest. JM had been staying in a shelter for three years. He was transported most mornings in a van pool to work at various suburban construction sites. With his minimum wage income, however, he could not afford an apartment.

One evening, as he had returned from work, JM had been jumped and robbed by two men outside the shelter. He had managed to get into the shelter. An ambulance was called, and he was taken to an ER. JM had a fractured jaw that required wiring for six weeks. He was given instructions to eat liquid or pureed foods only. Because of the difficulty in getting this type of nourishment, he had lost significant weight.

Ellen H, a fifty-six-year-old woman with a diagnosis of terminal lung cancer, was found living in a shelter. Her life was focused on shuttling between the shelter and the hospital so that she could receive radiation treatment.

EH's primary place for health care for most of her life had been ERs when she felt very ill. For some time she had noticed she had a cough. However, she remembered the long waits and negative experiences encountered during those ER visits and decided to wait and see if the cough would get better. When she began to have chest pain, she went to a public hospital ER, where a chest X ray revealed a probable malignancy. EH was admitted for surgery, which confirmed cancer.

EH lived in an apartment until she became ill. After the surgery, however, she could not work and eventually lost her apartment. She now lives in a shelter and goes to a hospital each day for treatment. The physicians tell her that this will help her pain but will not cure her. Social workers at the shelter are trying to help her get into a nursing home, but this will take some time.

David A is a thirty-year-old man with AIDS. He started using IV drugs when he was fifteen. DA went into a drug treatment program two years ago and has been drug-free since that time. He was living in an efficiency apartment when he began to lose weight and develop a cough.

One night he experienced shortness of breath and a high fever. DA went to an ER, where he was told that he had pneumonia and was admitted. During the hospitalization the diagnosis of AIDS was made, with Pneumocystis carinii pneumonia present. DA, who finally was discharged to his apartment, had hoped to return to work. When it became apparent that he could not work, DA applied for Social Security. It was not sufficient income, however, to pay his rent.

DA was admitted to the hospital again for pneumonia and, this time, discharged to a shelter. He continues to have fever and diarrhea and is losing weight. The shelter where he lives is open only at night, so he tries to go to a public library to sit and rest during the day.

Edward M is a forty-eight-year-old mentally ill man suffering from frostbite who was found trying to get to a soup kitchen. He is a Vietnam veteran who, since his military discharge, has become less able to function. EM has been hospitalized twice with a diagnosis of schizophrenia. After the last discharge from a mental hospital, he did not continue with his follow-up appointments.

For two years EM has lived on the streets. He slept most nights at the bottom of a subway train station, which afforded him some protection from the elements.

When transportation officials decided to erect gates around the station in order to keep people out of this area, EM began to sleep outside on park benches. One morning when EM awakened, his feet felt numb and he had difficulty walking. Eventually he went to an ER, was admitted for three weeks for frostbite of both feet, and then discharged.

A staff person from a shelter found EM trying to walk in the snow to a soup kitchen. He took him to a health service in one of the shelters. EM's feet were black, gangrenous, and oozing. He carried with him a small paper bag with gauzes and tape that had been given to him by the hospital on discharge. EM also carried a note in his jacket with instruction on how to care for his feet: "Change bandages daily." At the bottom of the note was the statement "Toes will eventually fall off."

Basic Policies for a Respite Care Unit

Before the opening of a respite unit, the following matters of policy should be considered.

Admission

It is essential to establish admission protocols before the unit is opened. Without these, the program could result in inappropriate discharges from hospitals and ultimately do more harm than good to the individuals to be served.

The respite unit must agree on the types of medical problems to be handled and the level of care to be offered before admission procedures are developed. Even with well-defined admission policies, however, there will be instances in which individuals require a higher level of care than the unit can provide. New patients, therefore, should be evaluated soon after admission, and the staff must be prepared to send those needing more care back to the hospital.

Medication

A policy concerning medication and its monitoring must be developed. For example, will guests be responsible for taking and keeping their medication, or will the staff? If staff members are involved in dispensing and maintaining medication, they should develop strict guidelines for proper storage and usage.

Medical Backup

There are many variations to medical backup for a respite unit. These may range from a fully staffed medical unit with registered nurses present on each shift and daily physician visits to a unit staffed primarily by shelter personnel with periodic medical team visits. In any case, the respite staff must be able to communicate easily with a medical practitioner. The respite unit should not attempt to duplicate a hospital. Admissions to a hospital can be expeditiously arranged, however, if the physician providing medical backup is affiliated with a hospital.

Discharge Planning and Social Services Support

Protocols for routine as well as emergency discharges from the unit should be developed. Further, persons admitted to the respite unit need to be made aware of the rules and behaviors that will lead to immediate discharge.

There is probably no greater stress for the staff than that arising around decisions for discharge. This issue can lead to splitting the staff because inevitably a guest will become closer to some staff members, while alienating others. Therefore, ongoing staff interaction around discharge decisions is not only helpful but necessary.

The respite unit also should define and determine the level of social services support that will be provided. Issues to be considered are:

- Entitlement acquisition
- Relationship of discharge to housing
- Patient retention pending nursing home availability

Relationships with Hospitals

Every attempt should be made for the respite care staff to develop positive relationships with local hospitals. This provides for good communication when patients are discharged from ERs and inpatient units.

Because hospital staffs are often appreciative of having a respite unit to which they can send homeless patients, they are more likely to readmit individuals if they know that the patients can be referred back to the unit after hospitalization. Good hospital communication also provides for continuum of patient care and information sharing.

Licensure

States vary in regard to requirements for licensure, particularly if dispensing of medication is involved. Regulations for respite care units are slowly being developed; however, for many states no such regulations exist.

Specific Problems Faced by Respite Care Units

Hospital Dumping

Hospital dumping of patients too sick or debilitated to be handled by a respite care unit is a common event. Even when there is consistent, good telephone screening of patients, respite care staffs will face this problem regularly.

A telephone call from an ER concerning a thirty-six-year-old male with cellulitis of his left leg was received by a respite unit staff after normal working hours.

The man had a prior amputation of his right leg because of frostbite. The ER physician thought that hospital admission was not necessary and prescribed a topical antibiotic ointment.

The respite unit agreed to accept the patient, and two hours later the man arrived at the unit. The respite care staff immediately recognized that he had severe frostbite of his left leg with blister formation and swelling. In addition, he had suffered from diarrhea for five days, and since there are few public bathrooms available in the downtown area, he now had raw, inflamed areas on his buttocks and in the genital area.

Arrangements were made for the patient to be admitted to a private hospital. He was treated in an intensive care unit for two days before his condition stabilized enough for physicians to perform an amputation of the left leg.

The staff must send patients back to a hospital when the discharges are inappropriate. To lessen the occurrence of hospital dumping, staff members should inform hospitals of inappropriate discharges and suggest that future respite placements will be limited should this situation recur.[1,2]

Hospice Care

The staff will need to make decisions regarding hospice care for terminally ill patients. If a patient's condition deteriorates to such a degree that the patient requires intense supportive care as well as narcotic pain medication, the need is beyond what can be provided in a respite unit.

The decision may be especially difficult for the patient and staff, particularly if the patient has stayed in the unit for weeks awaiting nursing home placement. Staff and patient may have bonded, and the staff members may be the patient's closest family. However, unless there is a well-thought-out plan of care for dying patients, it is best to think of readmission to a hospice unit.[3]

Elderly Dementia

Homeless people who are demented are a special challenge for respite unit staff.

Arnold G is a seventy-two-year-old man who walked into a shelter one night after apparently having been accosted several days before. He had dried blood with a small laceration on his scalp, as well as swelling and abrasions on his forehead. He also appeared confused; he had no idea where he had been living or how he had come to be at a shelter.

After being seen at a HCHP health service, Mr. G was sent to a hospital ER to rule out the possibility of a significant head injury. An ER physician called the HCHP staff to state that AG would be discharged back to the shelter and that a CAT scan of his brain was normal. The HCHP physician inquired whether the patient appeared confused and was told, "no more confused than any other home-less person that I see."

The HCHP staff believed that AG could not handle his daily needs, particularly in sub-freezing weather, and requested that he be evaluated by a psychiatrist to determine if he was a danger to himself. This was done, and the psychiatrist made a diagnosis of dementia. Despite this, AG was not admitted to the hospital but was discharged back to the respite unit.

AG presented a particular challenge to the staff. The doors of the respite unit are not locked, and guests may come and go at will. One day AG could not be found on the unit, and it was suspected that he had walked away. The police were notified, eventually found him, and returned him to the respite unit.

Although the process for nursing home placement has been started, it will take several months. And AG must be watched very carefully in order to ensure that he does not wander again.

All shelter respite units will be faced with caring for demented individuals. The adult protective services units usually have responsiblity in such cases; however, for most local agencies, no immediate housing is available. The Arnold Gs of the world, therefore, often end up in shelters, and respite staffs need to develop safeguards for them.

Mental Illness

Respite units are often presented with chronically mentally ill patients, such as schizophrenics. Psychiatric consultation can be provided for medication, intervention, and plans for treatment. However, staff members may find that they cannot handle mentally ill patients because they are too disruptive or threatening to themselves and others.

Habib M is a thirty-five-year-old man from Saudi Arabia who came to the United States to attend school. He was treated for cellulitis of his arm by the HCHP mobile van outreach staff one night and rode back with the staff to stay at the respite unit.

It was learned that HM, who had been living on the streets for a year, had been hospitalized in a psychiatric unit for ten days and had recently been discharged to the streets. He had been beaten and now carried a large knife to protect himself.

HM was agitated, paranoid, and demanding, and he angrily warned the respite care staff and guests not to bother him. He was taken to a mental health facility for psychiatric evaluation but refused admission.

There will be times when a decision must be made for the overall benefit of the staff and respite unit. There may be a degree of guilt or failure felt by staff members because they could not handle a difficult person with mental illness.

However, it should be recognized that the respite unit is not an inpatient psychiatric treatment unit.[1]

Substance Abuse

Dealing with people who have substance abuse problems is common. Naturally, as in any health facility, the policy in the respite unit is no alcohol or drugs on the premises. Friction develops around patients who do not adhere to the policy yet have medical conditions so severe that premature discharges because of drinking will exacerbate their illnesses.

Horace G is a fifty-eight-year-old man with pulmonary tuberculosis and cavitary lesions in both lungs. He has been on medication for four weeks and needs several more months of treatment.

HG has been told by the respite staff the rule of no drinking on the unit but has returned to the unit the past two evenings drunk. Although he goes quietly to bed, other patients and staff have become aware of his drinking. To discharge him back to the streets would almost certainly mean that he would not be compliant with his antituberculous medication and eventually become contagious to others.

Hector S is a sixty-four-year-old elderly demented patient awaiting nursing home placement. Although he does not leave the respite unit often, the staff believes that other residents of the unit bring him alcoholic beverages.

HS has been noted to be drinking nearly every day. To discharge him prior to nursing home placement would mean his return to the shelters or streets. However, the staff thinks that HS is too vulnerable to make it on the streets on his own.

Respite staffs will probably find it necessary to make exceptions for certain vulnerable patients. Such decisions may not appear fair when one resident is asked to leave immediately while another is allowed to stay. A psychiatrist consulting on a regular basis with the respite staff may be helpful in allowing staff members to share their feelings about these issues.

The degree to which a respite unit should become a substance abuse treatment program and whether residents should be required to attend AA or NA meetings are issues that need to be discussed. It is important to remember that the primary purpose of a respite unit is to provide care for those who are physically ill.

Detoxification of respite care residents requires written medical protocols. Because a number of homeless persons will be active substance abusers at the time of admission to the unit, medical detoxification will be needed.[4,5]

HIV Disease and Long-Term Care

Respite units will be faced increasingly with calls for admission of people who are ill with HIV disease. The difficulty this presents to the unit is that many of these patients will require long-term care and most likely will never be able to return to the streets or shelters.

A respite unit, therefore, could quickly fill all available beds with individuals needing long-term care and have little room for other residents with short-term needs. This situation, therefore, may demand an advocacy role for staff, to encourage government agencies to provide more respite and long-term care beds for homeless persons.[6]

Examples of Respite Care Units

Christ House

This is a respite care facility for the homeless in Washington, D.C. Initially it was constructed with private funds to renovate a deteriorated four-story apartment building of twenty-four thousand square feet.

The first year of operation, 1986, Christ House was entirely supported by private gifts. The District of Columbia government directly funded 42 percent of the cost for the second year. In 1988, through a subcontract from the HCHP, 70 percent of the operating budget came from local public dollars. The 1989 budget was $859,600, with an approximate cost of $69 per patient day. The 1990 budget is $1,150,000, with an approximate cost per day of $80 per patient. About 52 percent of the budget comes from local public dollars, and the remainder from foundations, individuals, and churches.

FACILITY

The first floor of Christ House includes a dining area, with an adjacent commercial kitchen that seats seventy-two comfortably; administrative offices; a living area for recovering residents; and a clothes closet and shower. The shower room can be used by persons who are homeless and living in the streets.

A small health clinic and pharmacy also occupy the first floor. This area is used by HCHP mobile van outreach team members to treat patients who have been referred to the clinic for more in-depth care.

Located on the second floor of the facility are eight rooms with beds for thirty-four guests. Each room has a sink and an adjacent bathroom. A nursing station is located midway and includes office space, a small lounge area for staff, and a receptionist area. Next to the nursing station is an examination room that has a small whirlpool, used for people with open wounds. Also located on this floor are laundry facilities and a lounge area for recovering patients.

The third and fourth floors of Christ House are the residences of some staff members and their families. In addition, there are rooms for volunteers and a community meeting area.

PROGRAM DESIGN

The original belief by those who planned Christ House was that the care to be provided would be similar to that given if one were convalescing at home. However, because many of the individuals arriving at Christ House—from both shelters and hospitals—were sicker than anticipated, it was decided to adopt a medical program model. Charts similar to those kept in hospitals are developed on each resident, including patient medical history, physical examination, order sheets, progress sheets, and consultant notes.

Eight-hour shifts are staffed by registered nurses. One nurse is primarily responsible for screening telephone calls for admission. If the call is from a hospital, the nurse requests that discharge medical and social services summaries, recent laboratory studies, chest X ray reports, and follow-up appointments be sent along with the patient. Nursing assistants provide care to the guests and are supervised by a registered nurse.

During the day a nurse practitioner serves as the clinical monitor of the floor and completes the initial medical history and physical for each patient. Medication initially is dispensed by the nurses. Most residents are responsible for taking their medicines by the time they are discharged.

Physicians residing at Christ House follow those admitted for care. One doctor is on call at all times, and a psychiatrist is on-site six hours each week for patient consultation and evaluation.

Christ House also offers nonmedical support to its residents. Social workers and a housing coordinator work with the guests to assist in postdischarge planning and acquiring entitlements. A volunteer coordinator and an activities coordinator help provide daily patient activities, such as arts and crafts and social events.

Four AA meetings are held each week. There is also an ego support group led by a psychiatric social worker. Attendance at unit community meetings is required. These meetings provide an opportunity for guests to share and discuss problems—i.e., who chooses what is watched on television.

ADMISSION AND DISCHARGE POLICIES

Admission criteria for Christ House are as follows: The individual is homeless with a physical medical problem, either acute or semiacute, that can be resolved in one week to two months, or the individual is too sick to live on the street or in a shelter but does not need to be hospitalized.

Consideration is also given to those who are elderly, vulnerable, and debilitated from living on the streets or in a shelter. An attempt is made to keep two emergency beds open.

Attention also is given to newly diabetic individuals, those with tuberculosis, and people with AIDS.

As a general rule, those admitted to Christ House must be continent and ambulatory with or without assisting devices, able to get along in a group, and able to follow admission rules and regulations.

Those who need oxygen, suction, feeding tubes, or IVs or are acutely psychotic or severely intoxicated and uncooperative are not eligible for admission.

Discharge policy for Christ House is that:

• Health problem or problems for which the individual was admitted have been resolved or improved enough to allow for movement to another environment.
• Health condition has deteriorated so that hospitalization is needed.

- Individual has been uncooperative with staff and not complied with the rules and regulations for admission.
- Person leaves against medical advice and discharges himself.

HEALTH CARE STATISTICS

There were 1,532 admissions to Christ House between December 1985 and June 1990. In 1989, 376 patients were admitted, with an age range of nineteen to seventy-nine years and a mean age of forty-five years. The average length of stay was thirty days.

In 1988, 334 individuals were seen. A summary of their diagnoses is shown in Table 11.1.

Table 11.1

HEALTH PROBLEM	NUMBER	PERCENT
Ear, eye, nose		2
Respiratory		16
Cardiovascular		11
Peripheral vascular disease		5
Dermatological		13
Neurological		12
Musculoskeletal		19
Gastrointestinal		13
Genitourinary / renal		5
Gunshot and stab wounds		4
Organic brain syndrome	45	
Schizophenia	29	
Amputations	10	
AIDS*	8	

*It should be noted that for the first ninety days of 1989, the number of AIDS patients was seven.

Sixty-two percent of the above individuals discharged were placed in alternative settings (e.g., nursing homes, group homes, their own apartments or rooms, alcoholism and drug treatment programs, and transitional housing).

LICENSURE

Currently Christ House is licensed as a boarding home because there are no regulations in the District of Columbia for respite care units. Prior to the establishment of Christ House, however, detailed descriptions of the types of patients to be served were provided to proper regulatory boards.

NETWORKING WITH HOSPITALS/OTHER AGENCIES

The respite unit staff makes the effort to maintain relationships with attending physicians and specific hospital staff for patients who are discharged to Christ House. This has been found useful, particularly if further admissions are anticipated or if follow-up specialty care is required.

One of the most helpful support systems in Washington, D.C., has been the Catholic archdiocese health care network. This is a volunteer network of more than two hundred physicians who provide pro bono treatment in their offices to low-income and homeless patients.

The staff anticipated that there would be occasions when violence would arise. However, this has rarely occurred at Christ House, perhaps because the facility itself is structurally sound, clean, well maintained, and decorated. Further, the staff has created a surrogate family atmosphere.

Persons who have arrived physically ill and withdrawn often begin to improve in a relatively short period of time.

It is easy to tell when guests are new arrivals at Christ House. They often lie in bed with covers pulled up over their heads and sleep. This is usually because they have been deprived of sleep while in a shelter or on the streets.

Another residual response from life on the streets occurs at mealtime. Often newly arrived residents heap their plates with food until they realize that each time they go for a refill, there is still food.

Another experience has been to see people discover or reclaim creative or artistic talents that have long been dormant, to see some who felt hopeless on arrival begin, little by little, to regard themselves as worthwhile individuals and start to express dreams and hopes.

A guest staying at Christ House after having lost parts of both feet to frostbite was sharing a meal with a visitor. In their conversation, the visitor expressed sorrow that the resident had lost his toes. The guest's response was: "No, don't feel sorry about my toes. It took me to lose my toes in order to gain my life."

The Shattuck Hospital Shelter Respite Unit—Boston

This unit was started in 1985 as part of the HCHP. The program provides care for homeless individuals who are too ill to be on the street each day but who do not need to be hospitalized.

The objectives of the program are to:

- Establish a facility where individuals can recuperate from illness and maintain regimes required to regain health
- Coordinate the operation of the facility with ongoing medical and shelter programs of the community
- Provide advocacy, counseling, and social services to assist individuals in the processes of stabilization and reintegration

A 20-bed respite unit was set up within the 180-bed Shattuck Shelter to provide a recuperative, supportive environment for homeless individuals. The unit staff consists of a nurse practitioner, a physician, a social worker, and three nurse's aides, working with the assistance of shelter employees—a psychiatric nurse, a substance abuse counselor, a social worker, recreational and expressive therapists, a physician assistant, and a coordinator.

A nurse practitioner and a physician make daily rounds and provide twenty-four-hour on-call coverage. Nursing aides give hands-on care under the nurse practitioner's supervision, and a social worker ensures that guests receive benefits and coordinates resources and discharge planning. Case conferences involving all providers are held weekly to review and update each patient's condition, exchange information, and discuss discharge plans.

ANCILLARY SERVICES

Ancillary services are provided through the Shattuck Hospital. They include outpatient diagnosis and treatment, physical and occupational therapies, an after-hours emergency clinic, dental and podiatry care, AA and NA meetings, and medical diets.

ADMISSIONS

Approval for admission to the respite unit lies with the nurse practitioner and the physician. Each referral is reviewed and the decision is based on established criteria and unit capacity to provide care.

HEALTH CARE STATISTICS

There have been more than 700 admissions since the fall of 1985, with an average stay of more than two weeks. During the period of January 1987 through February 1988 the diagnoses among 240 admissions were as shown in Table 11.2.

It is important to note here that although most of the listed categories have remained constant, the incidence of infectious disease has continued to rise with the increase in HIV-related problems.

REFERRALS

The largest referral source has been local hospitals. Other community shelters, detoxification units, and service agencies also have utilized the program.

Table 11.2

HEALTH PROBLEM	PERCENT
Orthopedic	30
Dermatological (cellulitis, ulcers, burns, frostbite)	23
Surgical	14
Infectious diseases	13
Chronic diseases	6
Cardiovascular	5
Neurological	4
Gastrointestinal and gynecological	2

Social services data from January 1987 through February 1988 indicate a placement rate of 42 percent of the 240 admissions. Individuals were placed in nursing homes, in halfway houses, in rooms in houses and apartments and with families and friends.

During the same period 42 percent of the homeless individuals received entitlements. Another 51 percent had benefits in place at the time of admission.

Denver Respite Care Program

STOUT STREET CLINIC (SSC)

The SSC, operated by the HCHP of Denver, Colorado, established the Respite Care Program in September 1986. The program, which is sponsored in collaboration with Samaritan House, the largest shelter in Denver, offers a clean, safe, and humane environment for homeless people needing time to recover from medical or surgical illnesses.

The SSC is a primary-care multidisciplinary clinic. It provides a full spectrum of health services to homeless men, women, and children and has had more than forty-five thousand patient encounters from its opening in May 1985 through July 1989. Samaritan House is an emergency shelter with a 250-bed capacity. It serves men, women, and families in a facility built for this purpose in 1986. Samaritan House offers twenty-four-hour-a-day housing, food, and social services support to homeless persons. Medical treatment and oversight for these individuals are provided by SSC staff.

PROGRAM DESIGN

The Respite Care Program began initially when Samaritan House agreed to reserve on a daily basis ten male and three female beds for respite patients. Persons admitted to the program include:

- Individuals who have been inpatients in area hospitals and are homeless. They must be able to use bathrooms, be capable of self-care, and not be violent.
- Persons who have a reasonable chance of recovery to full independence within four weeks.
- Individual who do not need oxygen or other specialized equipment or highly specialized diets.
- Stout Street Clinic patients who need rest and intermittent treatment—e.g., dressing changes or foot elevation.

All referrals for the respite program are through the medical staff at the SSC. In cases of posthospitalization care, a primary-care provider contacts the SSC medical staff to describe the patient's needs and present condition. If the Respite Care Program is appropriate, the patient is sent to the SSC with a discharge summary and other medical history. Transportation to the clinic is provided.

A historical review and physical examination are performed on each individual before admission. If the staff finds that the patient is not appropriate for respite care or has been discharged prematurely, the hospital is notified and the patient sent back with a written reason for refusal to the program.

It the program can be beneficial, the respite staff notifies Samaritan House that a new patient is being admitted. A respite care summary form, signed by a medical staff person, is sent with the individual to the shelter.

PROGRAM EXPERIENCES

Individuals placed in the Denver respite program have ranged from a three-month-old child post-heart surgery to a twenty-six-year-old dialysis patient; from a sixty-one-year-old man with unresectable lung cancer to a fifty-two-year-old man with compromised venous stasis disease; from a twenty-three-year-old patient with AIDS to a thirty-year-old man with severe frostbite of toes that eventually resulted in amputation; from an alcoholic waiting to enter a treatment program to patients with pneumonia, uncontrolled diabetes, and active untreated tuberculosis.

Summary

The development of respite care has evolved from recognition that neither the streets nor the shelters are an appropriate environment for those who are ill. Shelters throughout the nation have become the dumping ground for acutely and chronically ill individuals. Many of these people have health conditions that could be reversed with nothing more than rest in a protected environment where food and simple basic care are available.

Respite programs also demonstrate that a health crisis in a homeless person's life can be and often is the preceptor of change that moves a person out of homelessness. Time spent in a respite unit creates an opportunity for providers and homeless individuals to make extraordinary strides toward independence and breaking the cycle of homelessness.

BARRY BLACKWELL
WILLIAM BREAKEY
DONALD HAMMERSLEY
ROGER HAMMOND
MARSHA MCMURRAY-AVILA
CHRISTINE SEEGER

12

Psychiatric and Mental Health Services

Introduction

The relationship between homelessness and mental illness is complex. Public attitudes toward the mentally ill, the lack of expertise in community mental health centers, the minimal resources devoted to provision of services for the mentally ill, and the inadequate housing and income support for poor people all contribute to homelessness. So do the special characteristics of mentally ill persons, which render them vulnerable when times are hard. Helping the homeless mentally ill thus requires a variety of strategies, system-focused or client-focused. System-focused strategies include administrative, financial, and political efforts to create better systems of care for the mentally ill. The role of the health professional in informing public opinion, advocating on behalf of the homeless mentally ill, and empowering homeless persons to act on their own behalf is critical if system changes are to occur. Client-focused approaches deal with the personal needs of individuals for treatment, support, and rehabilitation. Clinical services for the homeless mentally ill are an essential component in any health service for the homeless, and the provision of these services is the focus of this discussion.

The discussion is divided into three sections. First is an overview of who the mentally ill and homeless are, an exploration of why they are homeless, and a brief description of how programs to assist them have evolved. Second is a detailed description of the contemporary mental health service delivery system that appears most effective for this population based on the authors' personal experience discussed in relation to a rapidly growing literature. Lastly, there is a brief summary and conclusion.

Overview and Evolution of Mental Health Services

Who Are the Mentally Ill and Homeless?

The accurate determination of who and how many are mentally ill among the homeless is difficult because of problems of definition and epidemiologic methodology.[1,2] There have been a number of surveys and research projects.[3,4] In addition, there are several excellent reviews on the topic.[4,5]

Diagnostically and demographically the mentally ill and homeless are a heterogeneous group, varying between cities and in duration of homelessness. The prevalence of psychiatric disorders in the homeless is many times higher than in the domiciled. Substance abuse, personality disorder, affective disorder, schizophrenia, and developmental handicaps are among the most frequent diagnoses, in declining order.[6] Comorbidity and complicating medical problems are common. Major mental illnesses such as schizophrenia and bipolar disorder occur in 30 to 40 percent, and as many as three-quarters of those with mental illness may have a history of problems with alcohol.[7]

A majority of mentally ill homeless persons are under forty and male, although females are an increasing segment of the population. Minorities are proportionately overrepresented.[4] The degree of transience is variable, may differ between cities, and can give rise to subpopulations that pose different treatment problems.[8]

Why Are the Mentally Ill Homeless?

Homelessness is multiply determined, contributed to by both socioeconomic and clinical factors. The former includes societal problems such as increasing poverty, reduced availability of low-income housing, and lack of affordable health care that are not unique to the mentally ill but that may affect them as a vulnerable population. Some socioeconomic factors have a more specific impact upon the mentally ill; they include stringent eligibility rules or long waits for disability benefits and neighborhood resistance to group homes.

Particular to the mentally ill have been several effects of deinstitutionalization.[9–14] Its impact has been debated,[15] but in one state hospital 35 percent of patients released became homeless within three months.[16] However, by no means have all the mentally ill among the homeless been institutionalized, and some have had no contact with the mental health system.[17]

Widespread closure of mental hospital beds led to a reduction of the hospitals' capacity to provide asylum to the disabled, with both good and bad connotations.[18] At the same time the provision of adequate community support has been limited by the failure of community mental health centers to attend to the needs of the chronic population, by failure to shift resources from institutions into the community, by failure to develop new support programs,[19] and by absence of attention to linkages between agencies.[20] The need for, but the lack of, community residential facilities has been clearly defined.[21]

From a clinical viewpoint it is possible to see how individuals with the psychiatric illnesses mentioned above might have difficulties obtaining support when both societal and medical resources are inadequate and poorly integrated. As a population they display poor social skills, thinking and judgment clouded by psychosis or substance abuse, behaviors that often appear bizarre, and impulses that may be poorly controlled. Not only do these difficulties diminish the capability to garner scarce resources, but they also invite discrimination and stereotyping.

Finally, the plight of the homeless who are mentally ill has been unwittingly worsened in some states by commitment laws that discourage involuntary treatment until violence is imminent or has occurred. It is easier to arrest those who behave bizarrely than to get them into psychiatric care. Coupled with the lack of mental health services, this has contributed to criminalization of the chronic mentally ill.[22,23] In Albuquerque, New Mexico, a survey comparing the mentally ill homeless with other homeless individuals found that the mentally ill homeless had more often been in jail (80 vs. 64 percent) or had been the victims of crime (77 vs. 58 percent).[7]

Whatever difficulties mental illness imposes or compounds, its presence is neither a necessary nor a sufficient cause for homelessness. Many homeless persons are not mentally ill, and only a minority of the mentally ill are homeless.

The process of becoming homeless involves disconnection from family or friends. Not surprisingly, a common characteristic commented on by those who work with homeless individuals is the problem of alienation or difficulty with affiliation evident in interpersonal relationships and in relationships with social agencies. This problem is contributed to by an overwhelmed social service system which often exposes the homeless to frustrating and dehumanizing experiences, by stigmatization and the social circumstances of homelessness, by psychiatric illness, and perhaps by psychological difficulties based on earlier developmental trauma.

Homeless persons are often easy to identify because of their poverty, the fact they frequently must carry all their possessions with them, and because of the difficulty they face in maintaining personal hygiene as the result of the lack of facilities. This high visibility and this low socioeconomic position isolate them and invite discrimination or stigmatization, manifested by their being banned from public places or simply objectified and ignored by the public and passersby.

Homeless persons are vulnerable to the dangers of crime and victimization. They often express fears of being beaten, attacked, robbed, or raped. This leads them to be careful of whom they talk to or where they stay. In some cities women prefer shelters to hotels because of the crime rate and isolation in the latter. Even in the relatively safe environment of a stable San Francisco shelter, women who have seen each other for months or even years avoid speaking to one another.

Although not peculiar to those who are mentally ill, an inability to affiliate is sometimes a component or product of psychiatric disorders. Psychotic conditions complicate family dynamics in the community, and certain personality types, such as borderline, antisocial, paranoid, or schizoid, occur relatively frequently among the homeless and are characterized by difficulties with attachment. Substance abuse often results in loss of affiliative supports through family rifts and unemployment. C. T. Mowbray and her colleagues found that in Detroit 70 percent of those who were homeless on admission to a state hospital had become so at a time of family breakup, rejection, or crisis.[24]

Problems of affiliation among the homeless may have a developmental origin in some cases. One study of the early experiences of homeless men[25] found a high frequency of separation and delinquency during childhood. A case control comparison of homeless with housed women[26] found that those who became homeless had been physically abused eight times more often than the control women (42 vs. 5 percent). Another survey found that 18 percent of homeless women in Albuquerque had histories of sexual abuse.[7]

Until this issue is examined more fully, the prevalence and cause of problems with affiliation among the homeless will remain speculative but may presumably stem from the realities of homelessness, from the manifestations of substance abuse and mental illness, or perhaps from an abusive or nonnurturant upbringing. A theoretical model has been proposed to explore these etiologic factors and study their therapeutic implications.[27] Based on three years of research in Austin, Texas, this model distinguishes between types of homelessness and describes the process leading from precipitating circumstances to weakening of resources, disaffiliation, and entrenchment. The model also identifies barriers to service delivery and makes suggestions to overcome them.

Evolution of Mental Health Services for the Homeless

Concern about the mental health needs of the homelessness began to mount in the early 1980's as managers of shelters and meal sites experienced increasing behavioral problems and untreated psychiatric illness among clients. Observers of skid rows noted that mentally ill men were starting to outnumber alcoholics. Another impetus at least locally was the National Institute of Mental Health epidemiologic catchment area study that exposed the scope of psychiatric problems in homeless men in Baltimore.[28]

Those concerned about the plight of the mentally ill homeless turned first to the agencies and institutions that provide traditional services, but the response was often hampered by the same difficulties that had helped create the problem. Access was impeded by long waiting lists and a catchment area mentality. The limited funds available were assigned to existing agencies for conventional services that restricted workers to selected sites or targeted assistance to segments of the population for specific interventions.

As individuals or groups began to appreciate the complex multiple needs of the homeless and their problems with traditional services, a few cities started to experiment with case managers and outreach teams. They began to identify the need for on-site multidisciplinary and integrated services.[29,30]

These pioneer efforts remained patchy and poorly documented until the RWJF/Pew launch of the HCHP in 1985. Initially the primary target for these projects was physical illness, and it was again assumed that psychiatric needs would be met from existing services. Experience proved otherwise. The mental health needs of homeless persons were often compounded and intertwined with physical illness, substance abuse, developmental handicaps, and social deprivation. For the teams examining and treating these clients, mental health concerns often were buried beneath, but interfered with, a hierarchy of more basic needs.

As data accumulated and were exchanged, a consensus began to develop. Supplemental local and state funds were sought to provide the range of services described in the next section. The availability of federal funds through the McKinney Homeless Assistance Act since 1988 should begin to make it possible to implement this system of care on a wider, national scale. Because of the variability among populations of homeless persons in different cities or states, accurate planning and efficient delivery of services can be facilitated by a local needs assessment survey of the type conducted in Albuquerque.[7]

Contemporary Mental Health Services

. . . one may reasonably expect that at some time or other the conscience of the community will awake and admonish it that the poor man has just as much right to help for his mind. . . . The task will then arise for us to adapt our techniques to the new conditions. Possibly we may often be able to achieve something if we combine aid to the mind with material support.
— Sigmund Freud, Address to the Fifth International Psychoanalytic Conference, Budapest, 1918

Among the more recent and rapidly growing literature on homelessness there remains a dearth of information or advice on psychiatric treatment. A task force of the American Psychiatric Association was appointed to address this issue in 1983 and published its recommendations three years later.[31] These included availability of supervised community housing and general medical care as well as comprehensive and accessible psychiatric services, a system of case management, and coordination between community agencies. The gap between these laudable goals and the reality is illustrated by an article on treatment planning[32] that describes the fragmentation of care and failure of traditional services to meet the needs of a mentally ill patient in a community shelter.

The lessons learned in the Johnson / Pew projects are just now being distilled[4] and are beginning to appear in print as specific guidelines for clinical care.[33] These pay attention both to the principles that underlie the provision of services and to the components of an effective service delivery system.

Principles of Clinical Practice

If a core characteristic of the homeless is disaffiliation, a key component to an effective program for the mentally ill is promotion of bonding or attachment to facilitate therapeutic and social relationships.

Several features of both providers and programs foster this. Involving clients in the self-assessment of their own needs is a first step.[34] Bonding often begins as basic material needs are met through attention to food, clothing, and a safe place to sleep while mental health needs may be low on the client's list of priorities. The providers who strive to get these needs met must possess a positive attitude toward the poor, mentally ill, and homeless that is free from stigmatizing or stereotyped thinking that blames them for their predicament. Empathy based on an appreciation of powerlessness is essential. Culture, social class, or professional status can create barriers unless workers are accessible and comfortable mingling with the homeless. An often extreme lack of trust is repaired only by extraordinary patience. Assistance may be perceived as an intrusion. First (second and third) offers of help are often rejected. Workers among the homeless present options, not solutions, and employ an approach that is respectful of the homeless person's need for space and distance. Acceptance of small goals and a high threshold for frustration are important. Creative, innovative, or unusual approaches are often a key to success.

The promotion of bonding is central to both personnel selection and program design. Workers who succeed have a deep commitment to serving the disadvantaged and display persistence, nurturance, and pragmatism. Those who persevere are often self-selected by these fundamental human characteristics and by resistance to burnout as much as by formal education or training. Programs that succeed are built on case management and networking principles that stress continuity and integration of services. They are best conceptualized as providing levels of care rather than by discipline or location.

Direct Clinical Services

As with the population at large, the bulk of mental health needs to the homeless are met by providers who are not specifically designated as mental health workers, such as paraprofessionals, nurses, physicians, and social workers. As is also the case with the general population, there may be a reluctance by the patient to seek or accept a mental health referral, possibly reinforced by past experiences of real or imagined harm at the hands of the mental health care system. More important may be the many barriers that exist to obtain psychiatric care. These include discrimination or stigma, assumptions of untreatability, and difficult or delayed access to conventional services, creating unrealistic hurdles for people living in chaotic circumstances and struggling to survive. What is different from the general population is the frequency and severity of psychiatric problems, the degree to which they interfere with an ability to meet basic health care and human welfare needs, and the extent to which mental illness is complicated by the existential predicament of the homeless person. Depression, anxiety, and sleeplessness may be reactive to or worsened by the loss and deprivation coupled with becoming or being homeless. Paranoid feelings, autistic withdrawal, and a secretive reluctance to share personal information are accompaniments of or amplified by the dangerous, hostile environment of the streets. Cognitive impairment may be exacerbated by malnutrition and untreated medical conditions.

All the above factors affect the function of the mental health professional, who must understand the role of the other health providers and support them as part of a multidisciplinary team through in-service education and on-site availability as well as by more traditional expert help on referral. The task is to care for the mental health of all the homeless, not just the mental illness of some.

Three levels of care can be conceptualized in meeting these mental health needs. First is a frontline outreach function that seeks people on the streets and at congregating sites; next are the multidisciplinary clinical services provided at clinics, shelters, drop-in centers, and meal sites; and last is a spectrum of psychiatric services available at clinics or on referral. These levels must be coordinated and integrated, and all must apply the same basic principles of care outlined above.

FRONT LINE (OUTREACH) TEAMS

Outreach was recommended by the American Psychiatric Association as the logical response to the reluctance shown by the chronic mentally ill and homeless to seek traditional office or hospital care.[15,35] The mobile outreach team in Milwaukee was among the first to be fully developed and studied carefully.[36] The team uses a mobile van which daily tours the shelters, meal sites, and other congregating areas around the inner city. Its members are chosen for attributes that lessen social distance from clients, and they use strategies of relationship building and power sharing designed to create trust. Team members function as case finders, case managers, and advocates, dealing with multiple problems, meeting basic needs, and providing linkages between the clients and disparate parts of the human resource system. Its members maintain sustained contact with clients placed in various outreach programs (such as the correctional services homeless program) and often organize and engage in social activities with their clients, such as movies, bowling, picnics, and shopping.

Of those individuals whom this team encountered on five or more occasions, 42 percent had substance abuse problems, 44 percent were chronically mentally ill, and 8 percent had dual diagnoses. Of a smaller and still more select group of thirty individuals who had been known to the outreach team for an average of six months, all but two had a mental disability. Eleven had major psychiatric diagnoses (primarily schizophrenia); ten, diagnoses of alcoholism; two, diagnoses of mental retardation; and five, dual diagnoses of chronic mental illness and alcoholism. Almost two-thirds had been treated previously for psychiatric problems.

The following illustrates the type of client found among this chronically ill population and the approach taken by the staff:

———————

Mike H was referred to the outreach team by a waitress from a coffee shop on the outskirts of the city. When he was first seen, his appearance was rough and dirty, his clothes were disheveled, and he emitted a foul body odor. Mike explained that he had been on the streets for almost twelve years and that he was trapped there by evil spirits and demons that made up the "masonry of the universe." They kept him from leaving the boundaries of a four-block area within which he slept in a sleeping bag on the steps of a local church.

The outreach team visited Mike two or three times weekly, taking food and candy, often buying him coffee. They sat with him on the sidewalk, listening, offering advice, and coaxing him to venture in the van outside his area. On one occasion a team member shared the food Mike had retrieved from a Dumpster.

Little by little over many months the team members gained his trust; he became more comfortable with them and seemed to look forward to their visits.

The team's next step was to obtain Social Security benefits. A field representative met Mike in the coffee shop and completed the paper work. Next the team found a psychiatrist willing to conduct an evaluation outside his office. Attracted by the possibility of obtaining income, Mike agreed, and they met on a downtown street corner within Mike's "safe zone." The psychiatrist confirmed a diagnosis of paranoid schizophrenia. Among other things Mike told him: "I see eyeballs and stuff; heads and eyeballs just hanging there. Spirits tell me the bodies are controlled by computers, just sad soul-destroying things. The bodies are preengineered."

As Mike's trust in the team grew, he ventured outside the boundaries of his domain and agreed to accept a community support program as his payee after Social Security was awarded. Once in the program, he agreed to take medication, and he is now stabilized and living in housing. The street outreach team continues to see Mike weekly and finds that he has now made other friends whom he visits regularly.

Sometimes the work with the chronically mentally ill involves families and children.

Shirley M and her husband, both white and in their early forties, arrived during the summer from out of state with their twin infant daughters and were first seen in a temporary shelter. Shirley had a history of chronic mental illness and was taking fluphenazine and lithium. The initial five contacts over the next six weeks were devoted to finding summer clothing, milk, and diapers for the children, obtaining food stamps and financial aid for the adults, providing transportation, and seeking low-income housing. Also included were a medical examination and a contact with a psychiatric nurse, who made a diagnosis of bipolar disorder and obtained a referral to the outpatient clinic at the country mental health center. A serum lithium level was elevated, and the client was counseled about dosage. As the family was placed in permanent housing, the outreach team maintained contact, ensured compliance with outpatient psychiatric follow-up, recommended parenting classes, and encouraged the spouse to enroll in a job-retraining program.

A particular concern of the outreach team is the problem of social distance presented by minorities who are mentally ill. Although members of the team represent the major cultural groups in our society, in order to provide expert care, they must interact with other providers who are almost exclusively white, middle-class males. This undoubtedly amplifies the existing problems of affiliation among the homeless chronically mentally ill.[37]

Luis R, a thirty-six-year-old Hispanic male, was first seen in a shelter after arriving from another city. Although he was bilingual, he refused to speak except in Spanish. Luis was obviously mentally ill but agreed to see the psychiatric nurse at the shelter site only after a number of contacts with the Spanish-speaking outreach worker, who acted as a translator. Eventually, after accepting treatment with medication, Luis moved out from the shelter when he became aware of the Hispanic community and found housing with Spanish-speaking friends.

As an index of the overall success of one outreach team, the status of the homeless individuals at the time of their first and last encounters with the mobile team was contrasted.[36] Of particular note is that one-third of the clients were placed in some form of community support program and that those refusing medical treatment had declined from two-thirds to a quarter. While these results are gratifying, this study provides a cautionary note concerning the limitations of outreach. It should not be regarded as a ruse for removing mentally ill homeless persons from the inner city and its success can be hampered by problems obtaining access to both acute-care facilities and long-term support in mental health programs which are often overloaded with existing patients.

One of the first experiences of the team was with Paul T, who frequented a variety of alleys, abandoned cars, and a freeway underpass. Neither worker was able to make headway, and when Paul did allow the workers to get close enough to talk, his speech contained a high level of delusional and paranoid thought. The workers continued seeing Paul over a period of several months until he revealed that he had been in a psychiatric hospital in the past, had taken medications, and remembered feeling better at those times. The team offered to accompany him to a local psychiatric hospital, and at the next meeting Paul said he was ready to go. Excitedly the team helped him into the van for the trip. The team explained the circumstances to the hospital staff and waited nearby while Paul was examined. That day was probably the low point for the team members as they heard, "Perhaps the man is mentally ill, but he doesn't need acute psychiatric care." Having no other option at this point, they returned the man to the alley where they had found him earlier in the day. When the team obtained administrative approval for admission, Paul refused to return to the hospital, but after several more attempts he agreed to try again. This time he was found to be in need of acute psychiatric care.

MULTIDISCIPLINARY CLINICAL SERVICES AT MEAL SITES, SHELTERS, AND DROP-IN CENTERS

Homeless health care providers may expect 40 percent of their patients to have mental illness, and many more will have emotional problems of some sort consequent to their homelessness.[6] A very significant mental health treatment role is played by lay workers in shelters and meal sites, by nurses and physicians in medical clinics, and by social workers who function as case managers. This includes recognizing mental illness and obtaining care, supervising ongoing treatment with psychotropic medications, and coping with the manifestations of psychiatric disorders in their day-to-day work, often by patients who refuse to accept traditional treatment. The latter involves providing support and counsel to those with anxiety and depressive disorders.

Although distinguishing the symptoms of mental illness from those that result from the predicament of homelessness is difficult, the extended contact afforded by casework function and the trust engendered by meeting the patient's basic needs often allow these distinctions to be made. Obtaining a more expert psychiatric assessment may tax the persuasive powers and persistence of nonmental health workers and often requires them either to be present at an on-site consultation or personally to accompany the patient to a psychiatric clinic or emergency room. In psychiatric terms, the primary care worker serves as a transitional object to bind the patient's anxiety at the entry point to a new or threatening situation.

Particularly difficult are the times when mental illness is so severe as to make it impossible to meet basic needs, establish a relationship, or obtain benefits. Often help comes only through ingenuity or when chance or disaster intervenes.

Alice N is a fifty-year-old white woman with chronic mania, known to outreach clinic workers for several years. She repeatedly declined offers of psychiatric treatment, was unable to use her benefits for self-care, refused to move from the streets, and was finally raped in a city park. Only then was Alice taken by the police to a psychiatric hospital for treatment. Once she was committed by the courts for treatment, major tranquilizers calmed her sufficiently that the caseworker who visited her on the wards and followed her back to the streets was then able to persuade her to use her benefits more wisely and move into housing.

Once ongoing psychiatric care is obtained, the primary care provider may play a vital role in supervising its continuation. This includes psychotropic drug taking, interpreting side effects, and facilitating compliance with both treatment regimens and keeping outpatient appointments. An important task is to explain and help simplify the treatment regimen to fit within the often chaotic life circumstances of the homeless individual. It is obviously important to have a safe place to sleep and to secure personal possessions before one takes a sedative drug. "Three times a day with meals" is a dubious instruction when a place to eat or even obtaining food is in doubt.

Apart from a role in seeking and maintaining psychiatric treatment, the primary care practitioner has to cope constantly with the emotional problems or manifestations of mental illness in clients, some of whom may decline treatment. Many workers possess the innate skills to do this while others benefit from in-service education, on-site consultation, and support groups provided by mental health professionals who function as part of the on-site multidisciplinary team.

The effective provision of such support by mental health professionals benefits from a healthy amount of common sense and creativity as well as experience with how primary care practitioners function. Approaches that have been developed in hospital or private office settings may not be applicable in an environment where resources are limited. For example, in-service education about the management of violence must deal with the reality that security guards, restraints, and adequate numbers of trained colleagues are not available. More appropriate is advice on how to defuse the threat of aggression in a dyadic encounter by shifting the focus of the patient's concerns to realistic origins. Other valuable topics for in-service education include the symptoms and manifestations of psychiatric disorders, the management of psychiatric emergencies, the benefits and side effects of psychotropic drugs, ways in which to foster compliance, commitment, and guardianship procedures, stress management principles for care providers, and the setting of limits for manipulative behaviors, substance abuse, or sexual acting out.

Support groups for primary care providers may deal with diverse issues. These include the danger of burnout, the difficult nature of the work with its minimal rewards, the value of humor in dealing with tough situations, and ways to mobilize personal support. The death of clients because of disease, violence, or exposure is a distressingly common topic and a source of anger and mourning. Conflicts among workers, teams, and hierarchical figures have been dealt with. Generally, health care workers among the homeless are sensitive to issues of power, value consensus building and shared decision making, but are wary and resentful of any arbitrary misuse of authority.

Finally, the availability of psychiatric consultation on-site is an invaluable asset to nonmental health workers, particularly around such issues as the degree of proximity that the patient will allow or the interpretation of transference situations.

Ken N is a fifty-five-year-old white male who never married and was first seen by a social worker at the meal site because he was the friend of another male client. After two months as an observer of his friend's interactions with the social worker, Ken ventured to discuss his own predicament. He had been on the streets for six years, sleeping in the daytime and spending nights in all-night cafés. He bathed once every three months, changed his clothes annually, and seldom attended to his inch-long nails or shoulder-length hair. The social worker preferred to meet him in the open and learned to breathe through her mouth. Despite his eccentric behavior and appalling hygiene, Ken was usually sober, conversed in a highly intelligent way, and gave no sign of psychotic thinking. Although he agreed to seek Social Security benefits, the agent had to come to the shelter in order to interview him. Ken agreed to talk to a psychiatrist only after seeing him several times at the meal site and sitting together with both the social worker and the psychiatrist. He revealed no evidence of psychosis, but talked of a disturbed childhood and a hostile, dependent relationship with an abusive single-parent mother. He appeared to fit the characteristics of a borderline personality disorder. While awaiting his benefits, Ken told his social worker that he had become enraged with his roommate, had slashed all his possessions with a knife, and had attempted to set fire to his own genitals with lighter fuel. The social worker felt frightened and discussed her concern with the psychiatrist. After Supplemental Security Income was awarded, the social worker was made the payee for benefits. Ken became increasingly angry in interviews, and the supportive relationship was quickly spoiled with control struggles. Ken was ultimately abusive and avoidant, disappearing for long periods on the street. The psychiatrist discussed the shift in dynamics resulting from the payee relationship and the displaced anger from Ken's disturbed upbringing. As a result, the social worker relinquished the payee responsibility, and Ken is now seen by male workers on the outreach team who maintain intermittent contact and supervise his health care needs. In a written explanation of his needs to Social Security, Ken stated, "I fear, at times, of not suppressing my extreme feelings of hostility and rage, which would result in violent external action. I don't have tolerance or patience for adverse circumstances and people."

THE SPECTRUM OF PSYCHIATRIC SERVICES

A fundamental aspect to adequate psychiatric care for the homeless is to provide and create access to a spectrum of services linked to each other and extending from emergency or on-site evaluations and acute care to outpatient and community support in a variety of rehabilitative programs.

Access and Linked Care: Access and linked care are facilitated by engaging mental health staff familiar with or employed by existing services with dedicated time available for homeless patients. This focus particularly is needed for those who have not yet obtained or are ineligible for benefits and care in the private sector. Health care agencies serving the homeless may obtain such services by independent contract or purchase them from existing state or county institutions and mental health centers.[38] The following example illustrates the difficulty of providing coordinated care for severely disabled people and shows how a psychiatrist with knowledge about the homeless can function in providing access to care and facilitating linkage between systems.

Bill W is a thirty-seven-year-old white male first contacted by the outreach team during a hot summer when he was living on a park bench because this was "his job." He wore a heavy coat and soiled clothes, was starving and dehydrated. After daily contact with an outreach staff had provided him with food and fluid for six weeks, Bill agreed to be seen at the county medical complex, where he was found to have active tuberculosis involving his spine, an organic confusional state of uncertain etiology, and schizophrenia. When his medical workup was complete, Bill was discharged back to the streets, still confused and psychotic with a complex regimen of antituberculous and antipsychotic medication. On his first night he returned to an emergency room complaining he had suffered a stroke and was admitted to a psychiatric unit. After two weeks Bill was still confused but less psychotic and was discharged into the care of the outreach team to be transported to a shelter. While the team was filling his prescriptions at a pharmacy, he wandered away and was lost for six weeks. During this time he was seen repeatedly in the emergency room but diagnosed as "malingering" and sent away. The emergency room was not aware of his inpatient admission and failed to notify the outreach team of his visits. Finally Bill appeared at the community support pro-

gram. He was agitated and crawling around the floor. The mental health outreach nurse accompanied him to the mental health center, where he was readmitted. The inpatient staff kept him for a brief stay and was preparing to discharge him again to a shelter when the psychiatrist for the homeless intervened. On the basis of information from the outreach team, the emergency rooms, the psychiatric nurse, and the inpatient unit, the psychiatrist insisted on and obtained placement in a long-term residential facility, where Bill's complex medical and psychiatric condition could be properly cared for in a protected environment.

On-Site Services: As discussed earlier, it is important to have mental health providers who are available to any of the shelters, meal sites, and drop-in centers or who can travel at short notice to meet patients or primary care providers. They conduct clinics simultaneously with internists, social workers, or nurses, facilitating immediate cross referrals and consultation. Between seeing patients and at slack times, the mental health professionals can mingle with lay volunteers and the homeless. Visibility and familiarity are important in facilitating a willingness to seek help.

In addition to providing support to the multidisciplinary team, mental health staff members who function on-site at clinics and shelters primarily serve a diagnostic or triage function to channel patients into existing services. However, they also inevitably provide a holding capability to buffer the long waiting lists at other facilities as well as to care for severely psychotic or indigent patients who refuse or are ineligible for treatment elsewhere. An important aspect in providing this care is the availability of an immediate supply of psychotropic drugs and special funds for their purchase. In treating patients who are unattached elsewhere the psychiatrist collaborates closely with whichever lay person or professional has developed a primary relationship with the patient, who may be able to foster treatment compliance.

Another virtue of on-site availability is the capacity to participate in crisis care and emergency intervention, either by making appropriate referrals or by direct involvement.

Betty W is a thirty-eight-year-old black woman with chronic paranoid schizophrenia who often traveled between cities in the state, living on the streets and in shelters. Her delusions made her distrustful of even the most dedicated caseworkers and clinicians. One day she collapsed on the library steps with a pulmonary embolus. In intensive care she refused all treatment, accused the staff of being demons injecting her with "ground-up black babies," and was placed in restraints to prevent her from ripping out her intravenous tubes. The psychiatrist working with the homeless knew of her admission and consulted on her care, participating in an emergency guardianship hearing. He recommended the use of intravenous psychotropic medication, along with anticoagulants, and this resulted in the gradual disappearance of Betty's psychotic thinking and delusional system.

Before discharge, contact was made by the psychiatrist with her caseworker at the shelter where the psychiatrist also worked. This ensured continued treatment, and the change in mental status and behavior was remarkable to everyone who had perviously known Betty on the streets.

A final possibility is the on-site provision of programs or groups for targeted problems or populations. Several authors[39–42] have emphasized the special needs of women, and in Albuquerque a women's support group has been formed.[7] Special attention has been paid to mothers with children,[43] to dealing with parenting, anger and conflict management, codependency, and addiction. Individual counseling is available to victims of incest and domestic violence. Other possible subgroups with special problems that can benefit from targeted support include HIV-positive clients,[44] adolescent youths[45–47] and the elderly.[48]

Acute Inpatient Care: Episodes of inpatient care are inevitable among the homeless but can certainly be minimized in frequency and duration if the patients are properly managed and effectively linked to outpatient services. In the time after deinstitutionalization, mental hospitals were blamed for creating too easy access for the homeless through a "revolving door."[49] Later the failure of deinstitutionalization itself was blamed, and the plea was made to "build a better state hospital."[18] More helpful than either of these extreme views is the program developed in Boston at the Massachusetts Mental Health Center.[50] Here a small number of acute inpatient beds are dedicated to short-term hospital treatment for the homeless during episodes of decompensation. The advantage of this arrangement is that it provides a staff dedicated to the needs of the homeless who do not regard them as incurable or hopeless and who can make effective referrals back into community support programs. The pilot project reports significant benefit for two-thirds of the thirty-one patients treated during its first year of operation. Included in the benefits was reduced conflict between shelters and mental health admitting facilities over the need for admission and access to beds.

It has also been argued that the homeless can receive effective acute care in a general hospital inpatient setting, provided there are effective linkages to a pluralistic service system.[51] Often a period of inpatient care provides the best opportunity to get a homeless person's illness and problems under control. This may come about through direct admission to a psychiatric service or after consultation on a medical unit.

Amy P was sixty-five years old and had lived at a small women's shelter for nearly a year. She was generally mute and could be found cradling and crouched over a doll she kept with her at all times. She occasionally smiled but refused all attempts of psychiatric or social service intervention. One evening, while she was waiting in line for her bed at the shelter, she fainted and was taken to the General Hospital, where it was found that she had a cardiac condition which was easily controlled with medication. During her medical stay she received a psychiatric consultation. With the help of psychiatric medication she agreed to be discharged into a geriatric halfway house and later to a co-op living situation. She continues to carry her doll with her; but she has a home and small community within the mental health residential system, and her quality of life is much improved.

Outpatient Care: The more routine aspects of outpatient care are best delivered by mental health professionals familiar with the problems of homelessness and willing to work with the patient's case manager. Prescribing practices must be tailored to the particular circumstances of the homeless.[33] Simplicity is essential. For example, it is best to use one-a-day-regimens and small amounts of drugs that are less likely to be lost, stolen, or sold on the streets. Intramuscular injections of long-acting medications have advantages.

Psychotherapy is generally directive, pragmatic, or problem-solving and is often focused on dealing with the realities of homelessness. It may include rebuilding self-esteem and morale eroded by the apathy, deprivation, and stigma associated with being homeless as well as advice and training in interpersonal skills to facilitate reconnection with families and resettlement in more conventional living situations. Friction with shelter mates and resistance to the recommendations of case managers and payees for disability benefits are other topics that may be dealt with in therapy.

Psychiatrists working with the homeless are sometimes asked to participate in evaluations for Social Security disability determinations. An energetic advocacy role is important at a time when the criteria applied are increasingly stringent. The secretive or withdrawn behavior of some homeless individuals may make it essential to seek information from case managers about day-to-day behaviors and disabilities. In some instances psychological testing can help establish an objective level of impairment that is difficult to substantiate on observations alone. An opinion concerning patients' abilities to manage their own funds must also be given. The psychiatrist's assessment and knowledge of personal dynamics may play a crucial part in this decision.

John H is a forty-four-year-old divorced white male with a twenty-five-year history of paranoid schizophrenia who was partially supported by his family until the delusions that his brother and mother had an incestuous relationship made life in the same house impossible. After he became homeless, social workers enabled him to apply for Social Security disability benefits to which he was entitled on the basis of earlier employment. When his brother was made the payee, John became enraged and threatened violence. The psychiatrist for the homeless met with John and his brother. An alternative proposal that a social worker case manager become the payee was equally unacceptable to John and provoked further threats of violence. After noting John's intelligence and general capability to manage his affairs but also his potential for personal violence, the psychiatrist recommended that John become his own payee. The threat posed to society at large was judged less than that to any individual assigned the task of administering funds to which John so strongly felt he was entitled.

Ron T. is a twenty-two-year-old white male who had been homeless for two years and was his own payee for Social Security disability benefits with a diagnosis of chronic undifferentiated schizophrenia. He first came to the attention of the psychiatric nurse for the homeless when he was seen in the emergency room complaining of a rash and was found to have the worst case of body lice the experienced physician had seen in twenty years. Ron denied psychiatric problems of any kind and claimed to have "plenty of money." He knew that he had Social Security checks but could not remember where. When transferred to a psychiatric unit because he was floridly psychotic, he was found to have fourteen hundred dollars in cash in his pockets. The nurse and psychiatrist for the homeless recommended that Ron be placed in the community support program, which would also assume payeeship for the Social Security benefits. After three weeks' treatment Ron was no longer psychotic. He was accompanied from the hospital by the psychiatric nurse for the homeless, who introduced him to the community support program staff member. They helped Ron collect his Social Security checks from the post office and gave him new clothes, arranged housing at a room-and-board facility, and set up a daily monitoring schedule to supervise his medication and dispense spending money. Several months later Ron is planning to move into an efficiency apartment to cook and care for himself. He believes the medication helps and states, "I was in terrible shape before. I couldn't even find a place to live."

Rehabilitation and Support Services: Rehabilitation services are essential for recovery from mental illness.[33] Structured psychosocial training programs in a "clubhouse" setting are highly effective in enabling and empowering mentally ill people to function to their maximum capacity in the community. Unfortunately for the homeless, the very structure of such programs is often a deterrent, so the principles of psychosocial rehabilitation must be brought to the shelters or residences where they feel at home. Assistance in the development of basic activities of daily living or prevocational skills are needed. Until such comprehensive service systems for the homeless are developed, clinicians must take advantage of those that are already in place in existing community mental health programs that serve the chronic mentally ill.

Dual Diagnosis: Any effort to provide services to the homeless leads inevitably to the issue of substance abuse. Repeatedly studies demonstrate that substance abuse disorders are the most prevalent of all the health problems encountered in the homeless. Any health care program for the homeless must confront this issue. Substance abuse patterns vary somewhat from city to city. In New York, for example, the most pressing problem is in relation to cocaine or crack; in Baltimore and Los Angeles it is alcohol. The mentally ill are not immune and are as likely to be substance abusers as other homeless people, so that programs focusing on the needs of the mentally ill are also compelled to address substance abuse problems. A relatively mild case of schizophrenia or bipolar disorder may be disabling because of the complications of alcoholism, and it may be the alcoholism that has led to the person's being homeless. Until the alcoholism is tackled, proper treatment of the mental illness or return to a stable housing situation will be impossible. Most cities have very inadequate systems of services for indigent alcoholics. Here again the mental health worker is forced to use great ingenuity and persistence in obtaining appropriate services for the patient.

Housing and the Continuum of Care

The provision of housing is a first priority for any homeless person.[52] This is particularly true for a mentally ill person for whom a stable and supportive environment is an important factor in recovery.[53] Treatment is seriously compromised when a person is unhoused and in an unstable and perhaps dangerous environment.[54]

Many regular shelter programs are wary of accepting psychiatrically disturbed individuals or cannot provide the special services needed. An essential step in treatment is therefore to obtain some type of housing. This varies according to the functional capacity of the person, ranging from emergency shelter to long-term residential placement.[55] A variety of supervised housing arrangements to meet these needs has been developed in the wake of deinstitutionalization. These programs are often more accepting of eccentricity and less demanding of adherence to rules.[56] They incorporate special supervision and support along with provision of a comfortable environment, food, or assistance with daily functions. Some provide twenty-four-hour supervision in a group living environment; others provide quite independent living with episodic visits from supervising staff. Some include foster care arrangements where a person can live in a family setting. When necessary, these programs provide supportive counseling by workers skilled in the rehabilitation of persons with mental illness and also maintain close linkages with psychiatric treatment facilities. Any program serving the homeless mentally ill should have access to such a range of housing options to meet the varying needs of its patients.

One successful example of this type of housing includes the use of inner-city hotels in San Francisco. Depending on the residents' level of capability, the staff may help create a community culture and provide basic support or structure. In some instances residents themselves form a cooperative organization to manage the hotel.

Another example of providing housing and completing the continuum of care is the Women of Hope Program in Philadelphia. This serves as an illustrative paradigm that incorporates may of the principles mentioned earlier. The program is administered by the Sisters of Mercy under the auspices of Catholic Social Services and is funded by the Office of Mental Health. The first residence for twenty-four women opened in 1985, and a second for twenty-two women in 1988.

Over the past five years outreach workers in this program have identified a hundred women who were mentally disabled and had been living on the streets for more than a year. These women became the target population for a carefully planned intervention, the goal of which has been to place them in a residence designed to provide housing with supportive psychiatric, medical, and social services. The program is housed in two former school buildings in the high-rent district of the center city, within walking distance of the Philadelphia Health Care for Homeless Medical Clinic, the local mental health center, the social rehabilitation programs, and the Social Security and welfare offices. There is enough space to provide each woman with a dignified, personal environment and to create a homelike atmosphere with several communal rooms. The permanent staff is made up of thirty full-time employees, including six with master's degrees in social work or counseling and twelve formerly homeless individuals. There is an additional full-time mental health practitioner (master's degree in counseling). Part-time psychiatrists are under contract from the mental health center with additional consultation provided by a doctoral-level psychiatrist and social worker. Health Care for the Homeless also sends a nurse practitioner to both sites each week.

Initial contact by outreach workers has focused on establishing a relationship around provision of basic needs for food, clothing, social services, and shelter. Each woman is invited but not required to comply with offers to shower, see a nurse, apply for income, and so forth. Over the first two to four weeks an assessment is made of all the individual's physical, mental, and social needs.

On the bases of this information a treatment plan is developed considering mental and physical health, social services, residential goals, and activities of daily living. These goals take into account the urgency of problems, their acceptability to the client, their potential to affect other residents, and services that facilitate secondary benefits (i.e., disability status to secure medical benefits and income).

The specific mental health goals include an initial evaluation by the mental health professional and interview with the psychiatrist, leading, if necessary, to ongoing treatment at the mental health center and assessment of ability to monitor medications if prescribed. For some women, short-term acute hospitalization may be suggested, using the mental health commitment laws only if the woman presents a physical danger to herself or to other residents. Social goals include seeking employment or participating in the day program or shelter workshop. Activities expected but not required from a resident include participating in house meetings, doing a chore, organizing and cleaning her bedroom area, paying rent, and participating in some recreational activity. Goals for daily living include regular sleep and healthy nutrition, physical hygiene, and appropriate dress.

The population served in the Philadelphia program has a mean age of forty-nine and a predominance of African-Americans (60 percent), almost two-thirds (63 percent) of whom have been on the streets for two or three years. Virtually all are diagnosed as schizophrenic (91 percent), with one or two individuals having developmental or personality problems. Less than a quarter (15 percent) have a concurrent alcohol problem, and somewhat more (18 percent) are dependent on drugs. Under half (42 percent) are deinstitutionalized, and 75 percent have significant medical problems.

In the period 1985–88 twenty-five women graduated to more permanent housing. Now each of eight women lives independently, in her own room or apartment. A few more have moved back with their families or into boarding homes. Two live in specialized care residencies, one is in the state hospital, and two are in nursing homes. Three have died. Factors contributing to success have included strong linkages to a mental health center and consistent health services, a committed, stable staff, and a program that is comprehensive but voluntary, based on mutual trust and individual attention that acknowledges a person's dignity and worth. Barriers to serving the mentally ill have included neighborhood resistance and the amount of staff time required to cut through red tape and prevent vulnerable clients form falling through the cracks between services. There are too few meaningful daytime activities and not enough affordable transitional housing for clients after they have achieved the goals set for them at the Women of Hope residences.[57]

Another example of the benefits obtained from specific attention to the problem of housing is provided by the increasing use made of Veterans Administration domiciliaries for young male veterans.[58] This population has a high incidence of alcoholism (70 percent), major psychiatric disorder (23 percent), and impaired cognitive function (77 percent), complicated by social and economic deprivation.

Conclusion and Summary

In the implementation of mental health care for the homeless a number of innovative programs have evolved to meet the needs of persons hitherto poorly served by traditional psychiatric services.

This system of care deals with a group of patients who often have multiple problems, contributed to by social and economic deprivation, the manifestations of both medical and mental illness, and difficulties in affiliation with other individuals, families, and health care agencies.

A central feature of the care provided is the way in which both personnel and programs attempt to promote attachment to services that are designed for easy access, to be well integrated and attuned to meet the entire hierarchy of human and health care needs. This is accomplished by nurturant, patient, and persistent nonmental health workers who use case management and networking methods. They are supported by mental health professionals who aim to provide on-site availability, in-service education, and linkage to the whole spectrum of specialized psychiatric services. Viewed within a historical and policy perspective, these new programs are part of a reform cycle that is focused on caring and community support rather than prevention of mental illness.[59]

The implementation of this system of care remains far from ideal. Better coordination could occur with correctional services and between mental health and substance abuse providers. Education of both the police and the public should be enhanced. Cooperative relationships with teaching institutions and training programs for different mental health disciplines are in their infancy.

Finally, the relationship of these new health care for the homeless programs with traditional psychiatric services needs to be defined. Ultimately the older established community programs might themselves implement effective mental health care for the homeless but only if they can assimilate and apply the lessons that have been learned.[60]

Acknowledgments: We are grateful to Sister Mary Scullion for contributing the part of the section on housing and the continuum of care that describes the Women of Hope Program in Philadelphia.

We would also like to thank all the co-workers, clients, and patients in Albuquerque, Baltimore, Milwaukee, and San Francisco who have contributed to our learning more about the problems of homelessness and how to help deal with them.

LISA THOMAS

MIKE KELLY

MICHAEL COUSINEAU

13

Alcoholism and Substance Abuse

*The Epidemiology of Substance Abuse Problems
Among the Homeless*

  Michael is a single, 31-year-old black male from the east side of Cleveland. He has been homeless for over one year, sometimes staying at his parents' home when the streets are especially harsh. His most recent bout on the streets lasted two weeks, following discharge from the residence program of the City Mission, Cleveland's second largest shelter for men. Michael was discharged for drinking. The Mission gave him a referral to the Cleveland Health Care for the Homeless Project (CHCHP) as they [sic] led him out the door. An appointment was made for him at the Downtown Drop-In Center, a day shelter operated by the CHCHP. Michael never kept the appointment.

  Three days later Michael came to the Drop-In. He had been sleeping outdoors and eating only one meal each day. He wanted food, a shower and a complete change of clothes. Instead, he was given a thorough assessment and review of his substance abuse problem by a chemical dependency counselor hired by the Project. Michael was assessed as being in the middle stages of chemical dependency for alcohol and cocaine. He had been drinking since the age of 15, and had recently started to smoke crack/cocaine. While he had been detoxed at least 8 times in the past, he had never followed through with treatment after discharge. His most recent detox program occurred only one month previous to his meeting with a substance abuse counselor of the CHCHP. Confronted with this addiction by the counselor, and given the choice of accepting a treatment program or returning to the streets, Michael chose a 28-day treatment program. He was enrolled with other clients referred by the CHCHP and participated in daily Alcoholics Anonymous (AA) meetings and weekly Cocaine Anonymous (CA) meetings. Upon successful completion of this program, Michael was accepted at a half-way house 50 miles outside of downtown Cleveland. For another 90 days Michael worked on the 12 Step Program fundamental to the AA concept of self-help. Michael found permanent work during his last days at the half-way house and remains sober 9 months later.[1]

Michael's story typifies the client profile of most programs working with the homeless. In Cleveland 88 percent of the clients seen by the Health Care for the Homeless Program are male, 70 percent black, 98 percent single, divorced, or separated; the average age is thirty-two. Many are cocaine-dependent with histories of alcohol abuse. Next to aches and pains, alcohol and drug abuse problems are the most frequently cited reasons for visiting the health care project.

The composition of the homeless nationwide has changed since the days of the skid row alcoholic, an older white male sharing a bottle of Sneaky Pete with his buddies. Skid row has disappeared from many cities through gentrification and the demolition of SRO hotels to make room for new condominums and upscale apartments in now-fashionable downtown neighborhoods. The bum, wino, vagrant—epithets for homeless persons of an earlier era—have been replaced by a younger more heterogeneous population. The new homeless represent all ages and ethnic groups; the employable and currently unemployable; the physically disabled, the mentally ill, and families with children.[2] Alcohol may no longer be the intoxicant of choice. Wine has been replaced by crack, cocaine, heroin, and speed. Polysubstance abuse is more common than pure alcoholism or drug addiction. Drugs are mixed and matched to slow the withdrawal, intensify the high, and prolong the experience. Treatment methodologies previously successful have been replaced by myriad programs, including acupuncture, medical detoxification, and self-help programs, all in an attempt to find a technique that works.

Earlier Studies

Studies on the prevalence of alcohol abuse and alcoholism date back ten decades. Since the early 1900's studies describing alcohol-related problems among the homeless indicate an abuse rate in the range of 30 to 33 percent.[3] Until 1986 the rate remained constant, indicating a much higher incidence of the disease among the homeless than the general population, but still involving a minority of the total persons homeless. Yet homelessness remained associated with drinking, providing the impression that all homeless men were alcoholics and derelicts. "Do men become homeless because they are excessive drinkers? Is there something in the condition of being homeless that drives men to drink? Where do the homeless men who do not drink and the alcoholics who are not members of the homeless population fit into the pattern? Finally, just who is the homeless man, and who is the alcoholic?"[3]

A 1987 study on alcohol abuse and dependence among homeless individuals form Los Angeles[4] discovered that the lifetime prevalence (the percentage of individuals who met criteria for either alcohol abuse or dependence at some point in their lives) was 62.9 per one hundred persons. Of the population, 18 percent had alcohol-only disorders, and 46 percent both alcoholism and mental illness. Of those in difficulty with alcohol (with or without associated mental illness), 41 percent also had drug problems. The alcohol-only group tended to be older white men who had experienced unsuccessful marriages and were currently unattached. They led traditional skid row lives, featuring a reliance on soup kitchens, day shelters, and missions. Many had military service records and work and family histories. They were more likely to be victimized and picked up by the police. Very few had received public entitlements over the course of their lives, and most cited the street as their usual sleeping place over the last year, having spent at least one night on the streets over the prior thirty days. Food was found on the street or obtained from soup kitchens. Overall their health was poor, and their ability to get around was impaired or prevented by ill health.

The report also described the incidence of the new homeless in Los Angeles: younger men with emotional disorders in addition to alcohol abuse; female heads of household who utilized public shelters to house their children but socialized with gangs on the streets; and single women with severe mental disabilities who drank to keep the voices away. Overall this new homeless group is younger, includes more women, has a greater percentage of blacks, has meager employment histories and educational levels, and is less likely to be in contact with family or friends.

James Wright in his April 1987 report to the National Institute of Alcoholism and Alcohol Abuse (NIAAA) found that among homeless clients seen as part of the national Health Care for the Homeless Program, the highest rate of problem drinking was within the homeless Native American population, and the lowest among Hispanics and Asians. Differences in the number of problem drinkers between blacks and whites were insignificant, for both men and women. Rates of problem drinking are low up to age fifteen but rise steadily through the middle years and then fall off among the oldest members of the homeless population. Wright also notes that rates of drug abuse and mental illness are significantly higher among alcohol-abusive homeless than among the nonabusers, especially for women.[5]

Treatment of Indigent Substance Abusers

Historically the public inebriate received treatment through the criminal justice system, primarily through time spent in the drunk tanks of local jails. In 1956 the American Medical Association first defined alcoholism as a disease, and more effort was placed on treatment methods. With the passage of the Uniform Alcoholism and Intoxication Treatment Act in 1971, sponsored by Senator Harold Hughes of Iowa, standards for the operation of programs for treatment and rehabilitation of alcoholics were established. The shift began from treatment in the jails to treatment in the health care system. The medical model of alcohol detoxification was born, and inpatient hospital-based programs to serve the alcoholic began. Who is to pay for this expensive form of treatment? Persons covered by health insurance plans and third-party payees are appropriate referrals to the health care system, but there is no room for an indigent patient who cannot pay. The social model of nonmedical detoxification began as a less expensive alternative, to meet the increasing demand for low-cost treatment, especially for homeless alcoholics.[6]

Edward is a 22-year-old single, white male, unemployed for the last two years, living in and around Cleveland. He began to visit the Downtown Drop-In Center in the late spring, looking for a place to shower and wash his clothes. Edward receives his General Assistance check at a friend's home not far from a crack house. Typically, during the first week of the month Edward is found in a continuous stupor due to his addiction to crack/cocaine. His July check was late in arriving because of the holiday and Edward resorted to theft to continue his habit. A fight with his partner left Edward badly beaten and he turned to the Salvation Army for help. After three days in their shelter, Edward was referred to the CHCHP.

Edward agreed to a test to assess his level of addiction. He was evaluated as a chemically dependent-poly substance abuser. Edward acknowledged the results of the test but refused to accept treatment, indicating a fear of sobriety. He wanted several days to think about his next course of action. Edward moved to the City Mission from the Salvation Army shelter, keeping in touch with his substance abuse counselor. When he finally agreed to treatment two weeks later, no beds were available in the treatment program that accepted homeless men. In frustration, alone and angry, Edward left. Two days later he returned and was immediately placed in the residential treatment facility. His treatment costs were paid from funds secured by the CHCHP. In Edward's case, the access to funds opened doors otherwise closed to him.

After his 28-day treatment program, Edward was ready for discharge. His August General Assistance check was being held for room and board charges at a local half-way house. Again, there was no opening and Edward was again frustrated by the unresponsiveness of the system. Through intervention by the Project's substance abuse counselor, Edward was allowed to extend his stay at the treatment facility until a half-way house bed became available. The check was held by the substance abuse counselor.

Once admitted to the half-way house, Edward made moderate progress re-connecting with his family, building for himself a support network. He found a job at a local restaurant and earned enough money to rent a room. He attends AA meetings and stays in contact with his AA sponsor. Edward admits to drinking but has not used cocaine in over 8 months.[7]

Edward's problem is that of every homeless person who chooses to enter a treatment program. Where do you live before entering treatment, after treatment, and (unless it is a residential facility) during treatment? It is one thing to be sober; it is another to be homeless. Sending a sober person back to the streets will only negate the positive aspects of treatment and put that individual back into the drinking / drug-abusive environment. Public beds are always full. Public policy does not allocate additional funds for more beds. Until public policy makers understand the need for treatment beds and halfway houses, more people like Edward will go without help, living on the streets. Research shows that patterns of substance abuse decrease as the residential status stabilizes.[8] The federal government's recently announced drug war strategy puts the onus back on the criminal justice system to handle the problem of drug abuse. It appears we are going backward in the treatment of the public inebriate.

Alcohol- and drug-free living environments are mandatory for persons desiring a sober life. Several model programs have been developed in the past three decades. These models provide low-rent alcohol- and drug-free environments for recovering substance abusers who wish to be independent but need time and training to make the transition from the streets.

Oxford House, Inc. is a useful example. This, is a multisite nonprofit corporation for recovering alcoholics who want to provide group housing for themselves. Members recognize that many individuals have dual addictions to alcohol and drugs. Persons recovering from a drug addiction are welcome into any Oxford House program. Most group living arrangements are only for men. The design is based on the self-help concept augmented by strict rules and regulations. There is no resident manager-counselor in any Oxford House program. Members govern themselves, and failure to comply with the rules means immediate expulsion. The first responsibility of Oxford House is to enforce sobriety. Other rules flow from the first.

Houses are financed through rental income and are self-supporting. Houses are usually located in neighborhood environments, to provide a natural setting. Each is initially assisted in establishing an accounting system to manage expenses, and members are asked to be accountable for themselves. Members must have incomes, but general public assistance (welfare) clients are accepted, provided they seek permanent employment to meet their share of expenses.

The Oxford House model requires at least a thirty-day period of sobriety prior to entrance. Coupled with an experience at a halfway house, this model works well. Oxford House is a good transitional or permanent housing alternative after primary treatment for alcoholism. Unfortunately there are not enough Oxford House programs to meet the need.[9]

Treatment Programs for Chemically Dependent Homeless

Helping homeless persons with alcohol or substance abuse disorders proved to be the most intractable of all the health care issues faced by the nineteen Johnson / Pew programs. Lack of community treatment resources was the primary reason. The Cleveland HCHP was among the most successful and is worth detailed consideration.

The CHCHP secured a Public Health Service grant to provide substance abuse services in addition to its primary health care program. Two employees of Alcoholism Services of Cleveland, Inc., were subcontracted to the project. The grant was designed to add a substance abuse counselor (also known as a chemical dependency counselor) to each of the two medical teams already working at emergency shelters, soup kitchens, and other sites frequented by homeless persons. The problems faced by the two counselors in the first six months of the grant were overwhelming.

The Downtown Drop-In Center, operated by the CHCHP, had been in operation two months when the counselors, both middle-aged white Irish Catholic males, began work. Both acknowledged their personal recovery problems and spoke freely of their past drinking.

An additional part of the Public Health Service grant was the availability of more than a hundred thousand dollars for nonhospital-based, inpatient residential detoxification and rehabilitation. In other words, the counselors had access to money to place homeless clients into treatment programs. Two facilities that met the federal specifications existed in Cleveland. One had been providing primarily alcoholism services to the indigent of the Cleveland area since 1948. The other, developed as a response to the cocaine epidemic, was better suited to the middle class. Service agreements were reached with each facility for a fixed fee per patient: a twenty-eight-day program at the alcohol facility for nineteen hundred dollars; a fourteen-day cocaine program for thirty-five hundred dollars.

During the grant design phase, it did not seem likely that many homeless persons would seek treatment for their alcohol or drug problems. Health care staff had repeatedly told clients to quit drinking for health reasons, to no avail. The staff consistently referred clients into public detox programs. One client had been through detoxification seventy-four times but continued drinking. With the implementation of the grant, however, the chemical dependency counselors were inundated with clients seeking admission into a treatment program. Referrals came from the Downtown Drop-In Center, the City Mission, and the Salvation Army. Almost every male homeless client seen by the CHCHP wanted treatment (fourteen or twenty-eight days of clean sheets, three meals a day, and a bed). Obviously this was not the way to run a program.

Clients interested in treatment had to complete two forms of assessment, the Michigan Alcoholism Screening Test (MAST) and a Chemical Assessment Sheet. The MAST distinguishes between chemically dependent and nonchemically dependent substance abusers. The Chemical Assessment Sheet requires a specific listing of the intoxicants used, how often they were used, with whom, and how the person's behavior changes as a result of use. Once clients are assessed as chemically dependent, they are referred to the appropriate treatment facility.

Two problems quickly emerged from this approach. Women were not being brought into the program, and the needs of mentally ill substance abusers were not being met. CHCHP counselors were unable to build relationships with women living in emergency shelters. Although two of the shelters ran chemical dependency programs and AA meetings were held at one, a link was not established. In Cleveland 60 percent of the women in emergency shelters are black. The substance abuse counselors are white males. A bond never developed between the counselors and the female clients, so few women sought treatment. Another roadblock to treatment for women was the lack of a facility for a mother and her children. A woman seeking treatment had to find an alternate place for her children. Children cannot stay at a shelter alone. Considering that a homeless woman has few housing resources available, the impediment of placing her children elsewhere while she seeks substance abuse treatment is insurmountable. In the first year of the program only seven women sought treatment with the help of the CHCHP. All were single without children.

The second major problem faced by the CHCHP was care for the substance-abusing mentally ill, those with dual diagnosis. A conservative estimate of the incidence of mental illness among the CHCHP clientele is 40 percent. In addition to the severely mentally disabled, such as schizophrenics, there are those with other affective disorders, including depression, manic depression, panic disorder, cognitive impairment, and antisocial personalities. Traditional alcoholism treatment programs do not address this concern, nor was dual diagnosis considered in the initial screening of clients. Patients were referred into treatment programs only to have an underlying affective disorder emerge postdetoxification. Without the experience or resources to deal with mentally ill substance abusers, the CHCHP failed to meet their special needs. They either left the treatment program voluntarily or began using substances while in treatment, knowing that the program was of little use to them.

For clients whose needs were met by the treatment program, 65 percent completed detox and rehabilitation in the first year of the grant. In addition, 80 percent were assessed as poly drug abusers. Cocaine was the obvious drug of choice among the homeless of Cleveland. Ninety people entered treatment the first year; fifty-four had their treatments paid by the CHCHP. Of the fifty-four, 40 percent were sober eight months later. Ten had medical insurance that paid for their treatment program, and 50 percent of these remained sober eight months later. The remainder (twenty-six) were treated free of charge. After eight months one-third maintained their sobriety.

The heavy demand for treatment and the prevalence of cocaine use mandated a change in treatment facilities used by the CHCHP. The fourteen-day thirty-five-hundred-dollar option was too expensive. Cocaine does not begin to leave the body until after the twenty-first day of abstinence. A fourteen-day program was too short to address the cravings a cocaine user experiences. A new program was designed for the twenty-eight-day facility, using proved methods in the treatment of cocaine along with well-established recovery programs aimed at the indigent.

The rehabilitation and treatment program is based on the Twelve Steps and Twelve Traditions of Alcoholics Anonymous. Clients are given the AA Big Book and additional literature to read during the twenty-eight-day period. Each day of the four weeks is rigidly scheduled from 7:30 A.M. until lights out at 10:30 P.M. Clients are assigned to chores, they share meals in the dining room, and they have homework most nights. Homework consists of readings from the Big Book or writing essays on their personal experiences with an addiction. The schedule during the day consists of lectures, group and individual counseling, art therapy, films and videotapes, and a group session on feelings. Issues addressed in lectures, films and counseling sessions include: the ego in recovery, signs of relapse, relapse prevention, reconciliation with self and society, and affirmation. Proper nutrition is taught, emphasizing the need for the physical body to heal. For homeless clients this can be a long process because of the problems caused by years of drinking and malnutrition. Stress management is addressed, providing coping methods for those accustomed to anesthetizing problems with alcohol or drugs. As the clients move from being aware of the substance abuse problem to other consequences, they enter four more phases, the importance of the physical, psychological, social, and spiritual aspects of life. By the end of the twenty-eight-day program they are ready to move from a sheltered, disciplined environment into a less restrictive residential setting.

We must remember throughout this discussion that the clients are homeless. Generally, this means they have few clothes, no personal items, no access to transportation or support systems. They need both a substance abuse counselor to handle the addiction and a case manager to untangle the other problems that contributed to homelessness. Clients need more than one set of clothes and certainly new underwear and socks. Shampoo, soap, a razor, deodorant, toothbrush, toothpaste, and a comb are coveted items that must be supplied. If they attend an AA meeting outside the rehab facility, transportation must be provided. Spare change for cigarettes and candy is always appreciated. A case manager is also required to trace identification (birth certificate) necessary for acceptance into the general assistance program. The case manager may be asked to find a former spouse to determine the status of the children or locate a friend who is storing a stereo or television. The case manager may have to unravel a problem with the criminal justice system. Pending discharge from the treatment program, the case manager will be asked to secure housing and furnishings, all at no cost or low cost. After treatment the client is sober, but all other problems associated with homelessness are still present.

Housing is a formidable problem confronting clients after discharge from a treatment facility. Halfway houses provide part of the answer, but there are not enough to meet the need. Oxford House programs are also a good answer, but they do not exist everywhere and can be costly. To remain sober, a recovering homeless alcoholic needs an alcohol- and drug-free environment in which to survive. The streets are not the answer.

Recovery

Recovery from chemical addiction is more than taking away the drug. Recovery is a journey, and after a while it becomes a way of life. The descent into addiction, homelessness, and poor health often takes years to achieve. The recovery process take years to practice. AA has a slogan heard at all its meetings: "'One Day at a Time." Recovery also takes one day at a time to practice before it becomes a habit and a way out of the morass of homelessness.

The person with a chemical dependency copes with life's problems by drinking or taking drugs. The chemical provides a temporary mood swing, close to euphoric. The chemical is consistent in providing this mood swing and can be trusted to produce the same effect time after time. Social drinkers control the degree of mood swing by regulating the quantity of chemical intake. The addict loses control and falls victim to dependency. As increased episodes of use occur, life-styles begin to change and revolve around the chemical. Tolerance to the chemical increases. The user develops more ingenious ways to get, use, and keep the chemical—e.g., sneaking drinks, stealing the drugs, prostituting for drugs. Projections of self-hatred onto others begin to ooccur as the user's whole life deteriorates and health, spirituality, emotional stability, and interpersonal relationships become adversely affected. The victim uses chemicals to survive rather than to feel euphoric.

Tammy is a twenty-three-year-old black woman. She quit school at sixteen. Her two children, ages seven and four, were taken away by the Department of Human Services. Tammy beat and abused her children while she was high on crack. Tammy had a public housing authority apartment but allowed her drug dealer to use it to manufacture crack. Within a week the apartment was taken over by drug dealers. Tammy lost control of her apartment but was allowed to stay and exchanged sex for drugs. She became superfluous after more women began visiting and living in her apartment. Tammy was forced out one month later. She began to sleep with friends and relatives before her referral to the CHCHP.

Tammy qualified for third-party insurance under her father's hospitalization insurance, and she was referred into a hospital-based detoxification program. She was discharged to her family five days later. An appointment was made with a CHCHP substance abuse counselor. No one was there to greet Tammy upon discharge. She never kept her appointment with the counselor. Tammy has been seen once by a former friend. She was living in her old apartment, selling herself for drugs.

Persons who are chemically dependent are always at risk for relapse. That is the reason people have to remain in treatment their whole lives. One of the most difficult jobs in treating addicts is to convince them that they cannot recover unless they avoid all mood-altering chemicals forever. The 10 to 15 percent of people in any society who suffer from addictive disease suffer greatly. Part of the reason is relapse. The AMA includes in its definition of alcoholism (chemical dependency) the fact that it is a disease characterized by a tendency to relapse. Of those who are treated, half to two-thirds relapse within two years, whatever their method of treatment.

There is only one proved way to recovery: abstinence one day at a time for a lifetime. Drug treatment cannot provide lifelong treatment, not inpatient, outpatient, hospital-based or nonhospital-based. No one could afford it. Yet there is a program that works for many people, and it is without charge. It is a therapeutic peer-group experience, following the "helper-therapy" principle whereby the helper receives as much help as the person being aided. It is known as Alcoholics Anonymous or Cocaine Anonymous or Narcotics Anonymous, and it works!

From Step 1 of AA—"We admitted we were powerless over alcohol, that our lives had become unmanageable"—the individual begins to address, along with others, the pathway to sobriety. Most treatment programs (fourteen to twenty-eight days) move the individual through the first four steps during treatment. The remaining eight steps are confronted over time during the course of AA meetings. Counselors suggest ninety meetings in the first ninety days of sobriety. The individuals should be as immersed in recovery as they were in addiction. Just as the chemical allowed addicts to cope with problems, so AA allows them to cope with life. Still, for the homeless, recovery can be all the more difficult because of the lack of a stable living environment. Inadequacy of resources for prolonged recovery has been identified as the most critical of all the problems facing homeless people in recovery programs. These resources include housing, access to a job, and entitlements. Tammy in the above case should never have been discharged alone. She should have been released to a counselor, who would have escorted her directly to a meeting with other recovering homeless persons. Arrangements should have been made for a halfway house, where she would have received an additional ninety days of intensive treatment and therapy. While at the halfway house, Tammy could have begun work on securing the skills she needed to get a job. She could have begun the process of recovery, or learning how to live independently without chemicals. She could have begun the process of learning how to be a parent, how to care for a home, how to be a responsible individual. Instead, left alone, Tammy returned to the only life she knew, the only action that produced a familiar response. As sober as Tammy may have been upon discharge, the treatment failed.

For a homeless person living recovery, the denial of housing and the opportunity to create a home may be devastating and may mean resumption of the chemical. To the well-known causes of homelessness—the lack of safe, affordable housing, the demolition of SRO housing, and the reluctance of communities to give zoning approvals to transitional living quarters—another cause can be added. How many public planners and managers include alcohol-free living environments in their housing mix? How many housing programs for the homeless support an alcohol-free environment?

The second difficulty is insufficient opportunity for jobs or jobs programs. Housing requires an income, and public entitlements do not provide sufficient income to support a home. For a homeless person in recovery, a job is very important. In addition to being a source of income, it is a source of self-esteem. Many people who are homeless have poor work records and meager work histories. Extra help to develop skills, good work habits, and confidence may be necessary. The substance abuse counselor should not be expected to act also as a job counselor. Existing service agencies in the employment field must be used, including the Private Industry Council, Job Training Partnerships (JTPA), and Manpower programs. Homeless provider networks should be expanded to include vocational programs. In Cleveland the county JTPA office operates a job-training and job-seeking skills program specifically designed for persons who have remained sober ninety days after completing the CHCHP chemical dependency program. Formerly homeless substance abusers are provided with two-week job evaluation workshops. Upon completion, each candidate is assigned to a job training program (e.g., diesel school or heating/air conditioning); to a remedial program (adult basic education or GED); or to a job. The employers of the first five graduates were happy to rehire their former employees once those persons had acknowledged addiction and a desire to maintain sobriety. The program in its first year successfully placed twenty-three graduates into full-time employment, with wages averaging $7.50 an hour and full medical benefits.

Social supports are also needed throughout recovery. The homeless client needs a bag lunch each day during job training, clean clothes to wear to an interview, transportation to the job site, and encouragement after a bad day. AA meetings provide the social setting to exchange feelings and a place to unload frustrations. AA suggests that each member find a sponsor within the organization with whom to build a relationship. Sponsors should have a longer experience of sobriety than the new member. Sponsors can also be useful in providing transportation to and from meetings.

Many pitfalls face the chemically dependent homeless person. Among them are the lack of treatment facilities, treatment methodologies culturally inappropriate for the indigent, lack of public resources, lack of successful programs in treating cocaine, and a lack of positive options after detox.

The current debate over cocaine and crack within the United States bodes ill for all sectors of our society. While attention is placed on drug dealers, there appears to be no overwhelming philosophical or moral movement (Just Say No) that will brake our society's drive to seek ecstasy through chemicals. New, more potent forms of drugs are introduced regularly. Cocaine becomes crack; amphetamines become methamphetamines, known as crank or ice; heroin is mixed with cocaine; and the beat goes on.

JOHN M. RABA

HERMAN JOSEPH

ROBIN AVERY

RAMON A. TORRES

STACY KIYASU

ROBERT PRENTICE

JO ANN STAATS

PHILIP W. BRICKNER

14

Homelessness and AIDS

Introduction

Acquired immunodeficiency syndrome (AIDS) is now the leading cause of death of persons between the ages of twenty-four and forty-four in major urban areas in the United States.[1] Still predominantly diagnosed in homosexual men and in whites, the demographics of human immunodeficiency virus infection, the cause of AIDS, are shifting to reflect a patient population increasingly minority, heterosexual, low-income, and intravenous drug-using.[2,3]

In many urban areas the incidence of AIDS and HIV infection in the homeless is or will soon be significant. The social and demographic characteristics of the urban homeless population indicate that many individuals have risk behaviors associated with high indices of HIV infection. Data from the Health Care for the Homeless Program reveal that 10 to 13 percent of the homeless persons seen in treatment sites are intravenous drug users and 10 percent are homosexual men,[4] although there is marked variation in percentages in different geographic regions. HIV infection in the homeless has been found predominantly in young, heterosexual, intravenous drug-using (IVDU) men and women and secondarily in homosexual men.[4]

The complex interrelationship between homelessness and HIV infection is yet to be fully explored. Some strongly maintain that the absence of stable domicile, disaffiliation, loss of support networks, and unemployment may predispose individuals to behavior (drug use, prostitution) that can lead to HIV infection.

For a subsector of the homeless population, drug addiction in itself predisposes to homelessness. It is also clear that the onset of a major physical disability such as AIDS can result in homelessness in an individual or family whose economic or social environment precariously borders on the edge of homelessness or disenfranchisement. In some cases homelessness can result from the forced impoverishment required to qualify for Medicaid benefits when illness has caused the loss of job and health insurance. In discussing HIV infection in the homeless population, we must avoid the labeling of the homeless with yet another stigma—i.e., AIDS— which would further isolate or create additional biases against this already disenfranchised group. ". . . all homeless are [not] at risk for AIDS, only those that engage in high risk activities or who are [sexual] partners of those who engage in risk behaviors."[5]

Here we present data concerning HIV infection and homelessness and discuss approaches to prevention, treatment, and support services.

HIV Infection in the Homeless Population

There are few published analyses concerning the prevalence and incidence of HIV infection in homeless populations. The exact number of homeless HIV-infected individuals is unknown. Indeed, fearing discrimination, many with known diagnoses (AIDS, ARC, HIV antibody seropositivity) conceal their conditions when they enter shelters.[6] Others live anonymously in the streets or transient hotels.

Most available data have been generated in large urban areas where the incidence of HIV infection is high in the general community and would be anticipated to be concomitantly higher in the local homeless populations. In fact, the information that has been collected reflects rates of HIV infection and an incidence of AIDS among homeless people substantially higher than in age-matched United States populations.

Using 1986 data from nine cities in the national HCHP, James Wright et al. calculated the incidence of AIDS in the homeless population to be 230 cases per 100,000 adults. This is significantly higher than the approximate 1986 national rate of 144 AIDS cases per 100,000 adults.[4]

Between 5,000 and 9,000 AIDS patients in New York City were homeless in 1988.[7,8] This suggests an approximate 13 to 14 percent incidence of AIDS in New York's homeless population. An ethnographic study of a public shelter for men on the Lower East Side of Manhattan completed in April 1989 showed that AIDS risk behavior was fairly widespread within the shelter population.[9] Of the 214 shelter residents interviewed, 78 (36.4 percent) admitted to shooting heroin or heroin in combination with cocaine, a practice known as speedballing. Shooting galleries discovered in the vicinity of the shelter were used by the residents. They also patronized prostitutes observed in the shelter neighborhood.

A retrospective study of 169 men tested for HIV antibodies at the Keener Building, a thousand-bed shelter on Wards Island in New York City, revealed an extraordinarily high seropositivity rate of 62 percent. Of those homeless men testing positive 53 percent were IVDUs, 23 percent were homosexual, 8 percent were combined homosexual and IVDU.[10] Although obviously from a biased sampling, this study confirms that at least some subgroups among the homeless have high rates of HIV infection.

A survey of all Boston Health Care for the Homeless charts from 1985 through February 1989 revealed a total of 30 persons with AIDS, 69 with ARC, and over 150 who have either asymptomatic HIV infection or present a compatible clinical picture but whose status was not known. This is a total of approximately 250 persons known to the team with documented or strongly suspected HIV infection. Approximately 20 percent in each of these categories were women. The vast majority (greater than 90 percent) had IV drug use as a risk factor.[11]

AIDS or ARC is diagnosed in roughly 5 percent of San Francisco's estimated 6,000 homeless people. While there have been no comprehensive seroprevalence studies within this homeless population as a whole, anonymous HIV antibody tests administered to 162 persons at a medical clinic affiliated with a soup kitchen and shelter between January 1 and March 31, 1989, showed that 21 percent tested positive.[12]

Studies on homelessness and AIDS have tended to focus on the adult population; however, since there is often a period of years between infection and onset of symptoms, many young adults with AIDS or ARC may have been infected during adolescence. There is growing evidence that homeless youths, because of a combination of high-risk behaviors and lack of social support, are particularly at risk for HIV infection.[13,14]

A study completed in 1985 in Los Angeles comparing behavior and social characteristics of runaway (110) and nonrunaway (655) youths between the ages of twelve and twenty-four shows that runaways are more at risk for contracting HIV than others.[15] Runaways had a greater prevalence of intravenous drug use (34.5 vs. 3.7 percent) and pelvic inflammatory disease (4.4 vs. 1.4 percent). There was also more street prostitution (26.4 vs. 0.2 percent) and homosexual (7.3 and 4.9 percent) and bisexual (9.1 and 4.9 percent) activity.

AIDS cases reported through March 1989 in New York City in 417 male youths between the ages of thirteen and twenty-four reflect risk behavior associated with three major risk categories: sexual activity with men at risk (63 percent), intravenous drug use (20 percent), and the combined category of IVDU and sex with men at risk (5 percent).[14] The 133 cases of AIDS reported among females aged thirteen to twenty-four in New York City for the same period fall primarily into two categories: sex with men at risk (44 percent) and IVDU (39 percent).

A major study of HIV seroprevalence among homeless youth, ages thirteen through twenty-three, known to Covenant House, New York, showed that 6.68 percent (74/1,108) of those tested were positive, 7.42 percent (52/701) of the males and 5.41 percent (22/407) of the females.[15] Seropositivity for HIV increased with age: Those eighteen and under showed a rate of 3.7 percent (19/510), while 9.2 percent (55/598) of youths over eighteen were seropositive. Hispanic runaways had the highest rate—9.06 percent (27/298)—followed by non-Hispanic whites—7.8 percent (15/190)—and blacks—5.35 percent (32/598).

AIDS Prevention, Treatment, and Support Strategies in the Homeless Population

Homelessness significantly complicates efforts to provide effective prevention, treatment, and support services. Lack of stable housing often undermines attempts to reduce high-risk behaviors or maintain a regular treatment regimen. In the face of these obstacles several cities, including those with HCHPs, have developed a base of experience in understanding the unique relationships between homelessness and AIDS and in providing a range of services that acknowledges and sometimes changes the circumstances under which the homeless live.

HIV Antibody Testing of the Homeless

As clinicians begin to focus on early intervention in the course of HIV-related illness, the temptation to test large numbers of individuals in a rapid and streamlined fashion will arise. It is important for practitioners working with the homeless to be aware of both the benefits and the potential dangers of testing in this population. HIV antibody testing should be undertaken only after sensitive pretest counseling of men and women, homeless or not, who comprehend the implications of the test results, who could benefit from the institution of treatment, or who need to know their HIV antibody status in order to modify their risk behaviors. If a patient is unable to understand the results or is at the moment unwilling to comply with therapy or change risk behaviors, then the indication for the test should be closely scrutinized. While news of HIV postivity can be devastating for anyone, it is particularly so for homeless persons with repeated losses and tragedies in their lives, who may be battling addiction and barely managing in the day-to-day struggle for survival. In the early years of the Boston Health Care for the Homeless program, two individuals committed suicide after being tested in situations where little or no counseling was given.[11] The Boston HCHP project found it essential to set up a safety net of services around the testing issue. In Boston, Project Trust, an addict advocacy organization funded by the Massachusetts Department of Health, accepts referrals of homeless individuals for pre- and posttest counseling, including frank discussions of what clients would do if they tested positive. Support and referrals for medical and drug treatment are provided. This kind of organization is one important element in a safe testing program; another is the availability of health providers with whom a relationship of trust can be established. The Boston HCHP staff assures newly tested individuals that they have a right to all the information that could affect their health, including details about new therapies. It must be made clear that the choice to accept a particular treatment is theirs and that their care does not hinge on their compliance with a therapeutic protocol.

Some advocates of large-scale HIV screening in populations such as the homeless have claimed that testing would reduce the spread of infection by curbing risky behavior. In fact, it has been observed that as long as they remain on the streets, those who are HIV-negative or do not know their HIV status are much more likely to stop using IV drugs and sharing needles than their counterparts who have tested HIV-positive.[11] Those who achieve a stable housing situation, even if they are HIV-positive, appear to have a somewhat better chance to remain drug-free long term. Virtually none of the Boston HCHP's HIV-positive individuals who remained in shelters have been able to stop using IV drugs completely, despite extensive attempts at education and support. Therefore, it seems irresponsible to undertake large-scale testing programs without providing a framework of services including counseling, medical care, and effective housing assistance.

Prevention

The essential element in the prevention of HIV infection is education, with demonstration of preventive techniques leading to modification or elimination of risk behaviors. However, the very condition of homelessness impacts on the potential for success of AIDS programs.

The foremost need in prevention of HIV infection in this population is permanent housing. Education programs about AIDS cannot be highly effective for those men and women whose day-to-day priority is finding a bed to sleep in and a meal to eat. A 1986 survey examined AIDS risk behavior in New York City residents in regard to injections of illicit drugs and use of heroin and cocaine.[6] The proportion of individuals who used needles for the injection of illicit drugs and who used heroin was about fifteen times greater among transients in the shelters and SRO hotels than in people in stable living accommodations. The proportion of those using cocaine among the transients was more than five times greater than that in the remaining population. Although this survey does not differentiate between homelessness as a cause or as an effect of ongoing intravenous drug use, providers of health care to the homeless have the strong impression that stable housing would improve the chances of homeless individuals to modify drug seeking and sexual risk behaviors. James D. Wright and Eleanor Weber have underscored the problems of AIDS education and prevention in the homeless population:

With no cure for the infection known or in sight, the public health emphasis has been on education and prevention, with "safe sex" and "clean needles" being the most frequently

Table 14.1 PERCENTAGE OF NEW YORK CITY
RESIDENTS IN DIFFERENT LIVING ACCOMMODATIONS
WITH DRUG-USING RISK BEHAVIORS ASSOCIATED WITH AIDS

	PERCENT IN SHELTERS, SROs, AND LOW-PRICED HOTELS	PERCENT IN OTHER ACCOMMODATIONS
Residents with any lifetime needle use	21	1.5
Residents with any lifetime needle use and use of heroin within last 5 years	12	0.8
Residents with any lifetime needle use and use of heroin within last 2 years	10	0.6
Residents with any use of cocaine or crack within last 6 months	25	5.0

urged preventive measures. One might wonder, however, just how successful a "clean needles" campaign can possibly be in a population of IV drug abusers where the simple act of washing one's face and hands, not to mention one's "works," is clearly problematic. Even to be seen with syringes would be grounds for immediate expulsion in many facilities for the homeless, and the street itself rarely affords either the privacy or cleanliness required for the task. With the going street price for sterile syringes in the range of $10 to $20 apiece, there are also obvious economic incentives to using the same needles again and again and to sharing them with less fortunate companions.[4]

Education of Homeless Persons

Education about the prevention of HIV infection and transmission which results in modified behaviors is the best means of controlling its spread. This is true for both homeless and domiciled populations. However, altering risk behavior is an enormously difficult undertaking. Much is known about education but very little about how to change conduct.[16] For this purpose educational programs must be tailored to the specific needs of the various overlapping groups within the homeless population with risk behaviors (IVDUs, homosexual men, heterosexual contacts, prostitutes).[16]

With the understanding that the homeless do not have access to or are not readily accessible to the usual educational channels, such as television or the printed media, educators must devise innovative formats that are attractive and comprehensible to the homeless. Videotapes, photo novels, and comic books have been used to augment presentations and group and one-on-one preventive counseling.[6]

Outreach efforts have been established in most urban areas. Here staffs go into the streets, abandoned buildings, viaducts, and shooting galleries where the homeless congregate or live. Education programs to give information about "safer sex" and make condoms freely available are well established and have been in place for a number of years in some cities. However, the distribution of clean syringes and needles continues to be controversial. Federally funded trial projects have existed in Tacoma, Washington, and New York City.[16] Free syringe and needle distribution occurs in various other cities as well, even occasionally under the guidance of local departments of health.[17]

Drug treatment and methadone maintenance programs combined with HIV counseling result in lower AIDS incidence and AIDS-specific mortality.[16] The nationwide deficiency in numbers of drug treatment beds and facilities hampers efforts to assist homeless men and women to enter rehabilitation units.

EDUCATIONAL EFFORTS: SEATTLE

In Seattle outreach education to street and shelter is coordinated through the AIDS Prevention Project (APP). Efforts have been made to reach all at-risk groups by surveying shelter directors and meeting with members of the Emergency Housing Coalition and provider representatives from the HCHP. The primary objective is to provide education at the larger shelters and then to spread out to the smaller sites as need and interest dictate. The APP staff gives monthly AIDS talks at the Downtown Emergency Service Center, the largest Seattle shelter, which houses an average of 235 men and women per night. Although videos, printed information, condoms, and bleach are available, the greatest draw is the opportunity for clients to engage on a one-to-one basis with staff and to be given a snack.

Street education efforts in Seattle currently include a needle exchange program and mobile outreach to various sites. The exchange program, started by the grass-roots organization ACT-UP (AIDS Coalition to Unleash Power), offers sterile needles and AIDS information six afternoons a week in a downtown heavy drug use area. This program, staffed by volunteers and APP outreach workers, has certain judiciolegal quirks. A person can be arrested for possessing drug paraphernalia (needles and syringes) that may have been supplied by the Health Department, which is mandated to do whatever possible to control this epidemic.

EDUCATIONAL EFFORTS: NEW YORK

New York City has numerous programs directed at educating difficult-to-reach groups (IVDUs, sexual partners of IVDUs, the homeless) about the prevention of HIV infection.

The AIDS Outreach and Prevention Program and the AIDS Mobile Outreach Project operate in selected areas where there is a high incidence of IV drug use. Former drug users serve as outreach workers and canvass the neighborhoods, locating drug users to educate them about AIDS, risk reduction behavior, and treatment. Referrals are made to drug treatment programs and to the Department of Health for HIV antibody testing.[6] Vans are used to contact especially difficult-to-reach individuals in the streets. Risk reduction materials, such as videotapes, pamphlets, photo novels, condoms, and bleach, are distributed. AIDS prevention education has been started in shelters, using on-site group and individual counseling and HIV antibody testing with pre- and posttest counseling.

EDUCATIONAL EFFORTS: SAN FRANCISCO

In San Francisco the Mid-City consortium to combat AIDS began an AIDS prevention program targeting IVDUs. After an ethnographic study of needle use practices, community health outreach workers (CHOWs) were sent to locations where drug users congregate to provide education about HIV transmission, how to disinfect needles with bleach, and how to adopt safer sex techniques.[18] The CHOWs distribute small bottles of bleach and condoms along with AIDS prevention materials. They specifically target the homeless in the streets and in transient hotels.

The San Francisco HCHP also gives AIDS education in its clinics in five city shelters and a drop-in center for homeless youth. Individual and group education, along with bleach and condoms, is offered by multidisciplinary teams of health care workers.

Education of Shelter Providers

Fear of HIV infection and misinformation about its transmission have occasionally resulted in the barring of suspect homeless men and women from shelters and drop-in centers. Education about this condition has been given to staffs of shelters, soup kitchens, drop-in centers, and SROs in an attempt to overcome ignorance. In Chicago, for instance, the Department of Health's AIDS Activity Office worked with shelter providers and the Mayor's Task Force on the Homeless to create brochures for drop-in and transitional shelters. The brochures reviewed HIV and its transmission, intake guidelines, standard precautions, routine house-keeping, confidentiality, and everyday living needs.[19] Shelter providers need to be encouraged to evaluate, during intake procedures, an HIV-infected individual's suitability for life in the shelter by the same criteria used to assess others seeking admission. No homeless person should be denied admission solely because of infection with HIV. Universal body fluid precautions are to be followed for all clients.[20] Disposable gloves and bleach must be available for use by staff during the treatment of open wounds and the cleaning of body fluid spills. Except in rare circumstances, confidentiality about health status, including HIV infection, of those in shelters must be maintained and in most states is protected by law.

The Seattle APP has formally trained employees of a number of shelters and drop-in centers about general AIDS issues. It has provided information on HIV transmission and assisted in developing protocols to decrease the potential for spread of infection. General housekeeping standards emphasize that all bodily fluid spills should be treated as if they could be infectious. Latex gloves are kept in easily accessible areas, and staff members are instructed to don them before dealing with any spill. Also, a one-to-ten-part bleach-water solution is used to disinfect any area soiled by blood, urine, or emesis. The mixture is made up weekly to assure potency.

General policy in Seattle is that no client will be refused service on the basis of HIV status. Seropositivity or an AIDS diagnosis may or may not be known to all shelter staff. Confidentiality is to be maintained. However, in certain circumstances medical, social service, and shelter providers have revealed and discussed an individual's HIV infection. Examples include a suicide threat or attempt, physical violence in which there has been bloodshed, the sharing of needles, and flagrant sexual promiscuity. In such cases the shelter administration may determine that a client is ineligible for services. Such decisions are made only with great deliberation during which possible danger to the individual is weighed against the threat to general safety and security. If these clients are denied further services, efforts are made to engage them with other appropriate agencies.

In San Francisco the HCHP has also developed AIDS education materials for shelter providers. In response to the same kinds of fears expressed by shelter staff, a registered nurse-health educator and the medical director developed infection control guidelines. These emphasize general precautions for all bloodborne disease rather than AIDS specifically, both to emphasize the universal need to adopt good public health practices and to minimize exaggerated fears. The HCHP also gives periodic educational sessions for shelter staff members about HIV transmission to increase their general knowledge about AIDS and enlist their support in prevention efforts among the homeless.

In Boston Pine Street Inn runs the oldest independent nurses' clinic in the country. The staff is currently at work on a manual of AIDS-related information and safety guidelines for shelters. Boston's Long Island Shelter has also taken a leading role in educational issues and has produced a video to educate staff about the difficulties of being HIV-positive in a shelter setting.

Treatment

Medical Complications of HIV Infection and Homelessness

Opportunistic infections are the major cause of morbidity and mortality of HIV-infected persons. Autopsy series report that 90 percent of deaths are caused by infections. Most of the remainder result from lymphoma, Kaposi's sarcoma, gastrointestinal bleeding, and suicide.[21,22] Homeless HIV-infected persons are susceptible to a variety of community-acquired infections more prevalent in shelters, in SROs, and on the streets than in stable housing settings. These include tuberculosis, bacterial pneumonias, soft tissue infections, and infestations as well as from ubiquitous pathogens like *Pneumocystis carinii*, cytomegalovirus, *Toxoplasma gondii*, *Mycobacterium avium-intracellulare*, and *Cryptococcus*.

PNEUMOCYSTIS CARINII PNEUMONIA (PCP)

PCP is the most common opportunistic infection in HIV-infected persons, occurring in approximately 80 percent of persons with AIDS.[23] PCP usually presents with some combination of fever, dyspnea, cough, decreased exercise tolerance, and malaise. Subclinical disease may be indolent in its progression. Thus, early detection requires aggressive diagnostic intervention, including gallium scanning, sputum induction, bronchoscopy, and hospitalization. Because the homeless are at risk for a variety of respiratory disorders that may mimic PCP, and since encounters with health care providers are often limited to serious illness, diagnosis may be delayed until the patient is clinically ill. Adequate follow-up of those with early PCP is crucial to determine if an insidious process is present. Homeless individuals not connected to a health care system may be misdiagnosed if evaluated on a one-time basis in a clinic or emergency room.

Outpatient therapy for PCP requires bed rest, antipyretics, close supervision for toxic reactions to antibiotics, and, occasionally, supplemental oxygen and infusions. Homeless persons with unstable housing arrangements cannot be managed adequately as outpatients and will require hospitalization in most cases. Prophylactic therapies, including oral antibiotics (trimethoprim-sulfamethoxazole, fansidar, dapsone) and aerosolized pentamidine (AP) require close compliance with prescribed regimens and, in the case of pentamidine, supervised administration to monitor for bronchospasm and other untoward reactions.[24–27] Oral sulfa drugs may produce rash, fever, leukopenia, hepatitis, or nausea, signs and symptoms that may cause intolerance in a large majority of patients. These must also be prescribed under close supervision.[24] Prophylaxis usually implies lifelong therapy. For homeless persons this is especially difficult because medications and prescriptions are often lost or stolen, and priorities are likely to be food and shelter rather than preventive medicine.

Mycobacterium tuberculosos (MTB) is a frequent cause of illness in HIV-infected patients, many of whom come from populations in which this infection is common[10,28–30]—i.e., intravenous drug users, Haitians, minorities, and the homeless. Tuberculosis can appear months to years before other clinical manifestations of HIV disease, although it can be a late complication of AIDS as well. Upper-lobe lesions and cavities common in those with reactivated disease are much less so among HIV-infected persons than are lower-lobe or diffuse interstitial infiltrates.[31] Extrapulmonary lesions involving bone, brain, lymph nodes, heart, and virtually any other site have been reported. PPD conversion rates among HIV-seropositive intravenous drug users were similar in one study to that of HIV-seronegative users, yet development of active tuberculosis was greater (4 vs. 0 percent) among the seropositives over a twenty-two-month follow-up period.[32] Among homeless HIV-infected persons, as distinct from those with overt AIDS, tuberculosis is probably the most common major infection, and detection relies on extensive case finding and periodic skin testing. Containment of infection within shelters involves isolation, use of tight-fitting masks, and compliance with chemotherapies. Hospitalization is warranted for most homeless persons with HIV infection and active tuberculosis to ensure containment and monitoring of compliance with antibiotic therapy until sputum conversion has been achieved. Adequate regimens for HIV-infected persons with pulmonary tuberculosis require two months of isoniazid (300 mg/day), rifampin (600 mg/day) and pyrazinamide (20–30 mg/kg/day), followed by seven months of isoniazid and rifampin.

Ethambutol (25 mg/kg/day) should be added to the initial regimen for patients with central nervous system or disseminated tuberculosis or when isoniazid resistance is suspected. Some experts suggest that persons with concomitant tuberculous and HIV infections should continue isoniazid therapy for their lifetimes.[33] In homeless persons, lack of access to care, prescription refills, periodic examinations, chest radiographs, and sputum cultures accounts for incomplete therapies, recrudescence of infection, and emergence of bacterial resistance. Issues specific to congregate shelter residents that affect the transmission of tuberculosis include overcrowding, inadequate ventilation, and communal sleeping accommodations (see Figure 14.1).

Candida infections of the oropharynx are a common initial manifestation of HIV infection, characterized by white plaques on the buccal mucosa, tongue, or palate. Candida infections predict the progression of disease and development of life-threatening opportunistic infection in many patients. In one series the interval between oral candidiasis and opportunistic infection was three months (range one to twenty-three months).[34] Candidial oral and esophageal infections interfere with nutrition and can lead to progressive weight loss. In the homeless these infections may go unrecognized until the patient is severely symptomatic. Oral hygiene is often inadequate in the homeless and may contribute to progressive infection and

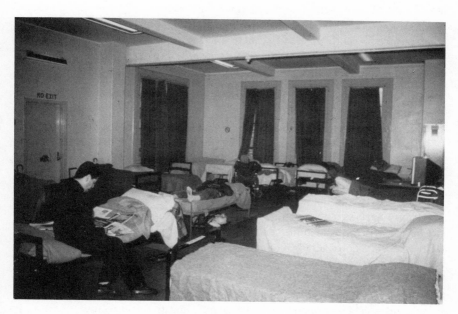

Figure 14.1 **Inadequate ventilation in communal dormitories may contribute to airborne transmission of tuberculosis.**

buccal and esophageal ulcerations. Diagnosis requires inspection, microscopy, and often invasive procedures (endoscopies) which may not be possible in homeless persons without access to hospital-based clinics. Therapies require chronic topical (nystatin or clotrimazole) or oral therapy (ketoconazole) which is needed for life to prevent recurrences.

Treatment Approaches

"The condition of homelessness among patients with AIDS and HIV infection presents serious problems that affect the delivery of medical and social services and the patients' welfare. . . ."[6] Homeless persons with AIDS may have concomitant medical conditions, such as trauma, peripheral vascular disease, physical disability, and mental illness that may interfere with their ability to sustain medical regimens and keep appointments.[35]

These patients appear to arrive for medical care later in the course of illness than do the nonhomeless.[11] Lack of trust in the medical system because of past experience, denial, confusion of symptoms with other entities such as substance abuse-related illnesses, and self-treatment of symptoms with escalating use of the drug of choice all are commonly seen.

Many people in shelters are unaware of the difference between HIV infection and full-blown AIDS. In addition, they may not be aware that new therapeutic developments can help patients live longer with fewer serious infections. If they have heard of new therapies, the homeless are occasionally concerned that the medical system will take advantage of their socioeconomic and educational status to "experiment" on them. Finally, there are fears of being discriminated against by shelter guests or staff if confidentiality was to be broken.

"Management problems of homeless AIDS patients as compared to non-homeless AIDS patients are more difficult. These problems include higher rates of signing out of the hospital against medical advice, refusals to complete diagnostic tests and undergo treatment for opportunistic infection, broken outpatient appointments, longer hospital stays, lost prescriptions, and patients lost to medical follow-up."[36]

It is not surprising that many clinical contacts involve individuals whose HIV status is not known but who are suspected to be antibody-positive. In these persons it is especially important to build up a relationship of trust in order to provide the confidence necessary to accept testing. In the meantime, it is crucial to take the same steps in health maintenance that one would follow for someone known to be HIV-infected. These include monitoring for sweating, cough, shortness of breath; routine measurement of temperature and weight; intermittent examination for oral candidiasis, lymphadenopathy, and changes in neurological status; frequent PPD testing; pneumococcal vaccine administration; serological testing for syphilis; twice yearly CD4 + lymphocyte or T4 counts; and frequent follow-up for early detection of infections. Prompt investigation must be initiated for weight loss, fever, respiratory disorders, and neurological complaints.

It is important for the provider to be vigilant about individuals who may not volunteer their symptoms. "The Boston HCHP reports that one man's only contact with the shelter clinic was a visit to request Nicorette gum to help him stop smoking. One-and-a-half months later he was hospitalized with florid Pneumocystis carinii pneumonia. We can only speculate that gradually progressive shortness of breath made him attempt to stop smoking."[11]

We cannot overstate the importance of a personalized approach to care that centers on a bond of attachment. The care provider must be an advocate; it is helpful to focus at first on other areas of assistance such as medical forms for welfare, transportation passes, and benefits; housing, clothing, and nutritional assistance; referrals for legal services and psychiatric and drug treatment as necessary. When the groundwork has been laid, the patient will feel much more comfortable accepting recommendations concerning testing or treatment. With proper support homeless men and women with AIDS and HIV infection return for appointments and can be followed with reasonable continuity of care.[6,10]

To this end, clinics located within the shelters are vital. Physicians, nurses, social workers, and other practitioners consistently present in shelter clinics can build up close relationships with individuals who might otherwise avoid medical follow-up. These clinics also offer crucial links and information for primary providers based elsewhere. The availability of a nurse or counselor who knows the individual patient well can sometimes be the deciding factor in convincing that person to enter the hospital or to follow through on medical appointments and diagnostic tests, and the staff can monitor vital signs, administer medication, draw required blood tests, and be alert for early signs of infection, often the most important facets of care for an HIV-positive person in a shelter.

Up-to-Date Therapies

A central feature of an integrated system of care for homeless persons with HIV-related illness is the availability of a clinic with access to the most up-to-date therapies. HCHPs in New York, San Francisco, Boston, and Cleveland have physicians who work both in shelters and in their backup hospitals' outpatient clinics. Patients can be referred to these clinics without interruption in provider-patient continuity.

For example, the Boston City Hospital Immunodeficiency Clinic provides a multiservice model. It includes primary medical care, continuity of nursing, connection to a major teaching center with access to clinical trials, expert social service support and pastoral counseling, nutrition, psychiatric and addiction services liaison, and a close relationship to the AIDS Action Committee. Without such a coordinated system, it would be easy for some needs of homeless patients to go unrecognized and unaddressed. This comprehensive model also encourages consistent follow-up in a population traditionally cited as difficult to engage. Boston currently places one physician from the HCHP project one day a week in the Immunodeficiency Clinic, to coordinate care between the hospital and the shelters. In 1990 a full-time physician and a nurse practitioner give HIV-related care in the inpatient, clinic, and shelter settings specifically for homeless persons.

In San Francisco the HCHP merged with the Tom Waddell, a freestanding clinic long known as a provider of drop-in medical services to the homeless. The merger brought to the clinic a multidisciplinary staff of medical, mental health, and social work practitioners as well as a commitment to aggressive outreach. To help the growing number of HIV-positive homeless in the central city area and those with AIDS or ARC, the clinic established a twice-weekly (soon to increase) AIDS clinic staffed by a physician, nurse practitioner, registered nurse, public health nurse, mental health case manager-therapist, social worker, and outreach worker. The on-site clinic is supplemented by staff members who go to key central city hotels, a rescue mission, and a residential program for the homeless with AIDS and ARC to give care on an outreach basis.

In Boston and New York, as in other cities, it has been possible to establish regular enough follow-up to maintain persons on potentially toxic therapies such as AZT with close monitoring of blood counts. The results have been encouraging. With the assistance of shelter staff members who awaken individuals for their nighttime doses, it has been possible to keep to an every-four-hour dosage schedule; timers have also been useful. Because AZT has street value, those carrying large amounts may be vulnerable, or this expensive medication may be lost; it is therefore prudent for shelter clinics to hold the AZT (or study drugs) in the clinic and dispense smaller allotments at regular intervals. There are currently twenty-five individuals known to the Boston HCHP project who have been treated with AZT, and others will be started shortly.

The need for prophylaxis for persons with AIDS or ARC who have low T4 (or CD4 +)[37] counts has led to speculation about the feasibility of administering AP in shelters or even in mobile vans. Although prophylaxis may also be achieved via oral medications such as trimethoprim-sulfamethoxazole, AP offers clear advantages in the homeless population. The simplicity of administration (bi-weekly or monthly dosing) eases compliance and monitoring. The low rate of side effects again makes this an attractive alternative to those with a basic mistrust of medications. Ten patients known to the Boston HCHP receive AP, most at Fenway Health Center, which has made this therapy available through energetic outreach and flexible timing.

Experimental protocols present a challenge to homeless individuals, who have many other demands on their time and often an underlying fear of experimentation. Once the alternatives are fully explained, however, and the provider is perceived as an advocate, many express a desire to know more about newer experimental therapies, even though the ultimate choice is usually AZT or other drugs with benefits and risks relatively well documented. It is important for staff members to stress hope for the future, and that any therapies which prove helpful could potentially be made available to patients. In Boston three homeless persons were screened for the dideoxyinosine (DDI) trial. One was accepted and has completed the first portion of the trial.

Support Programs

Substance Abuse Treatment

Entrance into a drug treatment program for illicit drug users is a necessary adjunct in the management and prevention of HIV infection in the homeless.

In a study of methadone maintenance patients that examined HIV risk behavior[38] it was found that time in methadone treatment is positively associated with reduced use of needles and visits to shooting galleries. Although methadone patients may continue to inject drugs, the longer they remain in maintenance treatment, the less the frequency of risky behavior.

Several studies suggest that methadone treatment if properly implemented can help prevent HIV infection in addicts who inject drugs.[39,40] Follow-up studies in addicts who entered methadone treatment during the past two decades show that opiate use was reduced upon entering but that the majority of the patients, about 80 percent, relapsed to drugs within a two-year period following discharge. Therefore, long-term or indefinite treatment is recommended for most addicts. The need for long-term therapy is especially required for homeless men and women whose living and housing conditions are generally in environments where access to street drugs is simple.

Drug treatment programs should educate patients about AIDS, provide relevant services, prescribe adequate doses of methadone to discourage heroin injection, and develop interventions to reduce or eliminate cocaine use, for which methadone is ineffective.

The shortage of residential and outpatient substance abuse programs is a major obstacle to decreased drug use and diminished risky behavior for HIV infection in both the domiciled and homeless populations.

Hospital Discharge Planning

Persons hospitalized with HIV disease who recover sufficiently to be discharged may face serious challenges in finding proper housing. For those few with ample funds and their own homes and family supporters, the issue may be moot. For the larger number, especially those who have histories of intravenous drug use, shelters or the streets may be their fate. Hospital discharge planners are generally aware of this point and usually strive to find reasonable placements for such patients, although that does not always occur.

A 28 year-old woman in a Boston area hospital with AIDS dementia and a platelet count of 30,000 was discharged at 2:00 AM via taxicab to an area shelter. There had been no consultation with shelter staff. She arrived without medications, information, or follow-up appointments. Investigation revealed that she had been at a community hospital for six weeks; this hospital, feeling that its resources for her had been exhausted, declined to take further responsibility.[11]

Hospital-based doctors, nurses, and social workers need to be educated fully about shelter conditions and alternative housing for homeless AIDS patients so that inappropriate discharges do not occur.

The Boston HCHP has found that it can avoid a substantial proportion of inappropriate discharges by frequent inpatient hospital rounds, close following of its primary care patients in the hospital, and development of good working relationships with resident physicians and continuing care workers at associated hospitals. The project staff has become known as a resource for advice about discharge planning as well as a possible source of primary care for those who have no regular provider.

The earliest of the few analyses to recognize that hospital discharge for such patients offered difficulties was done at St. Vincent's Hospital in New York City.[36] The medical records of all 231 patients discharged with the diagnosis of AIDS during the four-year period from November 1981 to October 1985 were reviewed retrospectively in order to learn the prevalence of homelessness.

Thirty individuals (13 percent) were homeless on admission. They had been living on the streets or in shelters. In contrast with the patients with homes, these persons were more likely to be black or Hispanic and to use drugs intravenously. Length of time in the hospital was longer for homeless patients than for others [sixty-two vs. forty days, respectively ($p > 0.02$)]. For this factor, homeless IVDUs and homosexuals had the same length of stay. This study was also among the first to recognize that IVDUs constitute the major pool of HIV infection among the homeless population of New York City.

A subsequent review at North Central Bronx Hospital (New York City) considered eighty-seven patients with AIDS hospitalized in 1985 and 1986.[41] Seventy-seven were IVDUs or their sexual partners. Ten were homosexual. Seventy-eight were members of minority groups. Seventy-two (83 percent) either lived with relatives or had their own homes. Fifteen (17 percent) were homeless on admission. Their fate upon discharge indicates that with effort, a variety of placement opportunities may be found. Of the fifteen homeless individuals, four were accepted into the homes of family members or friends, four went to hotel rooms offered by the city government, three went to hospices, three died, and one left the hospital against medical advice.

The imperative to help homeless patients with AIDS deal with housing issues is revealed starkly when we consider the children of these patients. The records of 108 individuals, all IVDUs from six hospitals in New York City, were reviewed by Ernest Drucker and colleagues at Montefiore Hospital (New York City).[42] They considered data on number, age, and custody arrangements for the children of the patients, along with the housing status of the patients themselves. At the time of hospitalization, 58 patients (54 percent) had a total of 117 children less than eighteen years of age. Twenty-seven of the children were in the patients' custody at the time of hospital admission. Drucker points out that IVDUs with AIDS who require hospital treatment have "profound deficits in social supports, child care arrangements, housing. . . . The progression of disease can be expected to intensify these needs, delaying hospital discharge and placing great stress on . . . already overburdened child care, housing and drug treatment services."

Respite Care

Many persons with AIDS or ARC have periods of recovery after acute illnesses during which they are too ill to be on the streets yet not ill enough for continued acute care hospitalization.

Therefore, facilities such as the Boston Shattuck Shelter Respite Unit have come to play an increasingly important role in intermediate care for those without homes. The Shattuck respite unit has twenty-five beds within a larger shelter. It is staffed by a nurse practitioner, a social worker, three respite aides, and a physician two days a week. The respite unit enables persons to stay inside twenty-four hours a day. In addition, taking vital signs, medication administration, dressing changes, and medical supervision are available. Social service support enables the time spent off the streets to be used to prepare papers for benefits, housing assistance, and referrals for drug treatment. The respite unit is also an ideal setting for initiation of AZT, for example, so that dosing time and blood counts can be closely monitored.

Residential Programs

The AIDS Resource Center in New York City was founded in 1983. Its purpose is to supply housing with support services and pastoral care for homeless persons with AIDS. The agency has developed three housing models and has successfully implemented two.

The scattered site apartment program, the first model developed, presently consists of twenty apartments for up to thirty-five persons. Bailey House, opened in 1986, is the second model and has forty-four residents. The apartment house model, similar to a small group home, is currently in the planning stages and will accommodate approximately twenty-five.

Public contracts fund about 70 percent of the annual budgets of the two existing programs. Private donations subsidize the public contracts to allow for expansion of services and begin new programs. The cost of the scattered site apartments is approximately $58 per day, and of Bailey House $125 per day.

The scattered sites can accommodate single persons and families with or without children. Apartments are rented by the agency, with the knowledge of the landlords, in buildings throughout the city. Support services include case management by a team of social workers, recreational therapy, pastoral care, and housekeeping. Medical and nursing care of the residents, coordinated by the AIDS Resource Center staff, is given by local hospitals and the Visiting Nurse Service (VNS) of New York.

Bailey House is the first supportive group residence for people with AIDS in New York City and the largest in the country. Residents are housed in private rooms with bathrooms. Three meals a day are served in a communal dining room. There is a large lounge area adjacent to the dining room and smaller lounges on each of the four resident floors.

Case management by social workers and a substance abuse counselor and recreational therapy, pastoral care, and housekeeping are available, in addition to kitchen staff, resident managers, receptionists, and security personnel. One of the major differences between the scattered site and group residence models is the availability of on-site nursing and medical care. The AIDS Resource Center funds a full-time nurse practitioner to coordinate medical and nursing care and refer residents to emergency rooms, clinics, and physicians when necessary. Assistants are available for personal care, shopping, and meals. When necessary, they accompany residents to the emergency room and clinic visits.

A physician from St. Vincent's Medical Center with experience in the care of AIDS patients consults at Bailey House two half days per week. Many of the residents receive primary care from him in his hospital-based clinic. Frequent contact between the nurse practitioner and consulting physician has allowed coordinated and consistent care of the resident.

The VNS, by referral, gives on-site intravenous infusions of amphotericin and ganciclovir, total parenteral nutrition, daily dressing changes, and injections. When residents need more assistance with activities of daily living than the Bailey House staff can provide, home attendants and home health aides are available through the VNS.

Individuals are referred to the AIDS Resource Center by the city's Division of AIDS Services. All persons considered for referral by the city must be homeless, have documented AIDS diagnoses, and be eligible for SSI and Medicaid. Those with histories of substance abuse must be drug- and alcohol-free and enrolled in a drug rehabilitation program.

These housing models offer homes to individuals with AIDS. Through an interdisciplinary team approach it is possible to help many such persons to live in a nonmedical setting. The residents of the AIDS Resource Center housing programs have cut down on drug and alcohol use, returned to school, reunited with families, made custody arrangements for children, and found clean, safe homes. Finally, when it is time, it has been possible for many to die in their own homes with dignity.

In San Francisco, the Shanti Residence Program offers housing to forty-seven homeless patients with AIDS in twelve apartments throughout the city. Beginning in 1983, the program targeted those able to live independently in a group setting. Also, the San Francisco AIDS Foundation provides emergency housing to the homeless with AIDS or ARC in a five-bed flat and in central-city hotels using a voucher system.

In 1986 a group of AIDS and homeless service providers began to discuss the growing number of homeless persons with AIDS and ARC in shelters, transient hotels, and encampments in vacant lots. Many were intravenous drug users, had mental health problems, or for other reasons were unable to live in the independent group housing provided by Shanti. The result of these discussions was the creation in 1987 of a residential program for homeless people with AIDS and ARC who also had mental health or substance abuse problems. Initially located in a SRO hotel through the city's homeless program, with funds for staff and operations provided by the Department of Public Health, the residential program has since relocated to a newly renovated facility, the Peter Claver Community. Operated by Catholic Charities, the program gives counseling, case management, and attendant care, as well as independent resident group sessions (including Alcoholics Anonymous and Narcotics Anonymous), in an environment that includes twenty-four-hour staff support. A contract with the AIDS Office of the Department of Public Health also offers home health care. Although case managers assist in maintaining regular health care, clinical staff members from the Tom Waddell Clinic come on-site as needed. The Peter Claver Community also has a contract with the California Department of Mental Health to work in a residential setting for people with mild to moderate dementia, a growing problem among the homeless with AIDS.

In 1989 the Department of Public Health, the Shanti Residence Program, and Catholic Charities received a state grant to provide residential programs for homeless families in which one or more members have AIDS or ARC. Located in two flats for up to eleven people, the programs enable homeless families to stay together for as long as possible.

Summary

HIV infection and AIDS are complex disorders with complicated therapies. The effect of AIDS on an already disadvantaged and disaffiliated homeless individual can be devastating. For at-risk men and women sensitive health care providers are indispensable in gaining patients' trust and establishing reasonable continuity of care.

Programs that bring medical services into shelters or are readily accessible to homeless individuals with HIV infection will be the most successful. Voluntary HIV antibody testing should be used cautiously in the homeless and only when patients are fully counseled. Homeless persons with drug addiction require admission into long-term substance abuse programs. Expanded respite care and residential living settings are needed in most urban areas for homeless patients with AIDS who have special care or housing needs.

Efforts to educate, prevent, diagnose, and manage HIV infection in the homeless population will not be optimally effective unless stable housing is available.

JOHN M. MCADAM

PHILIP W. BRICKNER

LAWRENCE L. SCHARER

JANET L. GROTH

DEBORAH BENTON

STACY KIYASU

DAN WLODARCZYK

15

Tuberculosis in the Homeless: A National Perspective

Tuberculosis in the Homeless

The incidence of tuberculosis has been declining in the United States since the institution of public health measures early in this century.[1] Decades before antituberculous chemotherapy became available, early isolation of active TB cases and improved standards of living resulted in dramatic declines in cases rates for all population groups.[2] However, although case rates improved dramatically, death rates of those with TB changed relatively little until the availability of effective antibiotics in the late 1940s and early 1950s. Drugs such as streptomycin, isoniazid, para-aminosalicylic acid, and ethambutol cured persons with pulmonary TB. Of almost equal importance, patients could now return to the community on treatment after a short period of respiratory isolation. Previously, TB patients were separated from the general population and their families in sanitariums for years. Most Americans alive today are too young to remember this means of treatment. The new, effective therapies and the continuation of public health measures meant that TB was no longer a disease to be feared. Between 1953 and 1984 the number of reported cases in the United States decreased by 73.6 percent (from 84,304 to 22,255) and the annual risk of TB decreased by 82.3 percent (from 53.0 to 9.4 per 100,000 population). In 1985 the decline in the annual TB case rate stopped, and there was a slight increase in 1986. Taking the rate of decline between 1981 and 1984 as a baseline, the Centers for Disease Control calculated that there were 9,226 excess cases of TB between 1985 and 1987.[3]

Significant differences exist in the overall risk of TB among various ethnic groups (Table 15.1). The largest increase in any age-group, 11.9 percent, was in twenty-five- to forty-four-year-olds. Men had nearly twice the case rate of women, and this did not change significantly between 1985 and 1987.

Table 15.1 REPORTED TUBERCULOSIS CASES AND
RISK OF TUBERCULOSIS, UNITED STATES (*JAMA*)
(*per 100,000 population*)

RACE / ETHNICITY	NUMBER OF TUBERCULOSIS CASES			CHANGE FROM 1985 TO 1987
	1985	1986	1987*	
White, non-hispanic	8,453	8,539	8,048 (4.3)	−405 (−4.8)
Black, non-hispanic	7,592	7,966	8,067 (27.6)	+475 (+6.3)
Hispanic	3,092	3,215	3,485 (18.7)	+393 (+12.7)
Asian / Pacific islander	2,530	2,572	2,477 (48.1)	−53 (−2.1)
Native American / Alaskan native	397	335	317 (20.0)	−80 (−20.2)
Other / unknown	137	141	123 ( )	( )

*The rate of tuberculosis cases is indicated in parentheses.

The national growth in tuberculosis cases since 1985 was reported from many localities but was most marked in New York City.[4] From 1984 to 1988 the number of New York cases increased 42 percent, from 1,629 to 2,317. The case rate increased from 23.0 to 32.8 per 100,000 during this period. In 1985 the New York City Bureau of TB began to identify active tuberculosis patients who gave either shelter addresses or no address. That year there were 150 such individuals, 8 percent of the total number of TB cases. In 1988 there were 240 homeless persons with TB, or 10 percent of the total.

Definitions of terms are important. Tuberculous *infection* is defined as dormant disease manifested by a positive tuberculin skin test. Infected persons do not have an active, contagious disorder but are at lifelong risk for development of active disease. Tuberculous *disease* is the active illness, manifested by clinical symptoms and usually by isolation of the causative bacterium (*Mycobacterium tuberculosis*) from sputum and / or tissue.

Boston

Prevention and control of TB among the homeless are difficult and complex matters. Issues of shelter, food, safety, and substance abuse may take priority, hampering efforts to screen, give prophylaxis, and treat for TB. Boston has long experienced this problem, and through joint efforts of the state health department, the Boston Department of Health and Hospitals, the Health Care for the Homeless Program, and individual shelter care providers, management of TB among the homeless has become a more attainable goal.

In May 1973, because of a significant number of active TB cases among the 350 guests of Boston's Pine Street Inn, the Massachusetts Public Health Department and the Boston Department of Health and Hospitals established a shelter-based TB control program. The purpose was to provide intensive and continuous surveillance within the shelter, identify TB cases, and perform related TB control activities. A chest radiography machine was installed in the clinic, and a pulmonologist was present one evening per week. Following institution of the program, the TB case rate within the shelter fell steadily. In 1980 the inn was relocated to a larger site, and between 1980 and 1983 the case rate continued to decline at this shelter, presumably because of improved space and ventilation.[5]

However, in 1983 and throughout 1984 a sudden increase in the number of TB cases was noted because of an outbreak at the Pine Street Inn. Many of the tubercle bacilli had a similar drug resistance pattern. Between 1984 and 1988, 85 cases of active TB were identified. Of these, 49 (58 percent) were with bacteria resistant to isoniazid and streptomycin. A consistent phage type was found in 43 of the 49.[6] A significant number of the earlier TB cases occurred in whites between the ages of fifty and fifty-nine who had histories of active or chronic alcoholism. By 1987, however, cases were concentrated in persons between the ages of thirty and thirty-nine, most of whom had documented risk factors for HIV infection. The isoniazid and streptomycin resistance pattern was still prevalent in this group, but in only 6 of the 16 cases diagnosed, while 9 were sensitive to all medications. The outbreak of active disease in these 9 cases was probably related to HIV infection.[7] The 1988 case rate for Boston's estimated 6,000 homeless was 267 per 100,000. This is slightly lower than the 1984–86 figures but still represents a significant problem when compared with the citywide rate of 24.95 per 100,000 in 1988.

The changing epidemiology of TB, along with the expansion of beds at other shelters around Boston, led the TB program staff to realize that managing cases among the homeless from one main shelter site was unrealistic. Early in 1986 the Department of Health and Hospitals' TB control nurses expanded their surveillance and control efforts. The public health nurses provided education at the four largest overnight shelters in the city. These facilities provide overnight shelter for an average of 1,315 persons on any given night. Boston's largest day shelter was also targeted for TB control efforts. It has an average daytime attendance of 350 persons, many of whom also stay at the overnight shelters. Information regarding trends in TB among the city's homeless, the need for screening, and modes of intervention were provided. Ongoing surveillance included TB skin testing, particularly of those exhibiting symptoms compatible with TB or seeking treatment for pulmonary complaints. All clients who initially tested negative to the TB skin test were encouraged to receive repeat testing every six months while in the shelters. Those testing positive received preliminary instructions regarding TB infectivity and an appointment for follow-up at the Boston City Hospital TB Clinic.

In the rare event that a symptomatic patient refuses conventional follow-up, attempts are made to intervene as needed in order to have a medical evaluation done. This may include scheduling a follow-up at another clinic of the person's choice or evaluating him or her in the TB clinic during nonclinic hours. If this fails, there is no recourse but to bar the individual from the shelter until seen by a physician. If the person is considered incapable of making sound decisions concerning care, then legal recourse may be the only option.

Because isoniazid- and streptomycin-resistant organisms have been common in Boston's homeless, TB prophylaxis and treatment regimens have been modified. Preventive therapy using isoniazid as a single agent is avoided when a person has a documented skin test conversion because of contact with a resistant case. If the contact cannot be identified, but the individual has resided in any of Boston's shelters since 1984 and has converted the skin test to positive, the modified treatment plan is used. Active tuberculosis patients are always started on three antituberculous drugs. Isoniazid usually is part of the regimen until there is information about bacterial sensitivities.

Close follow-up of clients on medications is stressed because of the common occurrence of isoniazid- or rifampin-related hepatotoxicity in conjunction with past or present histories of substance abuse or hepatitis. Baseline liver function tests and complete blood counts are obtained for all clients and then monitored every month or as clinically indicated.

Each client with active TB is evaluated for risk to the general shelter population. People who have shown noncompliance with medical intervention are treated as inpatients. Between 1983 and 1988 a total of fifty-one persons with TB spent an average of 135 days (range: 2 to 505 days) in a chronic hospital that provided TB care. Eight of these fifty-one (16 percent) required legal action to ensure their stay. Massachusetts law mandates inpatient therapy for those with evidence of active TB identified by a local board of health or two physicians as being a significant public health risk because they have earlier demonstrated noncompliance with recommended treatment.

Patients diagnosed with active TB who comply with therapy have other options. Some receive care at the Shattuck Shelter Respite Program, staffed by Health Care for the Homeless Program team. Adjacent to this shelter is the Lemuel Shattuck Hospital with its TB clinic available for follow-up care. Others may elect to receive medications within the shelters. Medication can be dispensed at any one of the four overnight or one large day shelter, all of which have fully staffed nurses' clinics. Before exercising either of these options, those newly diagnosed with pulmonary TB must be hospitalized until noncontagious (confirmed by three negative sputum smears). All clients are assigned to a TB control nurse for follow-up to ensure compliance.

One of the most effective factors in maintaining a surveillance and case management system is ongoing communiction between the shelter and health department staffs and the care givers. The public health nurses rely on the shelter staff to notify them if a patient does not appear for appointments. To make sure that patient care data are available, a global standardized information system accessible to involved shelters has been established. A computerized listing of patients and their TB status was first created in 1984. Data on that list included the client's name, date of birth, date and result of the most recent tuberculin skin test, chest X ray, sputum smear and culture results, and medication status. The list is updated to reflect changes in therapy. Distribution is limited, because of the need for confidentiality. By 1987 the list had grown to encompass data from the expanded TB surveillance and screening program. This computerized data system had limitations since it depended on the accuracy of the data sheets, the number of staff members available, and their motivation to carry on screening in the face of more immediate issues. Despite these problems, the list has proved indispensable for effective intervention. From 1985 through April 1988, 3,060 individuals have been screened for tuberculous infection and disease (Table 15.2), 1,686 receiving tuberculin skin testing and 1,950 receiving chest X rays. There were 12 cases of active TB found, and there were 115 documented cases of tuberculin skin test

Table 15.2 BOSTON: TUBERCULOSIS INFECTION AND
TUBERCULOSIS SCREENING DATA IN THE HOMELESS
(*January 1, 1985, to April 30, 1988*)

	NUMBER	PERCENT
Total number of screenings	3,060	
Skin testing		
Documented positive (≥10 mm)	696	41.3
Documented negative (<10 mm)	979	58.0
Anergic	11	0.7
Total skin tests given and read	*1,686*	*100.0*
Radiographic findings		
Normal chest X ray	1,713	87.8
Abnormal chest X ray	198	10.2
Suspicious for TB	39	2.0
Total	*1,950*	*100.0*
Total number of homeless TB cases	12	
Total number of documented converters	115	(24.5)

conversion from negative to positive while the homeless were in the shelter system. This suggests transmission in the shelter.

An additional vital resource has been Boston's Health Care for the Homeless team. Through regular visits to all the larger shelters, the team is often able to provide feedback regarding the location and health histories of clients. Difficult decisions about individual treatment plans are often clarified on the bases of the team's observations. Treatment failure and medication toxicity are often identified in a more timely manner.

Chicago

When the Chicago HCHP began testing homeless individuals for TB, it proved difficult to induce them to return for skin test readings and chest X rays. In 1987, therefore, a more intensive screening program was started, using incentives (McDonald's coupons) and prompt transport to the referral site. Through these modifications, the entire testing procedure was trimmed down and made more attractive, eliminating unnecessary waiting time and client paper work. The HCHP project also recognized the validity and usefulness of testing persons in SRO hotels. These individuals, less transitory in their life-styles than those in the overnight shelters, were easier to follow. The SRO population was similar to the currently homeless clients. In fact, most SRO residents had been homeless in the recent past.

Between March 1986 and March 1988, 227 homeless persons were screened for tuberculous infection and disease with tuberculin skin testing. Of these, 167 (74 percent) returned for a tuberculin skin test reading. Of those tested, 72 percent were men, 42 percent were black, 42 percent white, and 4 percent Hispanic. There was one Native American. Ethnic category was unknown for another 25 (11 percent). Of those who returned, 52 (31 percent) had positive tuberculin skin tests. No cases of active TB were discovered through this screening. All 52 individuals with positive skin tests were referred to the local Centers for Disease Control clinic for chest X rays. However, 23 (44 percent) failed to show up. Of the 29 who appeared, 20 (69 percent) had normal chest X rays, 8 others had abnormal chest X rays not consistent with TB, and 1 had a chest X ray consistent with old TB and was started on isoniazid (INH) prophylaxis, according to standard criteria.[8] Chicago has had no known outbreaks of TB within the shelter system, and drug resistance is almost nonexistent.

New York

St. Vincent's Hospital Department of Community Medicine has been involved in the problem of TB in the SRO hotel and shelter populations since 1979. A survey undertaken at that time evaluated tuberculin status and active TB among the residents of three SRO hotels.[9] Of a total of 250 individuals, 191 (76 percent) agreed to interviews and tuberculin skin testing. The result was that 98 (51 percent) individuals were found to have positive tuberculin skin tests, and of these, thirteen (6.7 percent) had positive sputum cultures for *Mycobacterium tuberculosis.*

In 1980 the department began health services on-site at a New York City men's shelter. Tuberculosis proved to be a common health problem in these men. A systematic survey of tuberculous infection and disease was begun in July 1982.[10] Tuberculin skin test screeningg and TB case finding results assessed in August 1988 showed that 1,853 men had been evaluated. Men were interviewed and, when these were indicated, had tuberculin skin testing, chest X rays, and cultures for acid-fast bacilli. A total of 1,671 (90.2 percent) men returned to complete interviews and have their tuberculin skin tests read. They were placed into one of four mutually exclusive categories to describe the presence or absence of tuberculous infection (see Table 15.3). When those who were tuberculin-positive as tested, those who were tuberculin-positive by history, and those with active tuberculosis were combined, 42.8 percent were found to be infected.

Age, race, intravenous drug use, and length of stay in the shelter system were studied, using a multiple logistic regression model to determine independent risk factors for tuberculous infection and disease. Increasing age, black or Hispanic race, IVDU, and time in the shelter system were found to be significantly associated with tuberculous infection. Most significant of these was length of stay. Those

Table 15.3 NEW YORK: SCREENING DATA
FOR TUBERCULOSIS INFECTION AND
DISEASE IN THE HOMELESS
(*1982–1988*)

TUBERCULOSIS STATUS	NUMBER EVALUATED	PERCENT
PPD negative	956	57.2
PPD positive	452	27.0
PPD positive by history	163	9.8
Active tuberculosis	100	6.0
Subtotal	*1,671*	*100.0*
Noncompliant with testing	182	
Total number evaluated	1,853	

in the shelter more than twenty-four months had a 65 percent infection rate (skin test positivity or active TB), compared with 31.5 percent for those in the system less than three months ($p > 0.001$).

Independent risk factors for active disease (culture-positive tuberculosis) included increasing age, IVDU, and time spent in the shelter population. IVDUs are known to be at risk for infection with HIV, especially in New York City.[11–16] Those using intravenous drugs were 2.9 times more likely to have active tuberculosis than nonusers ($p < 0.001$). This is presumably on that basis that HIV infection leads to activation of a previously acquired tuberculous infection.[17–20] Nearly 20 percent of those for whom data were available used or had taken intravenous drugs. The majority of these men used cocaine alone or in conjunction with heroin. It is notable that estimates of HIV antibody (Ab) seropositivity in New York methadone maintenance clinic patients range from 50 to 60 percent.[20,21] A survey of IVDUs in San Francisco showed that those who used cocaine alone or in combination with heroin had two to three times the HIV seropositivity rate of those using heroin alone.[22,23] Cocaine use was associated with more frequent injections and other types of high-risk behavior. In this New York City shelter study HIV Ab testing was done on eight of twenty-seven individuals with active TB who admitted to high-risk behavior. All eight were HIV-Ab-positive. Thus, nearly all intravenous cocaine users in this New York City population may be HIV-Ab-positive and at risk for activation of dormant tuberculous infection.

The study found rates of pulmonary versus extrapulmonary tuberculosis similar to those in the United States and New York City as a whole.[24,25] Eighty-two percent of active TB cases in the study were pulmonary. The remaining eighteen consisted of lymphatic (three), pleural (seven), and disseminated TB (eight). Treatment of TB was initiated in either the hospital or shelter clinic. By August 31, 1988, thirty-six men had completed therapy within eighteen months, and another thirteen were still on treatment. Thirty-eight men were lost to follow-up, both to the shelter staff and to the Bureau of TB. This usually occurred when the clients left the shelter. If they stayed in the shelter, men remained compliant with therapy. Thirteen had died. The causes of death were not known.

Compliance with antituberculous therapy presents a major challenge to both patients and health care providers. Most regimens require at least six months of uninterrupted therapy.[8] In the first weeks patients usually experience dramatic resolution of symptoms, and this reinforces the need for long-term compliance. After several months of therapy patients become asymptomatic, and compliance becomes more of a problem. This point shows why prophylactic treatment of persons with positive tuberculin skin tests but no active disease is often unsuccessful unless it can be tied in with another essential service such as a methadone maintenance program.[20] In addition, medications are frequently stolen and replacement is usually difficult, typically involving a several-hour wait in a clinic or emergency room while a medical record is pulled to verify the type and dose.

Risk factors for tuberculous infection and active disease are known to include increasing age and nonwhite race in the general population of the United States, and the study demonstrated these relationships (Figures 15.1 and 15.2).[26,27] Since the analysis found length of stay in the shelter system to be a disease risk factor independent of age, race, and intravenous drug use, one can assume that staying in shelters can lead to infection with *Mycobacterium tuberculosis*. Tuberculosis is known to be transmitted by the inhalation of aerosolized sputum droplets over relatively long periods.[28,29] Since TB spread is related to crowding and poverty, it should not be surprisiing that tuberculosis is found in congregate shelters.[30]

A flaw in this study is that the selection of patients could not be made randomly. Data were recorded while the staff gave health care to the residents of the shelter. Nevertheless, while the amount of active disease uncovered may be skewed because some of the men came to clinic with symptoms, the fact that so much

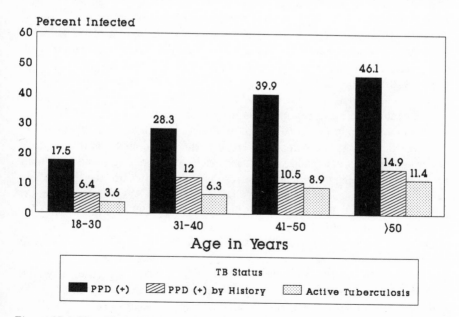

Figure 15.1 **New York: Tuberculosis infection and tuberculosis vs. age, 1982–1988 (n = 1,853).**

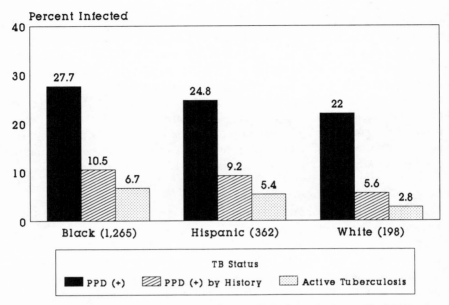

Figure 15.2 **New York: Tuberculosis infection and tuberculosis vs. ethnic category, 1982–1988 (n = 1,825).**

untreated contagious disease was found is significant. Those with positive tuberculin skin tests were representative of the able-bodied men in the shelter. The levels of infection found are far in excess of those for the housed poor in New York City. The last major survey of tuberculous infection in the city was conducted in 1973 and 1974, when more than 50,000 employees of the Board of Education were tuberculin skin tested.[31] The survey recorded both demographic data and socioeconomic status. In 1973 and 1974 New York City active TB cases were one-third more common than in 1989. Tuberculin skin test positivity (or dormant infection) was presumably similarly higher. Despite this, tuberculous infection rates in this shelter population study were nearly double that of the lowest socioeconomic group in the 1973 and 1974 survey of all age and ethnic groups (Figures 15.3 and 15.4). A major strength of the current analysis is that it was performed over six years and yielded consistent results during this time (Figure 15.5). It is interesting to compare these results with a study performed by the New York City Department of Health (NYCDOH) in 1988.[4] NYCDOH attempted to screen at several shelters with a total population of 13,997 clients. Either skin testing followed by chest X rays, where appropriate, or chest X rays alone were offered between September 1986 and March 1989. One-third (4,662) of the clients completed testing, but only 7 new cases of active TB were found. This yields a case rate of 150 per 100,000 successfully screened. Active TB cases may have been underrepresented in the NYCDOH screening survey for several reasons: Screening was broad and extended beyond homeless persons in a shelter clinic, those ill with active TB may have avoided the survey team because they mistrusted traditional health care systems, and the shelters involved may have housed younger and presumably more healthy individuals.

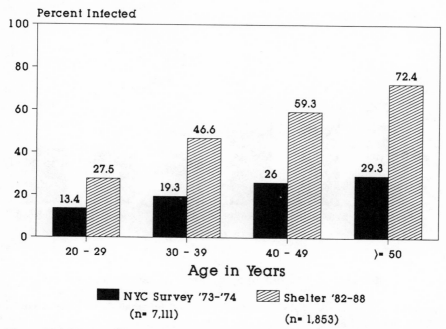

Figure 15.3 **New York: Tuberculosis infection in housed vs. shelter population, by age.**

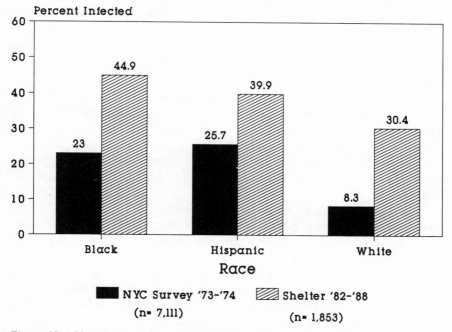

Figure 15.4 **New York: Tuberculosis infection in housed vs. shelter population, by ethnic category.**

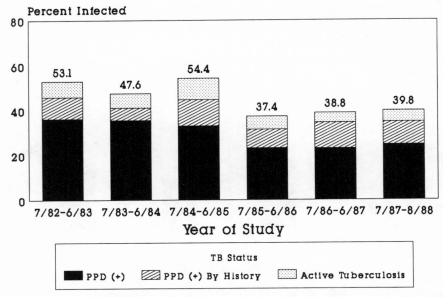

Figure 15.5 **New York: Tuberculosis infection and tuberculosis vs. year of study, 1982–1988 (n = 1,853).**

San Francisco

The San Francisco HCHP works with the TB Control Division (the TB Clinic) of the San Francisco Department of Health. The HCHP, through its shelter-based clinics, provides tuberculin skin testing and referral to the TB clinic for X rays, further evaluation, and treatment when indicated. If a homeless person at a shelter is found to have TB, broad skin testing follows. There are also periodic mass screenings, as well as testing of shelter and Health Care for the Homeless staff.

In 1987, 22 cases of active TB were found among the homeless of San Francisco, and 18 in 1988. This would yield an annual case rate of 180 to 360 cases of TB per 100,000 homeless, depending on estimates of 5,000 to 10,000 homeless persons in San Francisco. The case rate for San Francisco as a whole in 1987 was 43.8 per 100,000, or more than four times the national case rate.[32] Thus, the rate in the San Francisco homeless may be eighteen to thirty-six times the city case rate.

The majority of the 1988 active cases were in whites, while in 1987 blacks made up the largest group. Notably lacking among the homeless cases are Asians, who account for nearly half of all the active TB cases in San Francisco in general. In 1987 the mean age of a homeless person with TB was 38.8 (range 23 to 52).

In 1987 one case of resistant TB was found in a twenty-seven-year-old Nicaraguan man who had arrived in the United States in 1985. He presented to an emergency room with extensive bilateral pulmonary TB. The patient had a history of heavy alcohol and IV drug use. His sputum culture was positive, and the bacteria were resistant to isoniazid. He was treated with rifampin, ethambutol, and pyrazinamide on daily supervised therapy from January to September 1987. Sputum cultures became negative, and his chest X ray improved. He had probably acquired his resistant strain in Central America. In 1988 there were no reported cases of drug-resistant TB in the homeless.

Homeless persons with active TB are closely followed by the directly observed therapy (DOT) program. Patients come to the clinic five days week for medication, or alternatively, medication is brought to them. As a result of this program, in 1987 only two of twenty-two cases of TB in the homeless were lost to follow-up, and one in 1988.

HIV Infection and TB in San Francisco

As of December 31, 1988, San Francisco reported 5,834 cases of AIDS, and it continues to be in the midst of an epidemic. There are no reliable studies of HIV seroprevalance among the homeless in San Francisco. However, it may prove relevant that recent studies show an increased seropositivity among IVDUs. In 1987, 22 percent of the homeless with TB were infected with HIV, and in 1988 this had risen to 50 percent. It is not clear yet whether this increase represents a trend. It does make a strong case for tuberculin skin testing and treatment for those known to be HIV-seropositive or at risk.

From July 1986 through May 1988 the HCHP studied non-Asian-born persons between ages eighteen and sixty-five years with active TB. Risk factor data and HIV antibody status were obtained for consecutive patients willing to participate. Sixty agreed to the study. Of these, seventeen (28 percent) were HIV-Ab-positive. Positives were more likely to be male, black, homosexual or bisexual, and twenty-five to forty-four years of age. One patient had ARC, and another had AIDS.

The prevalence of HIV infection among IVDUs in treatment centers in San Francisco has been increasing. In 1984 and 1985 the overall prevalence was 10 percent. In 1986 and 1987 it rose to 13 percent, with 25 percent of blacks, 10 percent of Hispanics, and 7 percent of whites HIV-Ab-positive. In a sample of hospitalized intravenous drug users at San Francisco General Hospital, 21 percent were HIV-Ab-positive. Comparison of AIDS and TB rosters from 1981 to 1988 demonstrated increasing rates of correlation. In 1981 none of 30 cases of AIDS had TB. By 1988, 21 (1.7 percent) of the 1,218 cases of AIDS had TB. That year 20 of 313 cases of TB (6.4 percent) also appeared in the AIDS registry. These data confirm the relationship between the development of TB and HIV infection noted earlier.

Approximately 700 homeless persons have been screened for TB or tuberculous infection with tuberculin skin testing. An in-depth analysis is available for the first 403, done between march 1986 and March 1987. The first 279 persons completed extensive questionnaires including demographic data, pertinent medical histories relating to TB, and lengths of stays in "cheap" hotels. The questionnaire was subsequently changed to seek data regarding demographics and prior tuberculin skin testing or TB history. Women are overrepresented in the San Francisco sample because of screening at the Episcopal Sanctuary, a women's center. Also, the program staff wanted to target women because there had been a cluster of newly diagnosed TB cases at another women's shelter. Women had a 13.2 percent tuberculin skin test positivity rate, and men a 20.1 percent positivity rate.

Table 15.4 shows the results in the 403 persons screened. Of note is the continued loss of persons at each step in the screening process. Of the 403 individuals who received tuberculin skin tests, 296 (73 percent) returned to have them read. Of the 69 (23 percent) among the 296 with significant reactions ($>=10$mm), forty kept their appointments at the TB clinic for evaluation and chest X rays. One new case of active TB was diagnosed through this screening method, and four cases of previously diagnosed TB were encountered. For the first 279 persons screened there was no significant difference in mean age, sex distribution, or time spent in shelters or "cheap" hotels between tuberculin reactors and nonreactors.

Table 15.4 SAN FRANCISCO: TUBERCULOSIS
INFECTION AND TUBERCULOSIS SCREENING
IN THE HOMELESS
(*1986–1987*)

	NUMBER	PERCENT
Number tested	403	
Number read	296	73
Negative skin test	227	77
Positive skin test	69	23
No chest X ray done		
(lost to follow-up)	29	42
Chest X ray done	40	58
Current TB	1	
Previous TB	4	

During the March 1986–87 time period, a total of 303 cases of active TB were diagnosed in San Francisco. The TB Control Program determined that 23 cases were in persons who were homeless. The nurses in the TB clinic who have worked closely with the HCHP TB screening program made the determination of homelessness. They had access to the social service notes and also made their own evaluations. Clinical evaluation was used to diagnose 18 of the 23. Almost all of these came to the San Francisco General Hospital emergency room with symptoms and were admitted.

In November 1986 a longtime resident of a women's shelter was found to have extensive cavitary TB at the emergency room. Subsequent contact evaluation at that shelter showed high rates of tuberculous infection. Six cases of active TB were found among the residents and staff. In four cases, phage typing was done by the Centers for Disease Control. Of the four, only two were an identical match. This indicates three different sources of TB rather than a single source as suggested by the epidemiologic data. The index case suffered from a severe psychiatric disorder. She was unable to comply with treatment as an outpatient. At one point, after an appropriate court order, she was held involuntarily for a short period of time. Later, with the help of a social worker at the shelter, she faithfully took her twice-weekly medication, and she has successfully completed a six-month course.

Conclusions from the San Francisco Experience

- Tuberculosis is an important health problem among the homeless. One-quarter of the homeless shelter residents show evidence by tuberculin skin test of tuberculous infection. Since the average age of a homeless person in San Francisco and other large cities is between thirty and forty years, this high rate of infection may represent both a future and a current risk for the development of active TB. The prevalence of HIV infection among the homeless is unknown. Persons at risk or who are known to be HIV-Ab-positive should be tuberculin skin tested and, if they are positive, should be offered antibiotic prophylaxis regardless of age. Those found to have TB should be offered HIV testing and counseling.
- Noncompliance with random screening by skin testing is high. At each step in the screening process persons are lost to follow-up. Mobile X ray vans and sputum testing in select cases would be helpful.
- Transmission of TB is facilitated by crowded shelter conditions. This is clearly shown by the cluster of cases from the women's shelter. Proper ventilation, more space between mats or cots, and appropriately placed and maintained ultraviolet (UV) lights should decrease the rate of transmission.
- Thorough contact investigation is important and effective when a case is detected. Staff members, who may spend more time in the shelter than the average shelter resident, need to be evaluated. They are also at high risk for infection.
- In San Francisco random skin testing was not effective in finding current cases of TB. However, contact evaluation and supervision of therapy were highly effective. The HCHP plans to continue its screening program and increase its efforts to complete the evaluation process among the noncompliers.

Seattle

In January 1987 the Seattle, King County Health Department began investigating a possible outbreak of TB at a men's shelter. This particular site, an abandoned warehouse on the Seattle waterfront, is an evening residence for homeless men over the age of fifty. The shelter is financed and managed by Catholic Community Services with a professional and volunteer staff of twenty. There are approximately two hundred mattresses laid on the floor, arranged in rows an average of one foot apart. Ventilation is provided by open windows, weather permitting. The lighting system is a series of fluorescent mounts. On most evenings the shelter sleeps 150 to 175 men. It is open from 6:00 P.M. until 6:00 A.M. Those who sleep in the shelter spend their daytime hours at various locations in downtown Seattle.

This population of men is relatively stable compared with that in other shelters in Seattle. Approximately a thousand men per year pass through.

The shelter opened in October 1984, and the first case of active TB was reported in April 1985. There were five cases during 1985, six in 1986, and eleven in the first five months of 1987. Those eleven represent more than a doubling in the number in shelter residents over the two previous years. Three of the cases from 1987 were detected from the Health Department investigation; the remainder were reported by other health care providers during the evaluation of patients who were ill. Those with active TB ranged in age from forty-three to seventy-seven years. Twelve men were white, two Alaskan natives, and eight others Native Americans. There were no black men in this group. Nineteen had pulmonary TB, including four with cavitary disease. The three with extrapulmonary disease had miliary TB (two) and pleuropulmonary TB (one). Twelve cases had positive sputum smears for TB at the time of diagnosis. Twenty of the twenty-two active cases had bacteria susceptible to all standard antituberculous drugs. One specimen was resistant to INH and ethionamide and another to INH only. Previous treatment for active TB was known for five individuals. All had received multiple antituberculous medications, and one had also undergone a lobectomy. Two individuals had a history of INH prophylaxis, and another two a history of a positive PPD but no prophylactic treatment.

A survey was undertaken to determine the prevalence of tuberculous infection in those clients or staff members who might have been infected by the 22 persons with active TB in the shelter. In January 1987, 171 clients and 11 staff members underwent tuberculin skin testing. Of the clients tested, 140 returned for skin testing and 84 (60 percent) had significant PPD reactions ($>=5$ mm), according to Centers for Disease Control and American Thoracic Society criteria for "household contacts."[8] The proportion of patrons with significant skin tests was considered high when compared with an earlier skin test survey at this site. In May 1985, when tuberculin skin test screening was undertaken because of the recognition of 2 cases of TB in the shelter, 88 tuberculin skin tests were applied, 61 (69 percent) were read, and 22 (36 percent) were found to be positive. Further comparison of the results of the two screenings revealed that 12 clients were tested on both occasions. Of these, 4 who tested positive in 1985 also tested positive in 1987, 7 who tested negative in 1985 also tested negative in 1987, and only 1 individual's PPD converted between the two screenings. Of interest is the fact that 3 individuals screened in 1985 with positive PPD skin tests were among the 22 cases of active TB in 1987. In follow-up to the January 1987 screening, chest X rays were offered to all individuals tested, both positives and negatives. Those with suspicious X rays submitted sputum cultures to rule out active TB.

Following completion of this phase of the follow-up in May 1987, INH prophylaxis was offered to all clients with reactive tuberculin skin tests who lacked a documented prior positive test. Eighty-two individuals began INH prophylaxis. Medication is administered in a dose of 900 mg twice weekly. The second round of tuberculin skin testing was performed in June 1987 to extend the knowledge of skin test reactivity among shelter residents in general and to determine recent converters. Seventy-one (78 percent) of ninety-one persons tested returned to have the tests read. Twenty-three (32 percent) had positive ($>=5$ mm) tuberculin skin tests. Fourteen percent of those with positive skin tests were documented conversions from prior negative tests, suggesting transmission within the shelter. The increase in TB cases among shelter residents in 1987, the increase in tuberculin reactivity among clients in 1987 compared with 1985, and the finding of several skin test converters from January to June 1987 further strengthen the view that TB is being transmitted in the shelter.

Summary

Several threads run through the tuberculosis experiences in Boston, Chicago, New York, San Francisco, and Seattle. Tuberculosis is a disease of poverty and crowding. It should not be surprising that TB is found in shelters for the homeless where individuals sleep one to two feet apart for months at a time. These are the equivalent of crowding in nineteenth-century tenements. Several definitive statements can be made.

- There is a significant amount of tuberculosis infection and disease among residents of the homeless shelters in our major cities. Individuals staying in these shelters for a period of time risk infection with *Mycobacterium tuberculosis*.
- Many of those who acquire tuberculous infection (evidenced by a positive tuberculin skin test) are at increased risk for developing active tuberculosis because of concomitant HIV infection.
- Detection and treatment of active tuberculosis can be successful when coupled with other essential shelter services such as an on-site clinic or work programs.
- Close cooperation with local bureaus of tuberculosis control can help establish diagnoses of active tuberculosis and help ensure continuation of therapy when individuals leave a shelter or fail to show up for follow-up visits at a clinic.

Acknowledgments: The authors owe gratitude to M. Anita Barry, M.D., M.P.H., director of the Community Infectious Disease Epidemiology Program, Boston Department of Health and Hospitals, for her work in the Boston Tuberculosis Control Program.

OLGA PIANTIERI

WILLIAM VICIC

RANDALL BYRD

SHARON BRAMMER

MAX MICHAEL III

16

Hypertension Screening and Treatment in the Homeless

Introduction

Hypertension is the most common chronic disorder in the United States today.[1] It is well documented that high blood pressure, unchecked, leads to catastrophic cerebrovascular, cardiovascular, and renal diseases.[2,3] Hypertension screening programs initiated by state and local health departments during the last two decades have been successful in significantly reducing resultant morbidity and mortality.[4-6] The homeless, however, remain largely untouched by these efforts.[7]

Most of the alienating and isolating effects that homeless individuals experience originate from their debilitating poverty.[8] The homeless are forced into a survival mode of existence by a life of chronic crises and by the limited services and resources available to them.[9] The only medical help many homeless or nearly homeless persons can obtain is in overcrowded emergency rooms solely intended for giving acute care. Follow-up is virtually nonexistent, and chronic diseases are rarely recognized. Long-term health goals are not viewed as priorities by emergency room staff members, who may be awed by what seems to be the insurmountable difficulty of helping a homeless person, or even by the homeless themselves, who are concerned with relieving today's pain rather than with vague tomorrows.[10] As a result, the homeless remain enmeshed in a survival pattern of behavior, and the overburdened emergency health care system offers few options for long-term care.

The price of treating the later acute and disabling complications of neglected chronic disease, however, is many times that of preventive measures.[10] This is apparent both in monetary terms and, more important, in reduced potential and quality of life for those afflicted. Provision for chronic disease management and prevention must therefore be found to meet the long-term health needs of homeless individuals and families.

Specific strategies for the screening and treatment of the chronic disorder of hypertension in homeless populations living in shelters, drop-in centers, welfare hotels, and the streets are considered here, with data generated from such endeavors. This information results from the efforts of three health care programs committed specifically to the homeless and near homeless poor: the Downtown Clinic in Nashville, Tennessee, the Birmingham (Alabama) Health Care for the Homeless Program, and the St. Vincent's Hospital SRO/Homeless Program in New York City. The approaches these programs have developed for high blood pressure control have broad applications. The successful therapy of hypertension is a useful paradigm for health maintenance in general because it combines aspects of chronic disease management with secondary and tertiary prevention. Because it is an asymptomatic illness, hypertension challenges health teams to motivate patients to comply with treatment regimens.

The three programs employ aggressive outreach models for delivering medical services, coupled with a client-centered approach through the use of interdisciplinary teams. Some of their experiences have been similar. Others, based on regional and population differences, have differed considerably. A consistent finding was that homeless persons are deeply interested in their health and willing, when circumstances are not prohibitive, to comply with therapeutic plans.

Screening

Hypertension is the leading risk factor for cardiovascular, cerebrovascuular, and renal diseases.[2] Despite recent reductions in mortality rates, heart disease remains the primary cause of death in the United States, and strokes the third leading cause.[11]

Prevalence of hypertension among blacks has consistently been higher than for whites.[12,13] Recent studies confirm this and indicate that:

- The incident rates for blacks are at least twice as high as for whites independent of age or sex.[13]
- The years of potential life lost (YPLL) because of cerebrovascular disease are 4.5 times higher for black males than white males.[14]
- Black women with cerebrovascular disease have YPLL rates 3.9 times higher than white women.[14]
- Among black men *borderline* hypertension results in the same survival rates as those associated with *definite* hypertension in the general population.[13]

Most surveys support the conclusion that blacks are disproportionally over-represented in homeless populations.[15] By extrapolation, this finding supports the need for aggressive hypertension screening and treatment in the homeless.

New York City

In 1983 St. Vincent's Hospital started a Hypertension Screening and Treatment Program, funded by a grant from the New York State Department of Health. This effort was incorporated into the SRO / Homeless Program which was already in place, providing medical outreach services at shelters, drop-in centers, and SRO hotels. The majority of the individuals screened for hypertension lived at a large public shelter for eight hundred to a thousand homeless men.

In virtually all cases the medical personnel assigned to each site conducted the screening. The personnel included physicians, nurses, and medical and nursing students. Depending on the site, they took blood pressure recordings either as a component of a medical evaluation or as part of mass screening endeavors. As a noninvasive procedure blood pressure measurement proved useful for gently introducing shelter clients to the medical team. Often through the screening process other problems were uncovered, and on occasion potentially life-threatening situations were averted.

To ensure uniformity in screening, staff members were instructed to use identical equipment and to follow a specific protocol. A mercury sphygmomanometer was used for blood pressure measurements. Unless circumstances were adverse, readings were measured on the right arm with the patient in a sitting position.

Those with systolic blood pressures greater than 140 mm Hg or diastolics greater than 90 mm Hg were asked to return for rechecks. Individuals whose pressures remained elevated were referred to a physician for evaluation and treatment. Clients with diastolic readings greater than 120 were referred for immediate treatment.

In the four and a half years of the study a total of 5,197 persons were screened. Table 16.1 shows the demographic breakdown of the entire screened population. The distribution described here reflects the population of those shelters and hotels serviced by the St. Vincent's Hospital SRO / Homeless Program and is not necessarily representative of the homeless of New York City in general. As can be seen from the table, the largest group consisted of black males under the age of sixty-five.

Table 16.1 SCREENING POPULATION NEW YORK CITY

AGE	BLACK		HISPANIC		WHITE		OTHER		
	M	F	M	F	M	F	M	F	TOTAL
18–44	1,794	303	549	71	352	160	34	6	3,269
45–64	516	115	143	40	428	207	12	2	1,463
Over 65	67	24	12	6	204	147	4	1	465
Totals	2,377	442	704	117	984	514	50	9	5,197

The overall prevalence rate of high blood pressure was 25 percent.* Figure 16.1 illustrates prevalence rates with respect to age, sex, and race. High blood pressure was more prevalent in whites than in blacks, a startling finding. An examination of the mean ages of both groups offers a possible explanation. The average age of blacks screened was 37.5 years, significantly lower than the mean age (51.8 years) for whites (p < 0.01).

Additionally, a higher prevalence rate was found in women when compared with men. Again, the mean age of the women screened, 46 years, was significantly higher than for men, 40.4 years (p < 0.01). It is established that the incidence of hypertension increases with age for all sex and ethnic groups.[13] As can be seen from Figure 16.1, prevalence increases with age in the screened population. The unexpected prevalence ratios found therefore may have resulted from the age differences between groups.

When we consider these data and those following, it is important to recall that screening was conducted neither randomly nor with the purpose of carrying out a scientific study. Rather, the goal was to provide health services to susceptible individuals. Therefore, many variables operating on the selection of the clients screened are unknown or immeasurable. Findings cannot be legitimately comparted with studies employing random selection.

However, comparison with other New York contractors that used similar nonrandom methods but that were different because they served domiciled individuals reveals interesting findings. The St. Vincent's program was compared with twenty-eight programs, each providing hypertension screening for large, primarily indigent New York City populations during the same period, 1983 to 1988.

A caveat: All percentages cited below are based on the results obtained during the initial screening interview and are calculated according to standardized formulas mandated by the New York State Department of Health. Since data were collected at the time of entry into programs, these figures in no way reflect the efforts of subsequent interventions.[16]

- The hypertension prevalence rate in the St. Vincent's program was 25 percent. This was similar to the average prevalence rate of 27.4 percent found by other New York City programs.
- Of those persons with high blood pressures in the homeless program, 40.3 percent had no previous history of hypertension. This was almost double the 23.3 percent found in domiciled populations and was found to be significant (p < 0.01).
- In the homeless population at the time of screening, 17 percent of the individuals aware of prior hypertension remained untreated and uncontrolled, significantly higher than the 11 percent other New York programs included in this category (p < 0.01).
- Only 11.6 percent of the homeless who had been prescribed antihypertensive

*Prevalence rates were based on data generated during the initial screening and were calculated as follows: the number of individuals controlled on antihypertensive treatment plus those with elevated blood pressures (>140/90), divided by the total number screened.

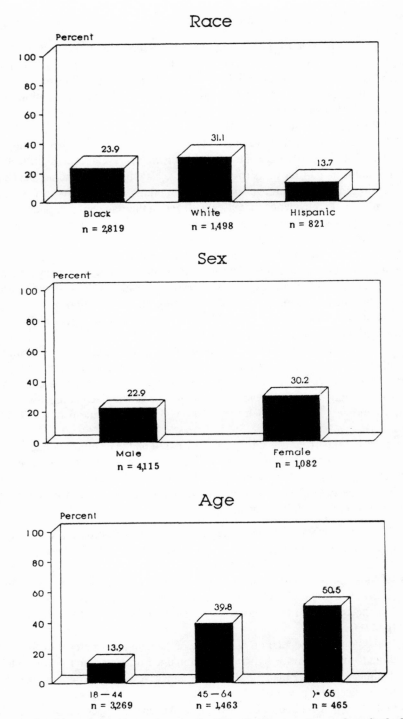

Figure 16.1 **Hypertension prevalence rates according to race, sex, and age in the New York City screening population. Prevalence is defined as the number of individuals controlled on treatment plus the number of individuals with elevated blood pressures (>140/90) divided by the total number screened. Blood pressure status was determined at the time of initial screening.**

treatment were controlled at the time of screening, compared with 29.8 percent in other programs. This, too, was found to be significant ($p < 0.01$).
- Of those with elevated blood pressures in the homeless program, 68 percent returned for a second reading at a later date. This was slightly higher than the 67.8 percent of the domiciled populations but not significantly so ($p > 0.01$).

These figures clearly substantiate the impression that the homeless are a medically underserved group and that without appropriate interventions existing disorders are likely to worsen. The return rate of the homeless for repeat blood pressure checks further demonstrates their willingness to take part in their health care when they are presented with appropriate options. In this respect they are comparable with other groups.

Treatment

The central and recurring issue in caring for homeless hypertensives is the aggressive pursuit of measures to improve compliance. Successful antihypertensive therapy in any population must reflect appreciation of the patient's life-style, side effect profile of drugs, and frequency of administration—in short, a client-centered comprehensive approach.[17,18] With this point in mind, it is crucial to recognize some characteristics of the homeless life-style in order to view treatment issues appropriately. The homeless are under stress from many factors. Those living outdoors are at risk of violent crime and suffer from exposure and other environmental hazards. Those in shelters and drop-in centers are subject to overcrowded sleeping arrangements, theft, rigid rules and regulations, and inadequate bathroom facilities. The chronic lack of privacy does much to undermine the dignity of the human spirit. Those who suffer from psychiatric illnesses, mental retardation, or substance abuse may have impaired coping skills that increase the impact of stress.

Because of a lack of funds or health insurance, homeless individuals tend to seek medical care only in acute emergencies. Storage space is limited if available at all; the homeless are therefore compelled to carry their belongings with them at all times. Medications are often lost or stolen, and multidose regimens confusing and impractical. The following history from the Nashville HCHP is illustrative.

_____

RW is a fifty-four-year-old white man who has had hypertension for at least twenty years. He first visited the Downtown Clinic in 1985, after referral from a local soup kitchen. RW lived in a car and had been unemployable for a year because of uncontrolled blood pressure. He admitted to poor compliance with medications because of side effects (weakness and dizziness), and he was hesitant to return to the hospital because of long waits and difficulties negotiating the system.

RW initially was asymptomatic and denied a history of significant complications from his blood pressure. It was learned later that RW had numerous hospital admissions, with diastolic pressures in the range of 150–180. He had a history of mild congestive heart failure, pulmonary edema, and noncompliance. A previous hypertensive intravenous pyelogram and a renal arteriogram were normal. He had smoked up to two packs of cigarettes a day for more than forty-five years, and he drank several cups of coffee per day.

RW had been prescribed long-acting propranolol, a thiazide-triamterene preparation, and two unidentified medications, of which he had samples. On examination his blood pressure was 190/130, with no venous distention, clear breath sounds, no abnormal heart sounds, and no dependent edema.

About one hour after RW was given 0.2 mg of clonidine by mouth his pressure was 140/100, and he remained asymptomatic. He was instructed to return after lunch. However, he wasn't seen again for about four weeks, when his medication supply lapsed.

Another complicating factor was RW's inability to understand and comply with recommendations. His performance on the revised Wechsler Adult Intelligence Scale, part of an evaluation for disability, showed an IQ of 58, consistent with mild mental retardation. Also noteworthy was that RW was illiterate and tended to anxiety or depression, probably aggravated or caused by his homelessness.

RW had complaints which were probably related to hypertension or to antihypertensive medication; in some instances it wasn't clear which was responsible. He had palpitations, dizziness, headache, fatigue, depression, bradycardia, epistaxis, leg cramps, and malaise. His symptoms did not parallel the degree of elevation of his blood pressure. RW had been asymptomatic with markedly elevated pressures, and markedly symptomatic with only moderate elevations.

In 1986 RW complained of angina for the first time (or what was interpreted to be angina since it was relieved within seconds by sublingual nitroglycerin in the clinic). There were no acute changes on the electrocardiogram, but he was referred for hospital admission because of unstable angina and severe hypertension (190/140). The clinic then lost touch with him for two years.

In 1988 he went to an emergency room during the night because of epistaxis and was hospitalized for twenty-three days because of difficulty controlling his blood pressure. Considerable time was spent adjusting and changing his therapy to find the right combination, and finally his attending cardiologist discharged him despite his inability to keep his diastolic level consistently below 120 mm Hg. He returned on his own at this point to the Downtown Clinic.

More recently there has been better hypertension control, for several reasons. First of all, social workers were able to get RW into public housing, which has substantially decreased his stress. Secondly, he was given a pillbox, with separate slots for hours of the day and days of the week. He has been able to do a better job of keeping up with his doses as a result. Thirdly, there was better control shortly after using transdermal clonidine. He does not feel comfortable changing his clonidine patches, so this is done at clinic visits, guaranteeing that he is seen often. The staff has developed a tremendous rapport with him, so he has some confidence and even enthusiasm in following health care recommendations.

RW's most recent blood pressure was 150/108. For four months he has had no change in his therapy, which consists of furosemide (40 mg every twelve *hours), atenolol (50 mg a day), minoxidil (2.5 mg every twelve hours), clonidine (0.2 mg twice a day), and a clonidine patch (0.1 mg once a week). Although there has been better than usual control in recent weeks, he remains a complex patient.*

Treating hypertensive homeless individuals involves specific problems. Patients often refuse diuretics a priori because of poor access to bathroom facilities. Also, the asymptomatic nature of hypertension has a detrimental effect on patients' motivation to comply with treatment.

Managing those who are alcoholics or concurrently drinking causes additional difficulties. Assessment of baseline blood pressure is complicated by the pressor effect of ethanol.[19] Treatment is further complicated by alcohol's potentiation of the hypotensive / arrhythmogenic capacity of some therapeutic agents. Chronic alcoholics often do not seek treatment for weeks at a time during episodes of heavy abuse. The poor water intake of patients during bouts of alcohol consumption, together with alcohol's inherent diuretic effect, may produce significant volume depletion, complicating the use of diuretics.

Nonpharmacologic treatments, such as weight reduction, low-sodium diets, and exercise, are especially difficult for the homeless to maintain even if they are sufficiently motivated. Food selection for the most part is out of their control, and exercise is limited because of the lack of space or equipment. Even an exercise as simple as walking is difficult for the homeless to manage because of the scarcity of comfortable shoes and socks.

As the above case demonstrates, medical plans must consider the realities and daily fluctuations inherent to the homeless life-style and respond with realistic approaches and alternatives. Continuity of care is an indispensable anchor for stabilizing treatment regimens and patient-practitioner relationships.

New York City

Analysis of antihypertension therapy in the St. Vincent's homeless health care experience centers on 290 individuals for whom full diagnostic and treatment data are available. Of the treatment group, 75 percent are men, and few are Hispanic. Most are black or white. Control of hypertension in this medical outreach project was arbitrarily defined as documentation of a normal blood pressure ($\leq 140/90$) at any time following treatment. Given the vagaries of living in the streets or at drop-in centers, many patients had blood pressure readings fluctuating between normal and abnormally high over months of treatment observation. Nevertheless, 71.7 percent of the group achieved hypertension control at one point. Among the ethnic-racial subgroups, white and (in small numbers) Hispanic patients had blood pressure control rates of 83.3 percent and 70.2 percent, respectively, while blacks had a control rate of 62.7 percent. Although these control rates may be considered good, the difference between black and white subgroups invites explanation. For blacks, diuretic treatment of hypertension was effective: In the diuretic-alone group the control rate was 68.4 percent, and in the diuretic-combination group the control rate was 64.1 percent. Only half the blacks achieved blood pressure control with nonpharmacologic maneuvers. In contrast, hypertensive whites who were prescribed nonpharmacologic treatments attained normal blood pressures in 80.8 percent of cases, and for those failing life-style interventions, pharmacologic therapy was effective in 82.4 percent. Recognizing racial differences in the biology of hypertension represents an advance in understanding of this common medical problem,[20] and among the homeless the current St. Vincent's Hospital approach to treatment includes nonpharmacologic prescriptions (weight loss, exercise as possible, alcohol avoidance) for white patients and, often, combined nonpharmacologic and pharmacologic prescriptions for black patients. In either situation a continuous and supportive interaction with a consistent health care team is crucial for treatment success.

Birmingham

For the homeless person with hypertension, a place for proper storage of pills is rare. Without this, pills are stolen and lost or, if kept in a pocket, simply pulverized by the movement of constant walking.[10]

Clonidine hydrochloride, a drug used for the treatment of hypertension, is available in a transdermal patch.[21] The patch delivers a steady therapeutic level of clonidine for seven days. For the homeless person with hypertension, use of the clonidine transdermal patch obviates the need to find storage for medications and can improve long-term blood pressure control, as the following case report demonstrates.

LJ is a black man who has lived in various Birmingham shelters for more than four years. A chronic alcoholic with known hypertension, LJ freely admits he does not take his prescribed medications.

When first seen by the medical team of the Birmingham HCHP, LJ was a thin man appearing twenty years older than his stated age of forty-seven. On initial examination he was intoxicated but cooperative. Blood pressure was 170/100 with a regular pulse rate of 78 per minute and regular. The rest of his examination was unremarkable.

Although LJ was given a once-daily antihypertensive, he was not seen again at the shelter clinic for two months. When he returned to the clinic after a month-long alcohol binge, he was in the early stages of alcohol withdrawal with a blood pressure of 170/110.

LJ was encouraged to try a 2 mm clonidine transdermal patch and was asked to return each week for a patch change. He was also given a few capsules of chlordiazepoxide, 25 mg, for his alcohol withdrawal symptoms.

During the next six weeks LJ returned weekly for his patch change. His blood pressure by the sixth week was 110/80 in spite of his continued use of alcohol. There were no side effects of the patch.

To evaluate the possible efficacy of the clonidine transdermal patch for other homeless men with hypertension, a study was initiated.[22] Between January and

June 1986 all homeless men seen by the program's staff with blood pressure readings in the hypertensive range ($\geq 140 / \geq 90$ mm Hg) were offered treatment with the patch in lieu of conventional oral medications. All medications were provided at no charge. Those choosing the patch were asked to return each week for a blood pressure check and a patch change. For those not opting for a patch, oral medications were also dispensed in a one-week supply. The 1 mm patch was initial therapy for most men. Aggressive follow-up was attempted for all those who did not return to clinic either to have their patches change or to receive their medication refills.

The twenty-one men enrolled were divided into three groups. Group I consisted of the ten men who used the patch throughout the twelve weeks of the study and two men who were discontinued from therapy because they were involved in motor vehicle accidents. Group II consisted of the five men who dropped out of the study, and Group III of the six men lost to follow-up (Table 16.2).

Table 16.2 TREATMENT RESULTS BIRMINGHAM

GROUP	AGE	FOLLOW-UP	MEAN BLOOD PRESSURE* INITIAL	MEAN BLOOD PRESSURE* TREATED
I (10)	44.4	7.5 weeks	164/108	140/87
II (5)	40.4	3.4 weeks	172/112	140/96
III (6)	41.6	NA	162/108	NA

*mmHg.

For the ten men in Group I who completed the study, the mean initial blood pressure was 164 / 108 mm Hg. With treatment the mean blood pressure dropped to 140 / 87 mm Hg, an average drop of 24 mm Hg systolic and 21 mm Hg diastolic. In Group II the mean initial blood pressure of 172 / 112 mm Hg dropped to 140 / 96 mm Hg. In all men normalization of blood pressure occurred within two weeks of starting therapy with the patch.

Men treated with oral medications did not achieve comparable levels of blood pressure control. Many did not return for regular follow-ups, making comparisons between those treated with the patch and those receiving pills impossible.

Twelve of the men (58 percent) were intoxicated during most of the medical encounters. Two additional men had intermittent problems with alcohol.

Comment: Over the limited duration of this study, the clonidine patch assured convenience and compliance with hypertensive therapy in homeless men. This is noteworthy in that adequate control of hypertension has been difficult to achieve.[19,23–25] It is important to recognize that the impressive blood pressure response with the clonidine patch could have resulted from the placebo effect or from the Hawthorne effect.[26] The men were indeed the focus of an unusual amount of attention, including aggressive follow-up. Certainly a combination of these factors may be ultimately responsible in part for the excellent blood pressure control achieved with the patch in more than 50 percent of the men treated.

Summary

The problems facing the homeless and the health care practitioners who care for them are myriad and complex but primarily contingent on the nature of homelessness. In order to meet the challenge, plans for chronic disease management and health maintenance must be multifocal and structured on a patient-centered comprehensive approach. Health care, perhaps the most personal of professional services, is most effective when it is built upon a foundation of trust between patient and practitioner. Consistency of personnel and continuity of care must therefore be constants in any therapeutic that attempts success. For hypertension, these measures are imperative if the harmful consequences of uncontrolled high blood pressure are to be prevented. The major tactical thrust against chronic illness, however, must attack the core of the problem—homelessness. Many obstacles to care would be eliminated or at least their effects contained if permanent residences, rather than "temporary" shelters, were available. All other remedies can be only palliative.

Acknowledgments: The authors owe gratitude to Christopher Maylahn, MPH, epidemiologist, Mary Lasker Heart and Hypertension Institute, New York State Department of Health, Albany, New York; and to Francisca Rodriguez, project coordinator, and Caridad Santini, secretary, SRO/Homeless Program, St. Vincent's Hospital, Department of Community Medicine, New York, New York.

The New York City Hypertension Programs were funded in part by a grant from the Mary Lasker Heart and Hypertension Institute, New York State Department of Health, Albany, New York.

PART III

PROGRAMS AND PARTNERSHIPS

ARMAND H. LEVIN

GARY L. BLASI

RICHARD W. HEIM

DONALD W. PARSONS

LAWRENCE I. KAMEYA

17

Governance, Program Control, and Authority

Introduction

The mission, development, and function of the Health Care for the Homeless Program stem from founding purposes. Specifics of programs differ, each expressing the interest of a diverse set of individuals, organizations, and staffs of preexisting efforts within a community. Many of the HCHPs derived from coalitions created to work with the local problem of homelessness, a community-based approach to ameliorating the problem. In most cases the coalitions themselves grew from the meetings of health professionals, major voluntary organizations, and religious groups dealing with the homeless. City, county, and state agencies related to health and mental health, welfare, and housing were frequently involved.

At some point the rather formless coalition was forced to become organized and responsible. An executive board was selected and in many instances became the governing entity, with a coalition advisory to the governing board and project. The governing board appointed a project director, staff was employed, and the work began.

The Coalition

The original coalitions developed overall strategies for giving health and case-work services to homeless persons in the local area. Transition from the period of creative energy first to the more reserved status of an advisory group and then to the governing board has been variously successful. While in general, the programs have been permitted to evolve in a healthy manner by the founding coalition members, in some instances founders have had trouble letting go, have interfered at a personal level with staff members or directors, or have bypassed the governing board. The opposite has also been seen: coalitions fading out, the spirit of mission leaving with them. This is perhaps even more harmful to program viability because without the moral foundation the project is likely to become just another clinic or even disappear, and all sense of the special needs of homeless persons is lost.

The Governing Body

An effective governing body often derives from the membership of the founding coalition. Members may be elected by the coalition or be selected by individual community agencies that believe they have the right to name a board member. Since the governing group has significant authority over the hiring and firing of the project director and is responsible for contracts and subcontracts, the members must seriously engage in the effort. They must realize that governing activities take time, both for scheduled meetings and also for subcommittee work and individual troubleshooting. The members are also expected to lead in fund raising.

For the nineteen HCHPs, good governance has been a painful evolutionary process. In almost every city twelve to twenty-four months passed before the membership was willing to take firm control, and during this time numerous challenges to effective program function occurred. Challenges were posed by board members who had conflicts of interest in subcontracts, who interfered with daily conduct of the program or undercut the project director, or who favored their own agencies over the HCHP, at times even diverting monies raised for the HCHP.

This discussion traces the evolution of governance in the projects, citing examples of common problems. It explains how the need to resolve issues improved the effectiveness of governance and identifies principles critical to program success and continuance.

Early governance boards of HCHP projects took various approaches to the task. For instance, the Cleveland Health Care for the Homeless Project originally had both a governing board and a coalition body. The former provided project oversight, and the latter a formal means for project input from the field.

In Los Angeles, at the outset authority was assumed by a Governance Committee composed of representatives for the city and the county and selected "neutral" individuals chosen for their special professional fields of endeavor. The composition of the Governance Committee clearly reflected a need to balance the interests of the city of Los Angeles with those of Los Angeles County.

The Denver project grew from an effort of a community task force formed in early 1984 to address the many facets of the homeless problem. The task force formed a new 501(C)(3) (not-for-profit) organization, the Colorado Coalition for the Homeless. This group completed the foundation grant application. The board included persons from the public and private sectors and was dominated by service providers. Upon receipt of the grant, the board established standing committees, among them the Health Care Committee, which was charged with governance of the HCHP project. The original committee was made up of coalition board members who had participated in the grant-writing and application process.

In Albuquerque the decision to apply for a HCHP grant was made by the Emergency Care Alliance (AECA), an already existing coalition. A committee of alliance members was commissioned to prepare the proposal. When a grant was awarded, a health care subcommittee was appointed to oversee day-to-day operations while the policy-making and operating authority remained vested in the AECA.

A coalition of various public and private organizations proposed Baltimore's project. The Health and Welfare Council, a United Way agency which had a major role in the grant application process, assumed fiscal responsibility for the project. Oversight was vested in the board of the Health and Welfare Council, but direct governing of the project was by a Governance Committee of selected coalition members. Linkage of the Governance Committee to the board of the council was accomplished by having a volunteer member of the council's board serve as chairman of the Governance Committee.

Implementation Leads to Change

All the programs have found it necessary to implement varying degrees of change in governance structure.

In Cleveland, while the project had a body called a Governing Board, it also had a Coalition. The role normally filled by a single governing body was divided between the two. The Governing Board was intended to concern itself with such matters as overseeing project operations, reviewing and approving program changes during the project's early development, and advising and assisting in the longer-term strategies for dealing with homelessness. The Coalition was to communicate to other public and private agencies and the community at large information about various aspects of the homelessness problem, advocate on behalf of the homeless, and develop strategies for sustaining the project beyond the four-year grant-funding period. At first, although it was intended that the Governing Board be composed mainly of laypersons, it consisted in fact mostly of service providers, as did the Coalition. While the division of responsibilities between the two was intentional, it did not have the intended result of separating the interests of those having a service provider orientation from those concerned with public policy, advocacy, and future funding. Confusion developed over the respective roles of the two bodies, and a satisfactory identification and separation of duties and responsibilities never developed. The most immediate result was that after several meetings the Coalition ceased to exist, leaving the Governing Board to carry on alone. The interest of the board had already waned, however, and efforts to rekindle it were not succeeding, despite the fact that it was asked to handle meaningful issues. It was decided to change the service provider orientation of the board, and at the end of 1988 it was reconstituted in an effort to meet the project's current needs.

Los Angeles illustrates a governance change more in form than in content. Composition of the project's Governance Committee was a balance of representatives from the city and county and nonaligned neutrals. At the outset an interim chair of the committee was selected from the city contingent, but with a clear understanding that a replacement would be chosen from among the neutral members. The same Governance Committee structure remains, but with one significant change. Recognizing its need to deal effectively with the challenge of identifying and attracting funding, the Governance Committee approved the formation of a new 501(C)(3) corporation. Membership on the board of the new corporation was offered to all Governance Committee members.

Governance in the Denver project has remained unchanged in form, but a significant change has been made in substance. A standing committee (the Health Care Committee) of the board of the Colorado Coalition for the Homeless remains. At the outset the Health Care Committee was composed of those Colorado Coalition members who had participated in the grant-writing and application process. Upon defining its mission early in its existence, the Health Care Committee recognized the need to change its character. To attain a balance of professional skills, it invited several community leaders to join. At present, six members, one-half of the committee, are representatives of the board of the Colorado Coalition while the remaining six are directly involved in various aspects of the delivery of health care other than through the Denver project.

The Albuquerque project was initially governed by a health care subcommittee of the Albuquerque Emergency Care Alliance, a coalition for the homeless. In an effort to sharpen the focus of the body charged with governance, the name of the subcommittee was changed to the Policy Advisory Board. It immediately assumed de facto responsibility for establishing and effecting policy. Subsequent annual reviews of the governance structure affirmed its appropriateness until September 1988, when in order to facilitate the acquisition of a desirable clinic site, action was taken to create a separate not-for-profit legal entity. Albuquerque Health Care for the Homeless, Inc. (AHCH), is a subsidiary corporation of the St. Joseph Health Care Corporation, which, at the request of the AECA, had earlier assumed operational responsibility for the project. Despite its subsidiary status, policy-making and operational authority is vested in the board of directors of the new corporation.

The Governance Committee of Baltimore's project functioned reasonably well in dealing with start-up operations and facilities. However, as it began to consider broader long-range issues, such as funding beyond the period covered by the grant, the need for change became apparent. The Governance Committee was comprised of representatives of the coalition that had submitted the grant application, some of whom were employees of service providers now under contract to the project. Those on the committee who represented service providers were loyal to the project, but with a somewhat narrow focus. A decision was made to appoint an ad hoc Long Range Planning Committee, whose mission was to consider and make recommendations for identifying and securing ongoing funding for the project. This committee was chaired by the vice-chairperson of the Governance Committee, who promptly solicited committee members from the community at large, including prominent professionals and lay leaders. As the committee pursued its objectives, many members began to identify strongly with the mission of Health Care for the Homeless. Some expressed interest in remaining involved with the project as Governance Committee members. The result was that over the life of the Long Range Planning Committee, a period of approximately eight months, the composition and focus of the Governance Committee were significantly changed. As it began to address the future needs of the project, it considered the advisability of converting Health Care for the Homeless to a separate and independent agency. A 501(C)(3) corporation was founded in March 1988, with the support and assistance of the Health and Welfare Council and pro bono legal services from a board member. This important action presented another opportunity to enhance further the composition of the board of the new corporation. Most previous members of the Governance Committee were elected to the new board, as were a number of new candidates with an attractive mix of professional skills and experience.

Change Does Not Always Solve Problems

Most of the projects found it necessary or desirable to change governance structure in order to meet different needs as the projects developed from their coalition-sponsored beginnings. Changes in the form or content of the governing mechanism, however, did not automatically provide solutions to a variety of knotty problems which persisted at a number of projects.

In order for any volunteer agency to function effectively, there must be a relationship between the governing body (the board) and the executive leadership through which each understands and respects the duties and responsibilities of the other. When there is a lack of understanding of the respective roles of the board and the executive, or a perception by either that the other is not filling its proper role, the tendency is for each to attempt to fill the void left by the other.

When the board fails to meet its responsibilities, it is the fault of the board leadership. When the executive leadership fails to meet its responsibilities, the fault at first is that of the executive, but if the failure is permitted to continue, it is also the fault of the board. It is therefore unlikely that an agency will be successful in the long run if the board fails in any material respect to fulfill its responsibilities.

One responsibility basic to the board is the need to be sure that members are well qualified and know what is expected of them.

In one HCHP project, board failure to deal promptly with the need to replace the executive, who was not assertive or a strong leader, ultimately caused the board to lose interest because meaningful issues were not brought to it. When the executive was finally replaced, it became apparent that the board itself needed to be reformed in order to achieve a desirable mix of talent and experience.

Even though the board has been reconstituted, there remains at this writing a serious question of whether or not it can be rejuvenated. Those close to the situation believe that the board was not qualified to deal with the real needs of the project and lacked a clear understanding of what was expected of it. Perhaps an assertive executive with leadership skills could have made a difference, but the combination of a board unaware of the critical need to examine its own effectiveness and an executive lacking the necessary abilities may prove to have been too damaging to overcome without a major dismantling and rebuilding effort.

Proper Board Function

What is the proper function of the board or other governing body of a volunteer agency? (The use of the word "board" will not be strictly applicable to all HCHPs, but for the purpose of this discussion, it should be taken to refer to whatever form of governance exists.)

This role has been defined as encompassing the duties and responsibilities to:[1]

- Act as trustees of the agency on behalf of its donors and/or funding sources
- Determine goals and objectives
- Establish policies, other general guidelines and limits for agency operations
- Be legally accountable for all aspects of agency operation
- Authorize programs sponsored by the agency
- Evaluate the results of the agency's operation

To what extent should these principles apply to the HCHP? All are important. A board that fails in any material way to exercise all the responsibilities set forth will place in jeopardy the future of the agency it is obligated to govern.

Act as Trustees of the Agency

The board of a not-for-profit agency must protect the public interest. Nonprofits receive preferential tax treatment because they offer a public service not otherwise available without subsidy, and the board should make certain that the agency serves more than narrow, selfish objectives.[2]

Has this principle come into play in the governance of HCHPs? Indeed, it has.

Some of the projects found themselves governed by representatives of the coalitions that had written the foundation grant proposal. As the projects moved from conception to operation, some members of the governance body were employees of organizations that had entered into contracts with the projects. Such an arrangement stands up poorly to scrutiny.

Faced with the need to eliminate the appearance of conflict resulting from the dual role of board member and service provider, a number of projects converted such board members to a nonvoting advisory status. This solution was not universally met with favor by the persons whose role was affected. However, it was generally accepted as necessary to the confidence and support of the various public and private constituencies to which the project was accountable. Leadership must be responsible for avoiding any suggestion that the board is not fully mindful of its fiduciary obligation as trustee of the agency.

Determine Goals and Objectives

Policy administration is a most important board function, one that can be divided into components. The first of these is that the board sets the goals of the agency.[1]

This point is particularly relevant to the HCHP projects. All were new ventures and, as such, did not have in place long-range plans setting out agency objectives and strategies for achieving them. The work of identifying objectives and strategies had to be done from scratch.

Not all project boards have engaged in a formal process of establishing goals, although every board would be able to agree on some by virtue of the basic aims of the HCHPs. On the other hand, some boards have adopted very specific goals and objectives, which are set forth in documents used as blueprints for project operations. One board has recently completed the development of a long-range strategic plan that will chart the agency's course for the next several years. In this case the board appointed an ad hoc committee to work with the project director to develop the plan. It retained as a facilitator a professional consultant experienced in working with medical institutions. The result was a well-conceived plan which the committee presented to the board at a special meeting. After thorough discussion it was adopted.

Developing goals and objectives should not be the exclusive responsibility of the board. The effort should be a joint undertaking with the executive director and staff.[2] The interaction between board and staff as they draft a mission statement and debate goals and objectives provides an excellent opportunity for strengthening their relationship and creating a mutual sense of ownership.

Establish Policies, Other General Guidelines, and Limits for Agency Operations

Policy administration also means the setting of guidelines and limits for all program functions.[1]

An administrative model developed by Richard M. Hodyetts and Max S. Wortman, Jr., identifies six policy levels:[3]

- Major policies: fundamental issues of mission or business definition typically involving questions of institutional direction, values, priorities, and principles that guide other decisions.
- Secondary policies: questions of primary clientele, types of services, delivery systems, which may focus on relationship of programs and departments to the overall mission. These issues often entail significant decisions about human, financial, and physical resources.
- Functional policies: concerns of major functional operations, such as planning, budgeting, finance, marketing, and personnel.
- Minor policies: decisions that govern day-to-day practices.

- Standard operating procedures: mechanisms and procedures to handle routine transactions and normal operations such as matters of form, process, method, and application of other policies.
- Rules: regulations that guide or prescribe everyday conduct.

The adoption of higher-level policies, their implementation, and their evaluation should be the ongoing concern of the board.[3] Minor-level policies, on the other hand, should not, unless a minor policy becomes a crucial factor in an important issue. For instance, the matter of permitting an employee to have time off from work to deal with a personal matter is a question of personnel policy which the executive should establish and is not a policy of the type the board should monitor. If in the implementation of the policy, however, it develops that the managers are applying the policy with discrimination, and this comes to the attention of the board, perhaps as the result of some action by an aggrieved employee, then the issue is transformed into one with much higher-level implications and should properly be a matter of board concern.

The danger of board involvement in the development and review of lower-level policies is twofold. First, concern with minor issues prevents the board from giving its attention to more important matters. Secondly, such a focus may have a damaging effect by causing a loss of perspective, a loss of talent, and a loss of institutional vitality.[3]

The HCHP projects were, and still are, vulnerable to the damaging effects of board concern with lower-level policies and procedures and the resultant involvement with day-to-day routine. This vulnerability is the natural result of board membership by coalition representatives and employees of service providers. The situation in many projects has improved as boards have changed their mix of members, but a number will continue to suffer the effects of their tendency to manage rather than govern.

Why do boards manage rather than govern? Richard P. Chait and Barbara E. Taylor[3] cite five reasons:

- Trustees may have specialized knowledge.
- Trustees may have specialized interest.
- Some trustees would rather act than delegate.
- Trustees tend to manage during an internal transition or crisis.
- Trustees may manage in periods of external turbulence and crisis.

In the case of internal or external crisis, board members may be called upon to assume some degree of control and become involved in administration. It is essential, however, to know when to disengage, pull back, and permit the professionals to manage the organization so that normality is restored quickly.

Such was the recent case in one of the HCHP projects. The project had previously been guaranteed in writing that it would receive substantial 1989 funding from the state. With no prior warning it was advised by letter, after the beginning of the fiscal year, that the funds would not be forthcoming. At the time of receipt of the alarming news, the executive head of the agency was out of the country. The crisis was brought to the immediate attention of the board president, who solicited the involvement of board members familiar with the state's legislative and executive budget procedures. They made immediate contact with the governor's office and the head of the department through which the funding would flow. Within several weeks, through these high-level contacts, the funding was restored.

A problem common to many of the programs was the need to resolve the question, Who's in charge? That projects had determined to provide health care by contractual arrangements with a variety of service providers created a situation in which staff members paid by different employers were required to work together as though they were employed by a single contractor. Each provider had its own employee policies, covering such matters as vacation, sick leave, and work rules. More serious, the employers found it difficult to relinquish to the HCHP executive the same degree of authority the executive would have over the staff if all worked for a single employer. Unclear lines of authority over hiring, discipline, and firing were common. These matters, while administrative in nature, were so important to the effective functioning of the projects that board involvement in their resolution became mandatory. In some cases the severity of the problem was lessened by direct hiring, as opposed to the earlier practice of transferring employees to the project from other unrelated assignments. Some projects dealt with the question more directly and more firmly, however.

In one instance representatives of the respective service providers were called together by the chairman of the board for a candid discussion of the need to clarify the executive's authority in personnel matters. The meeting was the beginning of a process which had its difficult moments. The service providers were asked to do what was necessary for the well-being of the program. The final result was a joint statement to the project staff from the chairman and the service providers that in order to correct the ambiguous line of authority, all had agreed, effective immediately, to vest in the project director full management authority for the program, subject to policies set by the board. Today the staff functions as a single unit, free of the tensions and frustrations attributable to the uncertainties of the earlier environment. Board intervention in resolving this problem was clearly necessary because of the serious threat to the project's well-being. Equally necessary, after the resolution of the issue, was the disengagement of the board.

The board should also establish or approve the limits of an agency's operations. This involves consideration of many significant factors, including financial and human resources, facilities, and, most important, the agency's primary objective or mission. The board, with input from the executive and the staff, should fix limits and enact policies that control and monitor the ability of others to take actions that will affect established limits of operations.

Be Legally Accountable for Agency Operation

We have referred above to the fiduciary responsibility of board members of a voluntary agency. We have also mentioned the need for board members to know what is expected of them. Nowhere are these aspects of board membership more important than when we consider the legal responsibilities of directors or trustees of voluntary agencies.

In general, board members of nonprofit agencies are legally responsible for the management and control of the organization.[1] The legal principle which should guide board members in this fiduciary role is frequently referred to as the Prudent Man Rule, a code of conduct incorporated in the statutory law of some states. New York's Not-for-Profit Corporation Law, in the pertinent part, reads: "Directors and officers shall discharge the duties of their respective positions in good faith and with the degree of diligence, care and skill which ordinarily prudent men would exercise under similar circumstances in like positions."[1]

On many occasions board members carry out responsibilities in accordance with the spirit of this rule without being aware of it. Giving consideration to the various aspects of an issue, choosing a course of action, and then voting or acting on it are one example. It is not necessary that every decision made by a board must be proved wise by future events. A director need not fear liability for every corporate loss or mishap. Board members are generally protected from liability for errors of judgment as long as they act responsibly and in good faith, with the best interests of the corporation as the foremost objective.[4] Problems arise when actions are taken without regard to available information that would lead a prudent person to avoid such action or when a person or board ignores other data that, if taken into account, would prompt prudent persons to act.[3]

Therefore, directors must be well informed with respect to the nature and extent of agency activities so that they make knowledgeable decisions.

The legal principle with the greatest potential to be a problem for governance in the HCHP projects is the prohibition of self-dealing. Directors of voluntary organizations as well as profit-making businesses need to be free of the implications of putting their personal or business interest ahead of those of the organization which they are bound to serve. Directors can with propriety engage in a business transaction with the organization on whose board they serve, but such activities at least need to be fair to the organization. The best course of action is to avoid self-dealing situations. Failing that, directors should carefully consider the appropriateness of nondisclosure or of not voting upon a matter in which they have an interest.

Many persons with governance responsibilities for an HCHP were, and some still are, employees of service providers under contract to the same program. In cases where there has been no action to eliminate the potential conflict of interest, attention should be directed to the elimination of any opportunity for the nature of the business arrangement to be seen as self-dealing.

Authorize Programs Sponsored by the Agency

The responsibility of the board to authorize agency services is an important one. The basic programs conceptualized in the funded HCHP grant proposals were authorized by the governing bodies of the initial projects. As a matter of fact, often the programs existed before governing bodies came into being and the boards initially authorized only *where* and *how* programs were implemented, not *what* programs would be offered. But as the projects have matured, opportunities for expansion have been presented. In responding to these opportunities, agency management must solicit the board's approval if the inclination is to expand or initiate a program. As in the case of the adoption of a mission statement or a long-range strategic plan, this presents another occasion when board and agency management can collaborate in the process of carrying out their responsibilities. When new or expanded programs are submitted for consideration, it is the board's responsibility to determine whether the initiative is consistent with the agency's mission and its long-range plan. If the matter involves a financial commitment, the question of whether resources are available must be addressed. There needs to be a determination of whether a proposed program would be redundant—i.e., whether a perceived need is already being met by other existing programs. While the responsibility of the board to authorize agency programs does not at first seem difficult, this is not always so. For instance, new program opportunities often carry with them the prospect of additional funding, which tends to obscure the possible costly side effects of program expansion. Such side effects may take the form of spreading management too thin or overburdening physical facilities or existing staff. Some opportunities for expansion come from funding sources with which there is already in existence a sponsor-agency relationship, thus making sensitive the matter of declining when that is deemed to be the appropriate response.

It is in the discharge of their responsibility to authorize agency programs that board members come to appreciate the importance of being knowledgeable about the agency's mission and long-range plans and of understanding the nature and extent of agency resources, human and financial.

Evaluate Results of Agency Operations

Board responsibility includes the need to evaluate the appropriateness, effectiveness, and quality of agency operations. Most boards have in place a process for evaluating the performance of the executive. In fact, to fail to assess the executive's performance is a serious omission. A performance appraisal should be performed annually, in writing, and thoroughly reviewed with the executive. The full board or a subcommittee may take on this task. Properly done, the evaluation of the executive's performance can serve, although to a limited degree, as an evaluation of agency effectiveness and quality.

Although most boards do appraise the quality of the executive's performance, few assess their own.[3] There are various ways for a board to get feedback on its effectiveness. One is to devote the closing minutes of its meetings to review the magnitude of issues discussed, the quality of discussion, and the patterns of participation. A second and probably more effective process is for the board to undertake an annual self-evaluation. Many boards have a periodic retreat to review and revise long-range strategic plans. If self-evaluation is not carried out at any other time, it would certainly be an appropriate item on the agenda of a board retreat. A third method of assessment involves the board in seeking comments from senior managers and others who may have informed opinions on a subject.

In the evaluation of performance, all aspects of board responsibility should be reviewed, including goals and policies, committee structure, board member selection process, the nature and quality of information presented at board meetings, and an examination of the agency's by-laws.

Governing bodies of the HCHP projects should embrace self-evaluation. The fact that the various governance committees and boards are still in their infancy and find themselves having to deal with varying degrees of change makes the present a uniquely appropriate time to undertake a thorough self-assessment. Is the board governing or is it managing? Has the board examined its committee structure? Has it developed a long-range strategic plan? Are agency goals and policies relevant? What is the mix of talent and experience of board members? Are meaningful issues presented at board meetings? Is the work of the board being done through standing committees which meet regularly, and are ad hoc committees appointed to deal with special needs? Is the board satisfied with the quality of performance of the agency executive? Is the board doing what it should to assure the fiscal soundness and stability of the agency? Should every board member make a financial commitment to the agency?

Conclusion

If HCHP governing committees and boards candidly answer these questions and others equally pertinent and then act to overcome any shortcomings thus identified, they will have fulfilled a most important board responsibility. In so doing, they will have contributed significantly to the ultimate achievement of the mission of the HCHP.

HOPE BURNESS GLEICHER
KAREN MCGEE
MARIANNE SAVARESE
ANGELA KENNEDY

Staff Organization, Retention, and Burnout

Staff Organization

GIVING HEALTH CARE to a disenfranchised, disaffiliated, and mobile group of homeless persons may seem a chaotic, perhaps an unmanageable feat. In fact, however, organization and structure are very possible within that context. Whether housed in an inner-city hospital in New York, in a small nonprofit organization as in Chicago, in a mobile health unit like Birmingham's Health Care for the Homeless Program, or in a freestanding clinic in Baltimore, HCHPs have developed staffs into interdisciplinary teams rather than into departments, speciality units, or other professionally fragmented groupings. For these organizations, form follows function—that is, organizational structure is intended to meet the needs of the homeless, rather than require these persons to suit the requirements of the organization.

The HCHPs emerged to meet needs that defied or exceeded the capabilities of individual providers. Most would agree that health care teams of several disciplines offer a solution to the problems of standard care,[1] such as fragmentation of services, exhaustive bureaucracies, and inflexible appointment systems. The phrase "interdisciplinary team" stresses a relatedness and dependence that cross the boundaries of separate, unique professions. This is particularly appropriate because the problems of the homeless rarely, if ever, fall neatly within the range of one provider. It is usual for HCHP staff to discover that the patient presenting with an acute respiratory infection also has a recent housing or job loss, marital conflict, or family violence.

There are several ways to define the interdisciplinary team. The team, in a loose sense, is "a functioning unit composed of two or more individuals with varied and specialized training who coordinate their activities to provide services to a client or group of clients."[2] In fact, some HCHP staff members may not view themselves as part of a team, but "if the basic mission or job requires that you and others must work together and coordinate your activities with each other, then you are a 'team' even though you may not formally call yourselves a team."[3] And the nature of health care for the homeless is such that if the efficacy of medical treatment is to be sustained, the services of an interdisciplinary team must be employed to treat the whole person.

While the makeup of interdisciplinary teams may differ between HCHPs, their composition should reflect the complex and diverse needs of the clients. For instance, at St. Vincent's Hospital SRO/Homeless Program in New York City, a team is a fixed group, usually composed of a physician, social worker, and registered nurse. The members of the team remain constant from day to day and site to site. In Baltimore teams are pulled together on a case-by-case basis. A nurse may work with a social worker and an addiction specialist when caring for an addict and with a psychiatrist and a health educator when working with a patient who has both schizophrenia and diabetes.

The team approach is valuable to the staff, the institution, and the clients. One of the its functions is to help its professional members overcome the stressful realities of working with a population whose health needs are overwhelming and likely to be overshadowed by the need for other forms of help, such as housing. In addition to giving mutual support, team members provide feedback, peer review, and objectivity in helping understand problems of difficult patients. Perhaps one of the most stressful by-products of treating the whole homeless person, whether "difficult" or not, is the ensuing feeling of responsibility for all of that person's problems. This can become overwhelming to an individual health worker.

―――――――

A withdrawn, evasive patient, cowering in a doorway, was drawn into treatment for leg ulcers by a medical staff person's continued offers of coffee and assistance. The weeks of attempts to engage the person in treatment caused the provider to become more aware of the patient's overall problems. The bottom line became obvious. There was a need for institutionalization in a mental hospital. This required weeks of working with police officers, judges, and mental health workers. The process became an incredible source of aggravation and frustration for the health worker.

―――――――

For the institution, teamwork is likely to prove itself in the world of cost benefits and cost-effectiveness.[4] The team brings a great number of resources to bear on a task and may arrive at a better outcome than one staff member can. This is true of administrative tasks as well. For example, in Baltimore direct service providers have input into the annual budget. This reduces strife between administrators and providers. Both groups are well informed about budget priorities and realities. In the Birmingham HCHP responsibility for fund raising, including that of obtaining matching local funds to meet federal funding requirements, is shared by all team members. The nurse practitioner agrees to solicit donated medical supplies from local hospitals, the medical director agrees to find peers willing to staff evening clinics on an in-kind basis, and the executive director works to secure United Way funds.

Teamwork benefits patients. Team skills decrease the frustration associated with multiple referrals to multiple sites and increase the likelihood of meaningful intervention. Homeless persons offer stories of referral from a medical provider to a pharmacist to a mental health clinic to a benefits determination office without having their problems resolved. This shuffle would frustrate (and most likely deter) even the most resourceful. Imagine the homeless person who leaves a hospital emergency room with an unfilled prescription (but with no financial means of filling the prescription) and instructions to get plenty of bed rest and fluids (but without access to a bed or fluids). Ultimately the goal of an HCHP would be to put itself out of business. Community resources would be available *and* accessible to all members of the community. However, the current situation evident from city to city is that there are limited resources available, and these go to those who are most resourceful. The homeless person who has lost everything, including self-esteem and affiliation with the whole of society, may find it difficult to be motivated toward resourcefulness.

Staff Selection

A common mistake is not putting enough time and care into hiring.[5] Because HCHP work is highly staff-intensive, success in staff selection depends heavily on the quality of hiring decisions. Susan Gross[5] cites three managerial traps:

- Hiring someone because you believe that having a warm body is better than not having anyone at all
- Redefining a job in order to get someone you like to take it
- Hiring overqualified people

Many of the HCHP project directors learned their hiring lessons the hard way as they set up their operations, but poor hiring decisions honed their abilities to identify the qualities that make a staff member successful (or not). In the case of the Birmingham HCHP, the medical director and Personnel Committee of the project's board of directors hired all project staff prior to employing the project director. On arriving for her first day at work, the director was introduced to the staff and was handed the project plan, a first-installment grant check, and best wishes from the board. Where would we be without a sense of humor?

In a list of the qualities that make an employee successful, it is important to state the obvious: No one staff member can possibly embody all the necessary traits. All of them can, however, be found in a team and, therefore, in an organization.

STAFF SELECTION

Sense of humor	Pragmatism
Creativity	Warmth
Resourcefulness	Open-mindedness
Sensitivity	Ability to solve problems
Commitment	Perserverance
Trust	Stamina
Tolerance	Patience
Compassion	Ability to set limits
Flexibility	Ability to measure
Experience	progress
	in small increments [6-11]

A quality commonly associated with failure is zealotry or an inappropriate overcommitment to the client(s) or the cause. Zealots are often on personal crusades that get in the way of their being team players. Further, their involvement may actually promote the patient's dependence on the provider or institution rather than foster independence on the part of the patient. Ultimately, in a healthy organization that frowns on this type of "treatment" for clients, the zealous staff member will be self-eliminating.

It may be equally instructive to mention what staff members in HCHPs are not. They are not saints, angels, selfless do-gooders, or people singularly devoted to their jobs, clients, and the pursuit of a messiantic age. While these terms are often applied to recognize the special purpose behind the staff's work, they may inadvertently diminish and separate staff members from their professional peers practicing in other arenas.

How do HCHPs attract employees who are both professionally competent and packed with the traits listed above? In addition to traditional means of finding job applicants, such as classified ads, many HCHPs cultivate potential future employees. For example, the Baltimore program offers placements or internships to students of medicine, nursing, social work, and psychiatry. In Miami and Birmingham, medical schools offer an opportunity to obtain "homeless health care" credits, which include both classroom and shelter clinic experience. In addition, although it has been so rarely in recent years, the National Health Service Corps may be a source of personnel; unfortunately the future scope of this program is uncertain.

Perhaps the singularly most important point in the staff selection process is the personal interview with each applicant. This is the one opportunity to explain candidly the organization's philosophy and structure. The applicant's responses throughout the interview, and the interviewer's skill in interpretation of those responses, disclose the personality of the applicant. A committed long-term employee will be in concert with the mission and structure of the organization, the most essential factor in job success beyond basic skills and experience.

Staff Sustenance and Retention

The HCHPs have experienced relatively low staff turnover. For example, almost five years after start-up, nine of the nineteen original HCHP project directors are still with their projects. Of the director positions that were vacated, five have been filled by existing project staff. Even in Birmingham, where hiring was completed entirely without the project director, six of the original eight staff members are still with the project five years later. Certainly staff turnover is minimized through meticulous recruitment and selection processes. A recently hired team social worker in New York at first perceived the elaborate interview process as indecision on the part of administrators, only months later realizing its value in the selection of health team members.

Once the staff is on board, the question becomes, Why does the staff stay, especially in an era of stiff competition for a diminishing supply of health professionals? Staffs of HCHPs point to a number of factors that contribute to job satisfaction. First, workers experience an enormous sense of purpose and fulfillment. At a time often characterized as empty, me-centered, or devoid of meaning, they take comfort in knowing that whatever their roles, be it nurse, social worker, physician, file clerk, dentist, or administrator, they make a significant difference in the lives of homeless persons.[11]

Employees may stay because they "fit," because they share values with the organization and their team members. They feel appreciated for being creative, sensitive, committed, flexible, open-minded. . . . Of course, these very traits drew the organization to hire them. The value of the opportunity to work in an environment which suits one's personality and beliefs is immeasurable. Individuals have their own "weights and measures" system against which they check job satisfaction. We know that the strongest individuals and organizations are those able to reap benefits from association with one another.

Staff members also cite more traditional reasons for job satisfaction, such as competitive salary and benefits packages and opportunities for growth. These are particularly noteworthy reasons in view of the scarce resources and relatively flat organizational charts that characterize much of the nonprofit sector.

Finally, many staff members reflect back on the support derived from the team approach. Highly developed and healthy teams are a tremendous source of encouragement and joy even in a challenging work setting. Institutions and teams skilled in caring for others have great potential to care for their own members.

Staff Burnout

A 22-year-old registered nurse read about our program in a professional journal and asked to work with us. She intended to pursue a career involved with the homeless.

Her motives were genuine, and her professional abilities in the first 6 months with us were considered superior. She tolerated poor working conditions well at the SRO hotels where she was assigned. At length, however, the fact that her patients rarely improved, and that several with whom she had developed a relationship died, disturbed her. She brought a birthday cake to a patient one day but found he had killed himself. She became depressed, resigned, and is now working in an inpatient service.[12]

A formal definition of "burnout" may serve us well: exhaustion from or wearing down by excessive or inappropriate use. While this definition does not imply that personnel are worn out by homeless people, burnout is a state often attributed to employees in the health and human services field. Those working with the homeless are certainly at risk.

The homeless, by the very nature of their needs and illnesses, are an extremely difficult group with which to work. The staff members who are attempting to provide services rarely enjoy the luxury of feeling that the problems they deal with have been solved. As a result, they may not be able to rest, physically or emotionally, after the stress of the day—or even the previous hour. The opportunity to resolve individual case problems is limited, and as a result, the staff may find itself in the position of operating with less and less energy.

The negative feelings produced by this descending spiral of energy find targets in the agency, the clients, or even the staff itself. The behaviors adopted to cope with this process impair the functioning of the staff and undermine the quality of service of the agency as well.

C. Shannon and D. Saleebey point out that burnout is indicated by:[13]

- Loss of concern for clients that in the extreme evolves into a cynical, hostile, and demeaning perception of them
- Deterioration of the quality and sometimes quantity of care offered clients
- Emotional isolation from clients and the job, expressed through savage joking, excessive use of technical jargon, increased involvement in outside work or increased time spent at work with little accomplished
- Correlations with drug and alcohol abuse, neurotic or psychotic symptoms, family conflict
- Lowered morale, higher absenteeism, lowered productivity, and a high turnover rate
- Physiological changes, such as higher blood pressure, poor appetite, insomnia, and psychosomatic symptoms

Organizational structure and process are responsible for many of the conditions that promote stress and increase the likelihood of burnout. Complex, confusing rules and regulations often hamper the ability to give clients adequate service. Other bureaucratic culprits are inexplicable and sudden changes in regulations governing client care and benefits, excessive case loads, lack of variety in the job, insufficient time away from stressful work, few safe outlets for emotional catharsis, and inadequate support groups.

The administrative and supervisory staffs can be a crucial defense against stress. It is not so much the personalities of the administrators and supervisors—whether they are warm or cold people—that matters. It is their approach to the staff members as they struggle to handle their work loads. Major stress reducers in the workplace are: feedback, public recognition for tasks well done, participation and input in operational or substantive decision making, supportive communication, adequate vacation time, noise control, provision of adequate supervision, orientation, and in-service training.

In-service training should give individual staff members ways to understand stress, their reactions to it, and techniques for combating the cumulative effects of stress and for improving their coping and stress management capacities. Through training, workers can develop individual programs involving cognitive, affective, and physical areas.

Because of the multiple causes of burnout and the individualized responses to the factors that produce it, no single approach or set of approaches will work across all settings. Waiting for signs of burnout to appear in a worker before taking preventive action will probably be doomed to failure. Once employees have become alienated from the job, they may not be able to recover their spirit.

In fact, clients, co-workers, management, social institutions or external systems, and workers themselves are potential contributors to burnout.[14] Patients who need but will not use the resources provided to change their lives contribute to staff burnout. So do those who present long-term problems when staffs have resources only for short-term solutions. Substance abusers who at last are ripe for full treatment cause frustration in the most resourceful of staffs when only detoxification services are available, and frankly hostile or extremely unpleasant clients wear down staffs.

A study by the Birmingham project revealed that 74 percent of the homeless showed clinical signs of depression. After years of ongoing employee contact with a people bearing this problem, in addition to their unkempt appearances, low intellectual aspirations, and poor grammar, it appeared that these characteristics were adopted by the staff. Some team members began to act and sound like the clients they were trying to assist. It was necessary to correct this drift. The problem was openly discussed; staff members were encouraged to take advantage of professional associations and training, to be aware of their dress and grammar, and even to get together periodically at "upscale" social events.

Within the work setting, personality conflicts or inadequate, incompetent, or unreliable co-workers can hasten burnout. In one HCHP project an employee who displayed many zealot characteristics created ongoing conflict during staff and management meetings. She disapproved if the staff questioned the need for services for a particular client and fought against the development of a case closure policy. Her open manner clearly communicated her disapproval of her co-workers for simply considering that a person might be terminated from services. Management intervention was essential to clarify staff roles, responsibilities, and resources. The management style had to be appropriate to correct this problem. In the case of the zealot employee, an autocratic decision maker style would have only eroded and eventually burned out worker morale. Discussion with all staff members about their roles and responsibilities resulted in improved understanding of the needs of the overly committed employee, as well as development of policies consistent with the mission of the organization.

Often the forces of burnout are external. HCHPs operate in a society that finds the problem of homelessness beyond comprehension and easy solution and thus often denies or minimizes it. Some overburdened social institutions impede effective responses to the problems. And HCHPs usually operate with inadequate budgets and supports. The ongoing struggle for problem recognition and unavailability of resources for a solution can prove the breaking point for a project director.

Finally, staffs often contribute to their own burnout. Some hold unrealistic expectations. Others lack political or personal vision about the work or are unable to value successes on a small scale. Problems in other areas of a staff member's life may lead to burnout. The task of taking each new day at a time, with an eye toward progress over the longer term, is extremely difficult.

Burnout prevention and treatment and optimizing individual and team functioning are required if the homeless, team members, and institutions expect to benefit. "It is naive to bring together a highly diverse group of people and to expect that by calling them a team, they will, in fact, behave as a team. It is ironic to realize that a football team spends 40 hours per week practicing for those two hours on Sunday when their teamwork really counts. Teams in organizations seldom spend two hours per year practicing, when their ability to function as a team counts 40 hours per week!"[15]

Burnout was determined to be a problem of such potential magnitude that burnout prevention plans were a requirement of the original Johnson/Pew HCHP grant applications. Three of the most common prevention strategies involved increased communications, access to problem-solving forums, and time away from direct service. In Birmingham staff members are given regular opportunities to debrief or ventilate, whether it be informal coffee times each morning, weekly staff meetings, or case management meetings. Those case conferences are recognized as an effective means for conveying information, reassessing goals and expectations, and discussing factors that provoke frustration as well as transference and countertransference issues that impinge on treatment.[15,16]

When staffs work with clients whose life problems absolutely defy simple resolution, problem-solving groups may be used to manage some of the forces that contribute to burnout. "Problem-solving groups offer staff an opportunity to identify the challenges of their work in an atmosphere that is nonjudgemental and supportive."[17] Such groups also empower staffs to develop creative solutions to obstacles which impede their work.

Time away from one's primary responsibilities, especially direct service work, can turn into the job-saving, burnout-saving break. Company-sponsored participation in a coed softball league has proven cathartic in Birmingham. Many projects make certain that staff members have a variety of areas of responsibility. This, for instance, assures that no one provides direct nursing or mental health care to homeless clients forty hours every week. Flexibility allows staff members to share their individual creativeness and resourcefulness across a wider range of skill areas. In one HCHP project, when dental care was recently added as a service, a medical aide was cross-trained as a dental assistant. She works in the medical clinic three days per week and the dental clinic two days. This satisfied her need for versatility and also provided an opportunity for medical policies to be shared as models by dental staff as they developed their own policies. Both the organization and the employee benefited from this arrangement.

Regardless of the strategies employed to prevent and treat burnout, managers must take care to tailor their approach to the needs of individual staff. What burns out one staff member may not even faze another. For instance, not everyone has difficulty recognizing and appreciating small, incremental progress. But, for those who do, burnout may be ever imminent.

Conclusion

Nonprofit managers often neglect one of the most important parts of their jobs: ensuring that purpose stays alive in the hearts and minds of their staff members and infuses their day-to-day activities. "Managers must periodically take the time to remind staff members why they are doing what they are doing, because restoring that sense of purpose can redirect or refocus their everyday efforts, revive their spirits, and lend new meaning and potency to their work."[5]

For the Health Care for the Homeless Program projects, staff participation in other activities for the homeless, such as housing rallies and shelter fund raisers, offers an opportunity to be in touch with the greater purpose of their work. The wise manager recognizes the need of all employees for fulfillment in their work and makes every effort to help them meet that need.

MARIANNE SAVARESE

THOMAS DETRANO

JILL KOPROSKI

CAROL MARTINEZ WEBER

19

Case Management

Tarantism: During the seventeenth century Giorgio Baglivi first described tarantism, a mental disorder common for many centuries in Italy. After being bitten by a tarantula, the victim would run to the marketplace, dance, and engage in riotous behavior. The only cure was music, especially the tarantella, which was written for expressly that curative purpose. This is an early example of a health system responding to the needs of a client.[1]

Introduction

Giving effective health care to homeless persons is challenging. We find a system fraught with fragmentation and costly misutilization. As we strive to ensure a modicum of health to those who have been neglected, it becomes apparent that the system needs help to respond better to the needs of the homeless. At the same time homeless persons need help to receive care within the system. Mediation is required between these disparate entities, the health system and the homeless individual. Case management helps us address the system and the client's problems at once. It has the potential to change the system from one into which clients must fit to one tailored to meet their needs.

Case management has been defined in a number of ways:[2,3]

- A process to link, expedite, facilitate, access, integrate, and coordinate services
- A method to affix accountability and responsibility for care

- A way to ensure that a community is maximally responsive to the client
- A mechanism to provide direct care in the absence of alternatives

These descriptions suggest that case management is a technique that can be learned and applied in the provision of health care to achieve positive outcomes. While this may be true, we have found case management to be more. In this discussion we describe case management as a tool and also illustrate its potential as a source of support for homeless persons.

Case management is the key element in any approach to service integration and has long been central to systems that heal.[4] In the care of the chronic mentally ill, for instance, it has been widely accepted as a way to orchestrate services and to create a unified system of care.[3,5,6] The need for "management medicine models"[7] has been recognized in response to the medicalization of social needs, in which primary care physicians are faced with the social problems presented by their patients.[8]

Historically, case manager models have been client-centered. The nursing, social work, and medical professions have always considered coordination, education, and advocacy inherent to their functions. Since its earliest days leaders in the community mental health movement have pointed to the need for a generalist to ensure continuity of care.[9] In 1968 Norris Hansell and associates described a "mental health expediter," trained in linkage, continuity, and counseling, who would focus on the needs of the patient and on the coordination of services.[10] Such an expediter was seen as valuable, analogously applied in other health and community service as an ombudsman. Ten years later Roger B. Granet and John A. Talbott proposed the "continuity agent," trained in continuity of care and functioning as an advocate for, educator of, and support person for the patient.[11] The expediter, continuity agent, coordinator, ombudsman, patient representative, systems agent, broker, nurse, physician, and social worker are versions of the now popular case manager.[9] Being client-centered is not new to health professionals. However, this point must be regularly rediscovered by systems that originally were established to meet human needs but may have evolved into self-perpetuating bureaucracies.

Case management has been touted but not proved as a solution to cost overruns and misutilization of services.[12] Some studies found it reduced hospital admissions and length of stay;[2,13] one study showed no effect on hospitalization.[14] Another revealed increased utilization, admissions, and costs per client compared with those not receiving case management.[15] Despite such evidence, health maintenance organizations (HMOs), third-party payers, state governments, and the federal government[2,12] all have seized upon case management as a way to save health care dollars.

A case management approach has been found to affect favorably the quality of life of its recipients. It decreases the social isolation of clients while improving their independence, occupational functioning, and ability gradually to integrate a return to the community.[13,14] These studies emphasize the importance of a familylike relationship between patients and staff which directly influence outcomes.

Major agencies have recognized case management as a significant process.[16]

In 1978 the National Institute of Mental Health (NIMH) promoted case management as a way to ensure comprehensive care. In 1983 the Joint Commission on Accreditation of Healthcare Organizations (JCAHO) suggested case management to coordinate services for continuity of care. In 1987 case management was federally mandated, permitting states to use Medicaid funds to provide home- and community-based case management for certain eligible populations.[2,15] In fact, the federal government cited case management as one of the five core services for the homeless mentally ill.[2]

Case management is both valuable and fundable. It reduces fragmentation, promotes a client-centered focus, may curtail costs, and improves the quality of life of its recipients. While the importance of service integration and cost-effectiveness must not be minimized, it is pleasing that such a basic, humane client-centered approach is promoted. Policy makers and health professionals often seem to be at cross-purposes. Perhaps now our purposes have truly crossed in a beneficial way. At one intersection, through a case management approach, we may have found a way to satisfy those who fund, those who provide, and those who receive health care services.

Leona L. Bachrach warns us not to introduce a new bureaucratic entity of case managers and persuade ourselves that the service system will now provide case management when in fact, case management exists in any successful program whether or not there are separately designated people called case managers.[17] Those committed to working with the homeless have always sought to improve the quality of their patients' lives by coordinating and integrating the services they need. Case management practice must be viewed not as the solution to system reform, but rather as the reflection of a system reforming to become more responsive to the special needs of its clients.

Since we *are* practicing case management as we create health care systems for the homeless, we must understand the field of case management in both a functional and conceptual sense. Our intent here is to define case management and the steps involved in the process and to illustrate the theory in terms of what it means to the client. We will discuss case management as a systematized way to provide health care, support, and asylum with the goal of improved quality of life for the homeless.

Health

The World Health Organization (WHO) defines health in broad terms: "Health is a state of complete physical, mental and social well-being and *not* merely the absence of disease or infirmity. The enjoyment of the highest attainable standard of health is one of the fundamental rights of every human being without distinction of race, religion, political belief, economic or social condition."[18] Aristotle defined health as "a necessary condition of a completely happy life,"[19] other ancient Greeks defined it as "a condition of perfect body equilibrium," and Native Americans view health as "being in harmony with nature."[20] The homeless share in this fundamental right to well-being, harmony, and happiness. As we provide health care, we must understand that any improvement in one's quality of life is healthy.

The person's subjective sense of health is paramount. While physicians are concerned with identifying and treating illness, patients are concerned with overall well-being and whether life activities are interrupted.[21] Case management must be distinguished from the practice of medicine.

Through this approach we are helping people live optimally; medical care is but one of the many services that our clients may need. Case management *is* the provision of health care in the broadest sense.

Pablo valued work and self-reliance. These were the essence of his sense of well-being. As a youth he sustained a traumatic amputation of his left leg below the knee. For him, using a prosthesis was quite natural, and he never perceived it as a handicap. He emigrated to the United States as an adult and carved out a modest life of relative comfort. He lived alone, had an apartment, and worked long hours as a cook in a small restaurant. Being an alien ineligible for amnesty, he wished to remain anonymous and kept himself isolated with few friends and no family. This, coupled with his inherent self-reliance, left him with a fragile network of support. He worked for cash, had little savings, and, of course, no health insurance. When his prosthesis broke, he could no longer stand without crutches. He lost his job, ran out of money, couldn't pay the rent, and wound up in a shelter for homeless men. He couldn't manage alone on the food line and needed a bed on the first floor in the "handicap wing." The shelter staff wanted medical proof that he "deserved special treatment," so they brought him to our clinic.

Pablo was pleased to meet us. Although he spoke little English, his objective was clearly conveyed. He rolled up the leg of his pants, pointed to his prosthesis, and said, "It's broken. I need a new one." His stump was swollen and bloodied, from months of rubbing and pressure on a crumbling prosthetic platform. Otherwise he was healthy. We treated his stump and referred him to the hospital-based Rehab Medicine Clinic for follow-up care. As a shelter resident he was entitled to this service. After his stump healed, he was measured for a new device, but all our efforts were stymied when we found that the "health care" to which shelter residents were entitled did not include prostheses. Pablo was determined to get "his leg," and we were determined to fulfill our promise, somehow. We were mindful of the limits to his entitlements, given his alien status. This was affirmed when a caseworker deemed him ineligible for Medicaid. But an experienced social worker, new to our team, knew more. She was sure that he was entitled to emergency coverage, despite his alien status, and set out relentlessly to prove it.

All the while Pablo waited patiently, planned the details of his departure from the shelter, and never lost his positive outlook. He lined up a job and arranged to share an apartment with friends he had met at the shelter. What was missing was "his leg." After six months of filing applications and placing phone calls on his behalf, the social worker struck the right bureaucratic chord; approval was granted. At his final fitting Pablo danced around the clinic on his new leg; he was exhilarated. That afternoon he returned to the shelter and sent word in to the nurse that he wanted to see her. She went out to the waiting room, and there was Pablo standing with his crutches at the far end of the hallway. He put his crutches aside, ran to her down the long corridor, and lifted her up with a big hug. "I can never pay you for what you've done for me," he said, "but I will remember you always in my prayers." The next day he was gone. He resumed the life he led before he became homeless, working for cash as a cook and sharing an apartment with a friend. What's different now is that he knows whom to turn to for help.

Support Systems

People do not prosper in an interpersonal vacuum. "Human needs are satisfied in relationships."[22] Support systems are defined as attachments, among or between individuals, that help people adapt to life's transitions, crises, and stresses.[23] Through guidance and feedback, support systems enhance problem-solving capabilities and emotional mastery. They also serve as islands of stability and comfort in a stressful environment.[24]

Such systems occur naturally among family, friends, communities, or religious groups. The essential elements of support exhibited by a functional family include sensitivity and respect for the needs of its members and an effective communication system. The family meets the continually developing biological, psychosocial, and economic needs of its members and, as an agent of socialization and control, mediates between society and its members. Through guidance, direction, and feedback the family unit practice provides collective strength, skills, experience, practical service, and crisis intervention to each member. The functional family unit is the traditional care management system.[16,25]

As we set up systems of health care for the homeless, we must recognize the essential nature of support systems and promote their development. In addition, we must recognize that the client-case manager relationship has the potential to become a support system. Just as the family mediates between society and its members, so the case manager mediates between community systems and clients.

What Marie wanted was a "room," but what she needed was protection. We met her in the winter of 1984. She was brought to our health station in the shelter by one of the caseworkers who had found her walking the streets at night. There before us stood a tiny old lady, about four and a half feet tall, wearing a floppy hat, beads, and a housedress that reached her ankles. Her legs were swollen to her knees, red and raw with weeping cellulitis. We soaked her wounds, and she accepted us readily. As she sat in our office all morning, we talked. Although her words were garbled and her head, arms, and hands writhed slowly and continuously, we understood her. "You call yourself a doctor?" . . . "you're a murderer"; "you're not a nurse, you're stupid," she said quite matter-of-factly, as if privy to some secrets of our past. "I want a room," she insisted, and became purple with rage when the social worker used the term "nursing home" much too soon!

Over the next few months we came to know Marie's story, and we became friends. At age sixty-eight, she is one of nine siblings estranged from her poor immigrant family. Growing up in this city, she completed high school, worked as a finisher in a sweatshop, went to the movies once with a boy named Sam, and had her own place. She spent ten years in a state mental facility and was deinstitutionalized after she secured legal aid on her own behalf. She had lived marginally in SRO hotels and on the street. She loved the movies and spent her days there, sleeping and safe from "the bad people who smoke." At night she walked the streets and terminals. She would flee her hotel room because of "mice" but thought nothing of striking tall strange men when angered by their approach.

Certainly this spunky woman was vulnerable and lucky to have survived. Medically she was relatively stable. We treated her cellulitis, bronchitis, and pneumonia, the sequelae of her life-style; had her eyes checked and got her glasses; and admitted her to the hospital on several occasions. She always complied. Psychiatrists confirmed a history of chronic schizophrenia and added that she was mildly retarded. Her mood swings were controlled with weekly Prolixin, but the tardive dyskinesia was irreparable. Still, our ministrations fell short, because what she really wanted from us was "a room . . . and a kitchen to cook spaghetti and meatballs." She wrote to government officials and agencies, begging for their help, and was spurred on by their replies. The health team, psych team, and shelter staff coordinated their efforts. We found SRO housing for her several times, but unable to manage alone, she kept coming back to the shelter. Much time was spent to convince her that she needed a more supportive setting. After one and a half years of interviews, visits, and setbacks, in 1986 she was finally accepted into a residence for the homeless mentally ill, run by a religious organization. She lives there still, spends her days at the movies, comes to the shelter for lunch, and visits the health team whether she is ill or not. She continues to correspond with the mayor and the governor, in her relentless quest for "a room." When we see her walking around town, we smile when she says she's "going home." If we ask her about her doctor, now she smiles when she calls him a "murderer."

Through team case management, Marie found a supportive network that eventually made provision for her needs in line with her capabilities. Marie needs a protective living arrangement and an undemanding life of comfort and dignity.

Asylum and Rehabilitation

Like a functional family that socializes each member toward adulthood, case managers provide support, asylum, and rehabilitation to each client toward the goal of improved health and well-being.

As we create systems of health care for homeless persons, the human need for refuge must be remembered. The provision of asylum, in a figurative sense, is the function of supporting and protecting a person.[26] It must be individualized. For some, the need for asylum is episodic; for others it may be lifelong.[17]

Asylums of the past failed as loci of care. Providing comprehensive services and support to residents within one small pastoral facility was an idealistic attempt to create systems responsive to their needs. The focus of asylums changed as they grew in size and scope and as inmates' needs were addressed collectively. Organizational values supplanted those of personal involvement, individualized service, and an attention to humanistic detail, all qualities required in systems of human service. The needs of the institution ran counter to and ultimately superseded those of its residents. As we devise systems of care for the homeless, we can learn from the failures of the asylum.

"Habilitation precedes rehabilitation."[27] As a function beyond asylum, rehabilitation cannot happen without support and protection. Human beings vary in their capacity for growth, and we must try to provide an undemanding life of adequate comfort and dignity for those who can be rehabilitated only to a limited degree.[26]

Why the Homeless Need Case Management

The most effective systems of care for homeless persons are those that recognize their special needs and characteristics.[28] Since we are not dealing with a discrete population, the notion that one program or approach will suffice is an impediment.[29] Despite their heterogeneity, however, homeless persons share common experiences in varying degree: They are poor, they are isolated, and they are in crisis.[30]

They Are Poor

Poor people slip in and out of homelessness. The boundary is permeable.[28] Most homeless persons are members of a multiply impoverished group in need of a wide range of services that includes but is in no way limited to a permanent living situation. The label "homeless" is actually a misnomer that focuses attention on only one aspect of their plight; they are jobless, penniless, functionless, and supportless in addition to being homeless.[6] They are impoverished of health by the life-style they are forced to lead and often by years of neglect.[31] They lack the resources and the relationships that would provide them with the "social margin" needed to survive.

F. L. Jessica Ball and Barbara E. Havassy surveyed homeless persons in San Francisco.[33] They found a serious mismatch between what these individuals needed and what was offered. Requirements for survival such as physical protection and housing along with material resources, financial entitlements, and employment opportunities were primary concerns; medical, social, and psychiatric issues were secondary. They "needed someone helpful to talk to . . ." and a "doctor was not what they meant."[33] Perhaps, through the individualized approach of case management, we will provide to the homeless "not only what we deem useful, but also what they deem necessary."[29]

Health problems of the homeless are inextricably intertwined with broad social and economic problems that require multifaceted and long-term approaches for resolution.[28] Given this wide range of problems in multiple spheres, they need services offered from multiple modalities and in different settings. Consequently, the homeless are particularly vulnerable to any lack of coordination, inconsistent treatment or philosophy, and disparate protocols and objectives.[29]

They Are Isolated

Kim Hopper stresses "the ordinariness of those on Skid Row. The distinction . . . is not their disability but their disenfranchisement."[34] J. Fernandez describes "the essential deficit of homelessness, namely, the absence of a stable base of caring or supportive individuals" and "the inability to establish . . . such a base."[35] Analogous to profiles of long-stay institution residents, the homeless are often unmarried and out of touch with family and friends.[28]

Studies have shown that homeless subgroups experience isolation in similar degrees. The social networks of the homeless mentally ill are impoverished and highly stressed.[36] Intimacy eludes them as they deny their dependency needs and drift in isolation searching for autonomy.[35] While living in a community, they fail to make contact with it, neither belonging to nor creating social groups of their own.[37] Young vagrants exhibit high degrees of familial estrangement and a minimal desire to return home; "they expect and ask little from their families."[32] Homeless aged men show a decreased sociability that distinguishes them from their domiciled peers.[38] The fragmented support systems of homeless families are illustrated in Ellen L. Bassuk and colleagues' survey: Single parents named "no one" or their "children" as their primary source of help.[39] Rural homeless, as well, were found to be suffering from the fraying fabrics of support in the farmlands.[28]

It is interesting to note that in disorganized societies, spontaneous support systems become strained and inadequate, especially for marginal people who need them the most.[24] Homelessness is one by-product of a disorganized society. In fact, some see it as a result of society's failure to care for those unable to care for themselves and as the consequence of a failure to develop significant support for those who suffer severe intrinsic impairment.[6] The absence of support systems is at once the cause and result of homelessness. Whatever the operant perspective, given the paucity of physical, social, and system supports available to the homeless, we must construct such networks from scratch.[6,40]

They Are in Crisis

Homeless persons must bear many crises. Indeed, a culmination of multiple crises is often the culprit. Both the event and the life-style of homelessness are the common crises shared by all of our clients.

The homeless are like victims of disaster. A disaster is an occurrence of such magnitude that normal patterns of life within a community are disrupted and people are plunged into helplessness and suffering; they need food, shelter, clothing, medical care, and other life-sustaining services.[41] Homelessness is a chronic disaster affecting people and families one by one, each of whom endures this crisis alone.

Recommendations have been made to improve the health systems' response to the homeless. In 1984 and 1986 the American Psychiatric Association's Task Force on the Homeless Mentally Ill[42,43] called for a comprehensive and integrated system of care to address their basic underlying problems, with designated accountability and adequate fiscal resources, the ultimate goal being a "true system of care, rather than a loose network of services." Housing, comprehensive care, crisis intervention, ongoing asylum, and case management were elements of that proposal. Stephen M. Goldfinger and Linda Chafetz stress that to serve multiproblem patients best, the system must be capable, comprehensive, continuous, individualized, willing, tolerant, flexible, and meaningful.[29] These attributes parallel those of effective case management.

Intensive Case Management

Systems of case management for homeless persons were studied by the NIMH in 1987[2] and the National Institute of Medicine in 1988.[28] In some cases it was a "critical link"; in others, another "bureaucratic barrier." Overall, case management services were found to be ill defined, with widespread conceptual confusion, lack of uniformity in practice, and little direction from the field. The NIMH addressed these problems by describing essential elements of the program surveyed and by convening an advisory panel. It concluded that homeless persons require a more aggressive, persistent, and comprehensive form of case management, beyond traditional systems. They need "Intensive Case Management." The NIMH advisory panel outlined specific initiatives to ensure its provision:

- Housing (both transitional and permanent as a key resource)
- Respect for clients' rights (to safeguard patients from the abuse of power by case managers)
- Formal interagency agreements (to integrate health and welfare systems)
- Empowered case managers (through training, certification, and supervision)
- Leadership (through research and system evaluation)

In addition, certain functions and qualities were described as essential to the success of intensive case management.

Functions

The distinct functions of case management help us identify, prioritize, and address the needs of homeless persons in an orderly fashion. They are elements of a problem-solving method, a dynamic process shaped by human needs, presenting problems, professional opinions, organizational constraints, and community resources. Adhering to these functions does not guarantee successful outcomes; rather, it serves to guide the case manager through the process of helping clients. They are:[2,3,25,28]

- Identification and outreach: to determine who needs services
- Assessment: to reveal needs, identify problems, and determine strengths and limitations of clients

- Planning: to prioritize objectives based on assessments and, in consensus with the client and team, to devise an individualized care plan with flexible and realistic goals
- Linking: to coordinate, to facilitate, and at times to provide comprehensive services in conjunction with the plan
- Monitoring: to evaluate progress and quality of linkages
- Evaluating: to determine whether or when changes in the plan are necessary
- Advocating: to act persistently on behalf of clients to access services; empower them to become their own advocates, effect policy and system change on behalf of all

As we reviewed the case histories of our clients, we could not always discern the functions of case management that had been applied. On closer look, however, they all were there. We were performing them automatically and had not appreciated the structure they lent our efforts. With the homeless, case management functions are often applied concurrently and in protracted phases. Much of our time is spent on outreach, ongoing assessments may remain incomplete, and plans are often thwarted. We link, monitor, and evaluate continuously, while maintaining an advocative stance.

Etta is a sixty-nine-year-old stately southern woman. She sought shelter when progressive blindness and difficulty breathing made life on the streets and in subways impossible. She always sat in isolation at a table in one corner of the shelter. Withdrawn and paranoid, she struck out whenever she felt threatened. Her need for health care was apparent, so the shelter staff identified her as someone we should meet. She would not enter our health station, so we reached out to her daily. As we gently and persistently offered care, she tolerated our presence at best and was steadfast in her refusals. During outreach, we assessed and monitored her from afar because she offered no history and would not be touched. Although limited by her obesity and shortness of breath, she was able to function. She was relatively clean, her layers of clothing were neat, and she ambled slowly with her cane to the toilet, the food line, and occasionally around the block. She seemed comfortable, so we continued our outreach, assessment, and monitoring.

By her behavior, we knew that she was fiercely independent. We wanted her to trust us and feel safe enough to make the first move. After two years she let us check her blood pressure. It was very high. She refused intervention but did allow us to check it now and then. This was the planning phase; she was in charge, and we were in conflict. Do we pursue her aggressively or allow her space? We chose to risk waiting again. Two months later she became incontinent when she was unable to reach the toilet. She requested medication, allowed one blood test, and revealed some history: Many years ago she had been treated for hypertension, diabetes, and cataracts. The linking phase began, albeit on her terms, and we coordinated services. The hypertension moderated as she complied with the medication and weekly blood pressure monitoring. Still, she had never entered our health station and would not allow us to address her other problems. We monitored her at that table in the shelter, a plan defined by her terms of time, space, and location. Eventually she worsened and was essentially chairbound. We could no longer safely respect her refusals. The shelter staff issued an ultimatum: She would be expelled from the shelter if she did not go to the hospital. She allowed our team physician to examine her at his hospital clinic session. This was done through several layers of clothes. She agreed to some tests that were performed over one month. The nurse escorted her each time. Two and a half years from the time we met, our assessment phase was nearly complete. The workup revealed that she had decompensated congestive heart failure, uncontrolled hypertension, diabetes, and cataracts. We added more medications to her regimen with her permission and monitored her at our shelter health station.

Suddenly she regressed and became increasingly paranoid. She rejected all interventions, stopped taking medications, and deteriorated dramatically. Her judgment was deemed impaired, and we had to commit her against her will. Interestingly enough, when the ambulance came, she was agitated but did not resist. Her shelter physician served as her advocate in the emergency room. During her hospitalization the outreach team supported her and provided linkage between her and the in-house staff. As she recovered quickly, her behavior and judgment improved. She planned her discharge with the social worker. She would not be placed and wanted "her own apartment" and "to manage her own money." Housing was found in an SRO; she travels the subway to see "her doctor" at the clinic, had her cataracts removed, and remains compliant with her care. Through persistent outreach and the coordinated efforts of the health team, shelter staff, and hospital staff, Etta was ultimately empowered to resume charge of her life.

In this case, applying the case management functions did not guarantee success. That was up to Etta. They did, however, serve as guideposts for us through a caring process that spanned more than three years.

Qualitative Aspects

Case management must be client-centered, comprehensive, and continuous.[2] These qualities transform the process into a truly supportive system of health care.

CLIENT-CENTERED

Clients should be involved in all aspects of decision making so that individualized goals are realistic and achievable.[44] The thrust of each plan should be rehabilitative. This focus serves to preserve function, limit disability, and enhance adaptive capacity while never demanding more achievement than is possible.[5,6,36,45] Assessments must be thorough and expertly performed, to determine clients' needs, skills, strengths, and weaknesses.[44] Ideally, evaluations should take place in the living and social settings of clients in order to formulate individualized and realistic treatment plans[6] and to assess their capacity eventually to assume their own case management.[3] Maintaining a delicate balance between doing what is technically possible while avoiding the frustration of unrealistic expectations is the key challenge.[5]

While rehabilitation provides direction to case management, advocacy is the bulwark supporting the process. The rights of the individual are paramount. They must be safeguarded when clients are unable to defend themselves.[2]

When we protect their rights, can we comfortably respect their right to refuse? They are not free to endanger themselves or others. As Leona L. Bachrach notes, "A patient's freedom also means freedom from psychological and physical harm, and from the deleterious effects of his own illness."[17] Case managers must determine when or whether clients are capable of informed consent. Therein lies the potential of the case manager to override client choice and client refusal through professional control and superseding influence.[4] The dynamics of this power must be recognized and understood as a force that could victimize. As Edmund Pellegrino advises, "to help an individual, there must be acceptance of the human being as he or she is, . . . authority must be handled in a humane way without extension into the person's belief and value system."[46] Case management is not about mastery and control; it is about assistance and advocacy. We must know our clients well to determine when to intervene on their behalf to keep them free from harm and when simply to remain available until they are ready, willing, and able to accept our help.

In order to maintain their objectivity and rehabilitative focus, case managers must recognize the potential for emotional overinvolvement in this intimate therapeutic relationship. They must temper expectations with patience and a sensitivity to each person's pace and progress. As case managers we often must be ready to help but not to treat,[40] to care but to not cure, and to maintain rather than to improve.[27]

Providing services in vivo, meaning on-site in shelters, streets, and soup kitchens, is essential for effective case management of the homeless.[2,40] We have found it a powerful way to communicate acceptance and our client-centered intentions. Caring for the homeless on their own turf helps the case manager perform realistic assessment and facilitates monitoring. Sometimes, however, clients may perceive it as an intrusion. A subtle presence, along with gentle persistent outreach, may be necessary to afford enough space to those who are guarded, allowing them to feel safe and able gradually to accept care.

COMPREHENSIVE

Case management must be as comprehensive as the nature of our client's needs. A good example is the New York State Intensive Case Management Program,[47] which was started in 1989 to serve the severely mentally ill, many of whom are homeless. A wide array of services is deemed legitimate and fundable: food, clothing, lodging, furnishings, utilities, homemakers, escorts, vocational training, and leisure time activities, along with medical care, crisis intervention, and transportation. This program illustrates the scope of comprehensive and relevant case management, providing "what they need, when they need it, for as long as necessary."[15]

In community health, arranging comprehensive services is a valued objective. However, "the tendency for each agency to be and do everything possible for each client can lead to incomprehensible comprehensibility",[4] confusing both staff and clients alike. In these settings, particularly with the homeless, case management is essential in order to integrate services, minimize duplication, and prevent mis-utilization. Case management should be an orderly process to help the professional staff and community agencies give comprehensive care while helping clients negotiate networks of services.

CONTINUOUS

Case management systems must be continuous. This qualitative aspect is three-dimensional, implying long-term commitment, day-to-day accessibility, and continuity of care. Being continuous or "non-time-bound" is a feature of case management that distinguishes it from other systems of health care provision.[2] For some the need may be lifelong. Given the chronicity of homelessness, almost all clients may need long-term care.

Being totally accessible is an ideal difficult to achieve. Case management is time-consuming. Those who need it may require extended periods of engagement.[2] Many mentally ill clients have low tolerances for closeness and are resistant to traditional treatment interventions.[35,37] Long hours, days, even months may be spent performing outreach, establishing rapport, and securing needed services.[2,37] Progress may be slow; crises and setbacks are predictable. Like a functional family, case management support must remain open to its clients. Certain measures, such as small case loads, twenty-four-hour on-call systems, and a team approach,[2] along with expert priority setting and realistic limit setting, enhance the accessibility of case management.

Any person who ventures into the fragmented arena of our modern health care system needs to feel a sense of continuity among providers. Case management, through effective linking, monitoring, and advocacy, will ensure a sense of continuity both for each patient and for the staff.[2] To implement continuity of care, certain measures may be applied, such as persistent monitoring of referrals, personal escort of clients, and devising patient tracking systems.[2,27]

The outreach team first met Doris in 1975. When the nurse and social worker approached her in the hallway of her SRO hotel, she was guarded but did accept them. The team visited her twice a week and formulated a plan with the following goals: to link her to medical care at the hospital-based clinic, support her daily functioning, and reduce her isolation and sense of loneliness. What Doris wanted was "someone to care about me now and when I die." Over the years the team came to know her well. Strong bonds developed, and the team became her surrogate family.

Born in Eastern Europe at the turn of the century, she emigrated here at the age of nineteen. While living with her aunt and sister, she worked in factories and sweatshops to earn a living. She married at the age of forty but soon left her abusive husband to move back with her sister. As she perceives it, her family had her committed because she was a "troublemaker." At age forty-nine she entered a state mental institution and remained there for twenty years until she met a "nice doctor" who told her, "You don't belong here and never did." At age seventy she was released to live in an SRO hotel room; widowed, without children, and rejected by her family, she was alone. Not actually homeless, she was certainly living in isolation on its margin.

Doris was an eccentric woman with her own garish style. She was always well dressed, donning bright red lipstick and costume jewelry. Her tiny room was cramped with furniture, but she kept it clean and colorfully decorated with curtains and plastic flowers. She spent her days in the park watching the children play. She loved children, and they responded to her. She was deeply religious and practiced her religion with fervor. Although she was often anxious, she derived strength from her spirituality and her newfound independence. Over the years the team promoted these strengths and intervened when she needed support.

Our program cared for Doris for fifteen years. This long-term relationship was sustained despite many changes of outreach team staff. She always felt comfortable with at least one team member and so was able to accept new personnel as they were acquired. With each change, the senior team member bridged the gap and eased the transition for Doris as she established new relationships. Doris was cared for continuously by the team entity and felt secure about this long-term arrangement.

The team was accessible to her daily. She relied on the team members and looked forward to their visits. They arranged medical care for her at the hospital-based clinic. She was relatively healthy, save for mild congestive heart failure and hearing loss. For Doris case management mostly entailed ongoing emotional support as she dealt with her loneliness and inexorable aging. She longed to be reunited with her sister but was rejected when the team attempted a reconciliation. Day-to-day interventions entailed monitoring her health status, escorting her to appointments, checking her mail, attending to her bills, and shopping for her groceries. In addition, team members accompanied her to religious services and celebrated with her on holidays. Eventually, as her health declined, she needed more help than the team could alone provide. While remaining her primary source of support, the team coordinated a comprehensive array of services for her as she became homebound. Continuity was maintained as the team served as liaison between Doris and the other agencies providing home care, "meals on wheels," and visiting companions.

Eventually she could not manage alone. Her room became cluttered, and she often left food burning on her hot plate. Her safety was in jeopardy, but she would not allow the team to intervene. The landlord initiated a process to have her deemed incompetent and ultimately removed from the hotel to a nursing home. The outreach team members were in conflict about her capacity to remain at home. They were torn, realizing how fearful she was of being again institutionalized yet appreciating the unsafe nature of her present state. Team members supported her through an ordeal that lasted six months. Advocating on her behalf, they secured *a lawyer as she wished and made plans for a second psychiatric opinion. But she was assessed, examined, and interrogated too many times. Exhausted and frantic, she seemed to sense her fate. She confided in a friend, the social worker whom she had met that first day in 1975, "I won't move. . . . I'll die first." On the day of the scheduled court hearing, Doris was found dead in her room. She was ninety years old. The team notified her niece, who assured them that Doris would be buried as she wished in sacred ground. For Doris, case management support and interventions spanned fifteen years, providing what she needed, within the realm of what she wanted—independence.*

Life Space of Case Management

As homelessness is intertwined with broader social issues, case management is both influenced by and dependent upon adjacent systems. It cannot be divorced from its setting,[15] which includes organizational support, case manager skill, client involvement, and community resources.[2] The concept of case management is sound; when it fails, it is a systems failure.[4]

Organizational Support

To sustain case management programs, funding must be available on a long-term basis, along with deep personal and agency commitment.[44] Just as case managers support their clients, so organizations must support the overall case management system.

A distinctive feature of case management is that it clearly affixes responsibility to one person or team.[2,15,28] Accountability must extend with the same clarity to the organization providing the service.[2,5,44] Organizations are accountable to regulatory agencies and funding sources as well as to staff and patients. They are responsible for proving the value of their case management systems. John A. Talbott urges systems that care for the chronically mentally ill to "reward quality not quantity; funding must reward ambulatory and preventive services; and leadership must be drawn from those who value people and quality, not from those who thrive on paper and quantity."[27] Case management programs must be evaluated from new perspectives that measure the quality-of-life outcomes of clients and the level of commitment of staff, in addition to productivity.

Organizations must empower case managers by legitimizing their roles and affording them sufficient authority to advocate and care for patients effectively.[2] Better outcomes result from case management programs that are less bureaucratic, where staff members have greater latitude to make decisions and greater access to administrators.[48] Small case loads give case managers more time to support clients and teach them the skills that they need.[14] Ideal staff-to-client ratios are less than 1:40.[2] Because caseworkers come and go, the system must provide the necessary backup.[5] Team configurations can ensure this while preserving continuity of care.[49] Supervision must ensure that a flexible, action-oriented, human-centered approach is maintained.[2] Forums to discuss realistic case outcomes enhance supervision and reduce frustration in the staff.[14] Regular supervision also safeguards the patient's rights by detecting early any potential abuse of power and control by case managers.[2]

Teaching all personnel about the field of case management is important.[2,5,10,42,44] Besides improving the skills of the case manager, such training promotes adherence to the concept throughout an organization and acceptance of the process within the community. Systems must also offer career structure, mobility, and reasonable reimbursement. Otherwise case management will be performed by young, inexperienced practitioners and be plagued by attrition.[5]

The Case Manager

Case management may be performed by an individual or a team. Each approach offers advantages and disadvantages.[2]

INDIVIDUAL

Using an individual case manager makes it easier to designate responsibility and fix accountability,[44] facilitates supervision and interagency collaboration, and may be less confusing for each client. Individual case managers must have comprehensive skills. Surveys of practice have found that while the qualifications, backgrounds, and educational preparations varied widely, all case managers were required to have had some clinical or mental health experience.[2] "Interdisciplinary Cross Training" is necessary for persons assuming this role.[11] They must be knowledgeable about health, mental health, welfare, rehabilitation, and other community resources and must possess the skills to assess, gain access, coordinate, and advocate on behalf of their patients.[10,11] Anyone who performs case management alone faces a formidable challenge.

TEAMS

We cannot expect one staff member to possess all the time, resources, and skills required to address the complex array of interrelated health needs presented by homeless persons.[49] For the homeless, case management is facilitated by interdisciplinary teams. This approach makes better use of available resources, overcomes fragmentation of services, and promotes individualized care.[50] Simply having enough people present to meet the numbers seeking help and to share the multitude of follow-up tasks generated are reasons enough to use this approach. Because assessments are made from the various perspectives of each team member, complete patient profiles can be developed in a timely fashion.

With teamwork we can reach out farther, assess more thoroughly, plan more comprehensively, monitor more persistently, and advocate more powerfully. Teams provide the depth and breadth of case management required for homeless individuals.

Teams are client-centered. The patient is part of the team and the reason for its existence. With teams, clients have more options because they are less dependent on any one practitioner.[51] In addition, through the use of teamwork, staff members derive the feedback and mutual support that preserves the energy the team needs.[49]

Continuity of care is achieved through teamwork. Patients have greater access to the case management process because team membership is contiguous, leadership is flexible, and roles are often reciprocal.[49] While teams may be altered by absences and staff turnover, the case management entity remains constant and continuity is rarely disrupted. As team members pool their time and share responsibilities, they can address the needs of more individuals. Continuity is preserved while productivity improves. By collaborating with other agencies and advocating on behalf of patients, extended teams form networks. Such liaisons enhance continuity and facilitate the implementation of care plans.

Although the team approach seems ideal for the practice of case management, it has some drawbacks. The value of collaboration is offset by the "process loss"[51]—that is, the time and energy it takes to collaborate. Great effort is spent on developmental tasks, establishing group norms, and maintaining effectiveness.[49] While this may momentarily divert a team's focus away from client care, collaboration is essential to prevent team dysfunction and maintain communication within the case management entity. Another drawback is the diminished sense of satisfaction that staff members may feel because responsibilities and rewards are shared.[51] Issues of territoriality, role misconceptions, duplication of effort, and competition among team members are potential sources of conflict that drain energy and spirit.[49]

The disadvantages of a team approach are also felt by clients. Anxiety may be heightened by expectations that they become part of the team and participate in planning, and they may become confused when inconsistencies or incongruencies occur between members.[51] Successful case management depends upon how well the team resolves internal problems.

Resources

Case management can promote official interagency interdependence. Case management success is, in fact, directly dependent upon the social, health, and mental health services found within a community. The case manager must collaborate with other agencies to coordinate and gain access to care. Without formal interagency agreements at local, state, and federal levels, the success of such orchestration depends solely on the skill of the case manager.

"A primary cause of fragmented services is fragmented funding."[52] To correct this tendency, the NIMH recommends that collaboration be supported through funding inducements.[2] The National Health Care for the Homeless Program induced formal interagency agreements through its requisite coalition building in each city.[53] Ideally, if we could reduce service fragmentation and redundancy through interagency collaboration, the need for case management would not be so urgent. Patients could wend their own way through a more orderly community system.

Case management can shape the nature of resources available. By helping clients select the most appropriate and affordable services and identify unmet needs, case managers help create a more responsive community system.[3,52] What Talbott has proposed for systems of mental health could be applied to the homeless as well: "to pull together the disparate patchwork of services and to effect change toward a unified set of services; unified at the bottom not at the top, through a system of vouchers shaping the nature, location, and funding of services through consumer choice and option."[27] The impact of demand is powerful. Certainly, it is one way to create a more responsive system of health care.

Measuring Success

The future of case management as a system of health care delivery depends on studies that can prove its value in terms of measurable outcomes. Research has suggested that case management limits costs, maximizes appropriate utilization of existing health services, promotes the reintegration of clients into the community, and improves the quality of clients' lives.[12-15] Such studies must be validated.

Client Perspectives

As we evaluate programs, the perspectives of clients provide valuable insights. What these people find most beneficial is relating to a caring person and improving their own functional abilities.

The relationship between the client and case manager has great potential. In one study "the relationship alone was found to be the key therapeutic factor" because of the sense of partnership, continuous personal support, and decreased social isolation that each client derived.[14] When case managers established "peer-like" and "friendly" relationships, their clients felt respected, more comfortable, and less threatened.[9] Clients valued "having one person who cared and helped them through the maze of programs" available.[54] The experience of feeling that someone cares is inherently therapeutic.

Clients value the basic skills they learn and the strength they derive from the case management relationship.[14] What H. Richard Lamb proposes for the chronically mentally ill, is applicable in case management: "expand the remaining well part of the person and thus his functioning . . . focus should be on the healthy part of the personality and the person's strengths."[55] For clients, being empowered and supported within a therapeutic relationship is the essence of case management.

Conclusion

Case management is more than just an orderly process that assists practitioners to coordinate comprehensive services. Its application can shape the nature of health care systems so that they become more responsive and relevant. Moreover, case management models have the potential to become a source of human support for those who have none.

The concept of case management is not new to those of us who work among the homeless. In fact, we have been practicing it all along. To us, the needs of our patients are paramount. We struggle to orchestrate multiple services for them as we face the barriers of fragmented systems. We strive to create programs that address their expressed needs. Daily we remain supportive of them as they overcome crises and stabilize their lives. Through the Health Care for the Homeless Program we have begun to shape the orientation of an overall system into one uniquely responsive to the needs of homeless persons. Now we must build upon these principles to create a field of practice for humane, client-centered health care—entitled case management.

ROLANDO A. THORNE

CATHERINE ZANDLER

JOHN B. WALLER, JR.

LINDA KEEN SCHARER

MARSIA CANTO

20

Entitlements

Introduction

The homeless in the United States are the poorest of the poor, below any recognized, structured level of our society. If a safety net exists to catch those at risk, homeless persons are already below it. They have either fallen through or were in the depths before the net was erected.

Government entitlements are ill designed for this group of persons. Even the rudimentary documents that serve as the entrance key for most very poor individuals, such as birth certificates, are not available to the homeless. When entitlement programs can be effectively distorted in order to obtain basic benefits, the process demands an intense effort on the part of trained staff members. Results from four years of effort by the nineteen Johnson/Pew HCHPs prove that even with assiduous, highly motivated effort, results are poor. In most projects attempts were made to seek Medicaid income, for instance, but the cost in employee time of obtaining Medicaid funds usually surpassed the dollars received.

The three programs discussed here are among the most successful and offer valuable lessons in technique and perserverance. First, a few definitions of terms are needed.

Medicaid

Medicaid was created in 1965 under Title XIX of the Social Security Act. It is a means-tested program through which the federal government shares costs with the states to give health care services to the poor. To receive benefits, people must be virtually impoverished. It is noteworthy that Medicaid is protected from reductions under the 1985 Gramm-Rudman-Hollings Act.

Medicaid law mandates that states provide medical services to all those who receive assistance under Aid to Families with Dependent Children (AFDC) programs and, in general, to those eligible for Supplemental Security Income (see below). States otherwise have a great range of choice in the Medicaid benefits they offer. The portion of state Medicaid costs borne by the federal budget ranges from a minimum of 50 percent in states with high per capita incomes (for example, Alaska, California, Connecticut, Delaware, Nevada, and New Jersey) to a maximum of 77.4 percent in low-income states (Mississippi).[1]

To unravel the strands that form Medicaid, it is first necessary to understand that it consists of fifty different programs, one for each state.[2] The matter of Medicaid eligibility is a prime example. The states have discretion about the degree of poverty, income standards, and coverage for varying groups of people. In recent years, for instance, the ratio of Medicaid recipients to the numbers of those below the federal guideline poverty levels ranged from highs of over a hundred (Hawaii) and eighty (California) to lows of twenty or less (Texas, Idaho, South Dakota).

Supplementary Security Income (SSI)

SSI is an income assistance program administered by the federal government through the states. In its basic form SSI gives cash, not services. Federal SSI benefits are in the range of $325 per month for an individual and $500 for a couple if they have no other income and live outside an institution. Some states increase this by adding funds from their own budgets.

SSI came into being as Title XVI of the Social Security Act amendments of 1972 and was designed to provide some equity across the states for benefits offered to the aged, blind, and disabled poor. The federal government has established uniform national eligibility standards, including those for income and assets. In recent years this standard has been in the range of about 70 percent of the federal poverty level. SSI is thus distinguished from Medicaid, where fifty different state standards may exist. Nevertheless, it is generally true that SSI recipients are also Medicaid-eligible. The fact that federal standards apply offers those seeking SSI benefits a degree of protection from arbitrary state cutbacks in Medicaid designed to balance budgets. The federal component of SSI is not at risk during current budget negotiations in Washington because it is protected from cuts under the Gramm-Rudman-Hollings Act. However, state eligibility rules vary widely.

Social Security Disability Income (SSDI)

In recent years the process of obtaining disability benefits has been challenged by politically driven decisions to deny such benefits through arbitrary abuse of the application process. Proving disability from mental illness has been made particularly difficult, but no disease or disability has escaped excessive, perhaps illegal scrutiny. Challenges to the present system have been partially successful in restoring some equity to the SSDI benefit process, but obstructive guidelines remain. Eligibility determination continues to be a multistage phenomenon and unfavorable administrative decisions remain common. Appeals often lead to a fair decision, but the appeals process is onerous, time-consuming, and expensive and has a freezing effect. Thus justice is denied.

The Road Map of Social Security Disability Benefits illustrates these points well.

Veterans Affairs (VA) Benefits

Eligibility for VA care is based on three criteria, variably enforced by the Veterans Affairs Department: veteran status, degree of disability, and service connection of the disability. Access to care for veterans age sixty-five and older was made easier in 1970 through passage of Public Law 91-500. Since then, older veterans are deemed eligible for service in VA hospitals, nursing homes, and domiciliary care programs for disabilities that may not necessarily be connected with service duty, regardless of ability to pay.[3]

For younger veterans, such as those of the Vietnam War era, providing service-connected disability requires preparing a comprehensive package of data and papers to present to the VA. For those without documents, for those with mental illness, for those whose lives are utterly disorganized, legitimate VA benefits can be obtained only with help.

Phoenix—Advocates for the Disabled, Inc.

BR, a paranoid schizophrenic man of uncertain age, was originally approved for SSI in 1984. However, he moved around extensively, and often his checks were returned to Social Security. He came back to us intermittently for help in getting his checks replaced. Our social worker's notes state that he continues "to feel that people are after him and that he must keep away from them." He refuses mental health treatment, food stamps, and housing assistance because he wants "to roam." He is now in jail in the state of Washington, charged with assault. This makes him ineligible to receive his monthly checks. Somehow we think we may see him again.

Advocates for the Disabled is a community-based agency serving destitute persons since 1974. Clients include about two hundred homeless persons each year, individuals who have been denied entitlement benefits or whose benefits have been halted.

Homeless clients are referred from a wide variety of sources, primarily other agencies that serve the homeless. Upon referral, appointments are made for intake interviews at homeless clinics, at shelters, or at Advocates' own office. The staff member and the client develop a case plan at intake. They complete all forms,

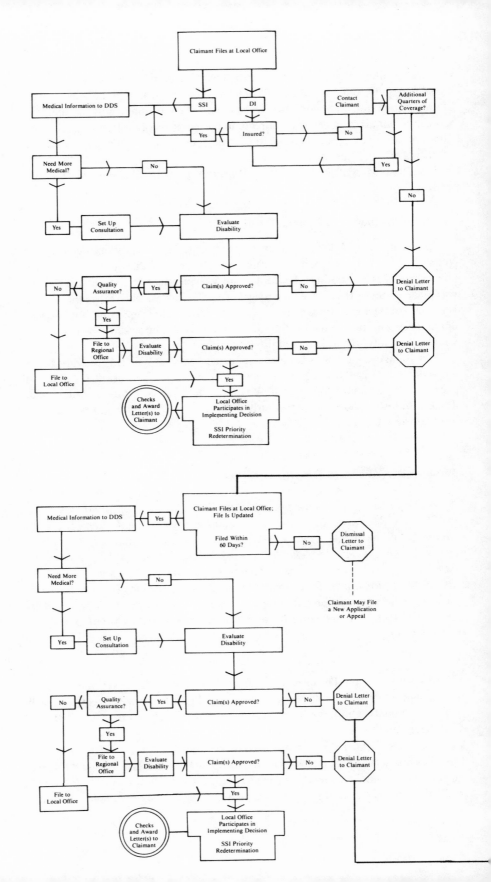

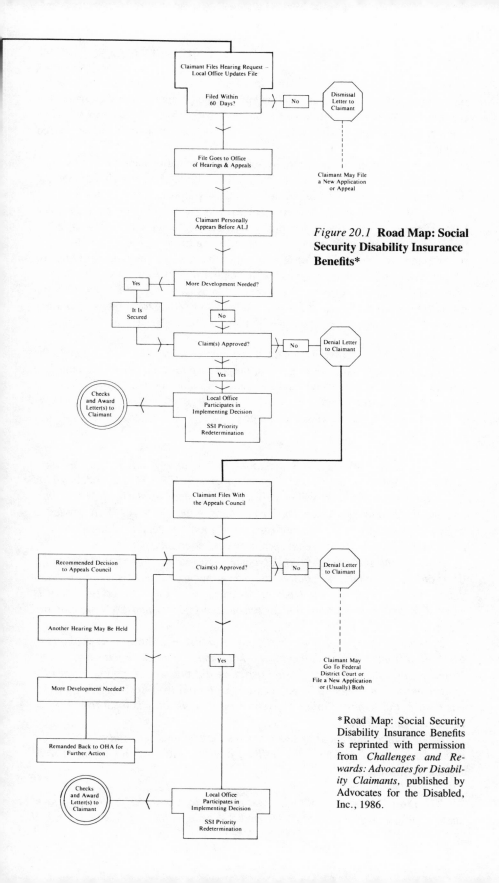

Figure 20.1 **Road Map: Social Security Disability Insurance Benefits***

*Road Map: Social Security Disability Insurance Benefits is reprinted with permission from *Challenges and Rewards: Advocates for Disability Claimants,* published by Advocates for the Disabled, Inc., 1986.

including those for release of information, for gathering of work and social histories, and determining basic survival needs. Medicaid application documents are collected at Advocates' office and submitted to the Arizona Health Care Cost Containment System (AHCCCS) offices (see below) in a uniform, organized manner.

Most forms of entitlement require medical examinations and proof of illness or disability. Advocates has a close relationship with the Phoenix HCHP, and the program physician is available promptly for these purposes.

If the claim is denied at the initial application, a common event, Advocates helps in the appeals process. Medical records are gathered and reviewed, additional examinations are conducted by the program physician or psychiatric consultant, and legal representation is secured. Advocates has negotiated refusal of the government to accept applicants who lack permanent addresses. All agencies now acknowledge the organization's own address as satisfying address requirements for homeless clients, and it also offers them a secure location for important documents and welfare checks. Through Advocates, a post office box is also available.

A representative payee is obtained for clients, if needed and allowed, for subsidized housing applications or other purposes, enrollment in vocational rehabilitation programs is pursued, and assistance in returning to a family in another state arranged in some cases.

The following histories span the range:

FF was a fifty-four-year-old alcoholic white man who left Indiana six days prior to his disability hearing and came to Phoenix in 1984. He was robbed of his few remaining dollars shortly after arrival in town, ended up at a homeless shelter, and was referred to Advocates. During the ensuing months he regularly needed to borrow $15 to $20 to survive until his $173 monthly general assistance (GA) check arrived, loans always repaid promptly. He continued to drink.

After twenty months of effort Advocates assisted him to obtain a successful decision on his SSDI claim before the Social Security Administration, a claim dating back to 1980. On the basis of his earnings in the auto industry he was entitled to and received $44,000 in retroactive benefits and $631 in monthly income.

Beset by chronic pain from an earlier cervical fusion, arthritis, and alcoholism, FF showed from first contact that he was not capable of managing his own funds. However, the Social Security Administration did not require appointment of a representative payee, and thus Advocates was barred from serving this purpose. His family, thousands of miles away, was out of contact. His local friends were no more capable than he.

FF died nine months after receiving his claim funds. His only assets at his death were several broken-down trailers, one of which was his home, a shell without utilities or plumbing.

BL, a forty-seven-year-old man, was referred to Advocates in 1987 by a local shelter because Social Security, GA, and SSI benefits had been denied. BL had suffered permanent injury to his right hand, arm, and shoulder when the limb was caught in a paper winder twenty-five years earlier. He also had a congenital hearing disability. BL had managed to work intermittently until 1981.

Through Advocates BL received GA and was accepted for vocational rehabilitation (VR) services. He entered a local college, is working toward a degree in accounting, is living in Section 8 housing, and is able to manage on his own with a VR allowance, GA, and food stamps. When his SSI and Social Security claims reached the hearing stage, he was already well into his VR program and opted not to pursue his disability claim. Advocates supported his decision. In this instance, a disabled homeless man was given temporary help that allowed him to work toward self-sufficiency.

JR, a sixty-year-old man, came to the agency in 1987, referred from a local shelter. He had been fired as a candy vendor for the circus. Advocates helped arrange a move to the transitional shelter and, after several months, to subsidized housing. In late 1987 JF's concurrent claims for SSDI and SSI were denied at a hearing. The Case was then brought before the appeals council, where it was remanded back to the local office of hearings and appeals. A favorable decision was issued nearly a year later.

JF's ability to work had been compromised by an auto accident in 1981 that caused back and knee problems and impaired his ability to stand for extended periods. He had had a year of college and worked for decades as a salesman. However, after the accident he found it difficult to hold a job, even one selling candy at the Phoenix Zoo, because of a combination of impairments, including visual limitation, a hand tremor, and anxiety.

This man came to Advocates with zero income. He progressed to $173 monthly GA and food stamps and subsidized housing. The happy ending includes remarriage to the wife from whom he was divorced during the years of financial difficulties. They have purchased a mobile home with his retroactive benefits and are financially secure on his Social Security disability benefits and his wife's retirement income.

Evaluation of the quality of its own services offered to clients is pursued vigorously by the Advocates program. All social workers at the staff level meet weekly with supervisors to review each active case. A written summary for each client is completed every six months and reviewed by the supervisor, as are case closures. A quarterly printout of services provided and of outcomes is maintained, based on each staff member's daily log. This information is used, in part, to determine the ratio of success for clients who follow through on service plans.

Problems

Lack of proof of citizenship has proved a major obstacle in establishing benefit status for homeless disabled persons. A characteristic instance is that of a twenty-seven-year-old homeless man approved for SSI benefits who, because he had spent much of his life in foster care, could not track his birth records. More than eight months passed from the date of his favorable SSI decision until he actually received payment. He had no income during this period other than the state of Arizona's $173 per month GA benefit, which also requires a current medical statement. A delay of eight months, it should be noted, is a substantial improvement over the situation faced by Advocates when it first started. By organizing data for submission, including all medical information, Advocates has reduced the average time delay prior to the initial hearing in half from the earlier maximum of eighteen months.

The transition from homelessness to mainstream life is obstructed by lack of commonly acceptable identification, such as a driver's license. Food stamp ID is not accepted by banks, and therefore, a client who receives a benefit check and lacks other proof is unable to open a bank account.

Arizona is the only state without a Medicaid program. As a substitute, the state has created AHCCCS to function as the state and federal health care program for the indigent. Under AHCCCS it can take more than a month to obtain an eligibility appointment. All documents supporting income and residency requirements must be available at the appointment time, and once approved for health care, the homeless person has no control over the geographical location of the assigned primary care physician. A ten- to fifteen-mile trip is commonplace. Appointments may end after city buses stop for the day, leaving homeless clients no option but to walk back to the shelter. Transportation thus becomes a critical issue.

Acceptance by the staffs of many agencies and businesses, such as Social Security, welfare, physicians, banks, and housing managers, is often poor, sometimes strikingly so, when clients appear dirty and unkempt. This reaction, while compatible with our understanding of human nature, clearly reduces the quality and quantity of services available to homeless persons.

Overall Success Rate

The rate of successful claims for homeless clients of Advocates who have followed through on the entire process is nearly 100 percent. It is striking that only 2.5 percent of the homeless seen by Advocates lack work histories; 20 percent of disability claimants have been helped to receive SSDI based on their previous earnings; another 33 percent have received concurrent benefits, both SSDI and Social Security. The remaining 47 percent received Social Security only. The aggregate *retroactive* benefits that Advocates obtains for clients during a typical year total $1.2 million, and continuing monthly income an additional $1.0 million. Total cost per client for all Advocates' services averages $137.50.

Detroit

Detroit, a city of more than one million, continues to suffer from the effects of the recession of the early 1980's. Unemployment for the city during this period rose from 13 percent in January 1980 to 20.4 percent in January 1983. The percentage receiving unemployment benefits dropped from an average of 70 percent in 1980 to 20 percent in 1983. The Detroit Homeless Health Care Coalition concluded that unemployment insurance was a public benefit that played a minimal role in the lives of Detroit's homeless, an assumption borne out by a continuing unemployment rate of over 19 percent in 1987.[4] In that year it remained true that less than 20 percent of the unemployed received benefits.

Entitlements

Entitlement benefits for Detroit's homeless were limited by regulations of the Michigan Department of Social Services that required applicants to have permanent addresses in order to apply. This, coupled with the lengthy waiting period to be certified for some benefits, became top priorities for change by the Detroit Coalition. Here, note that for GA, the program for which many single men are eligible, the waiting period was forty-five days. Another major concern was the complicated process and high rejection rate for SSDI. This particularly impacted on Detroit's large mentally ill deinstitutionalized population, persons released into the community without adequate housing, financial support, or community mental health services.

Wayne County is the provider of last resort for medical care to indigent persons. GA recipients, mainly single men, receive vouchers from the county when they need medical care. This involves visiting a caseworker for each episode of care. If specialty services are needed, special approvals are necessary, often taking forty-five days. Detroit HCHP has usually ended up giving care to these individuals without reimbursement. If hospitalization is required, and if it is not deemed a life-threatening emergency, clients must be placed at a county-approved secondary (smaller) institution, where the Detroit HCHP physician often does not have privileges. Therefore, unless the homeless patient voluntarily returns to the Detroit HCHP team after hospitalization, no follow-up or continuity of care is possible. In the case of those with tuberculosis a lottery system assigns clients to one of two hospitals with TB wards.

James D. Wright and Eleanor Weber in *Homelessness and Health*[4] show that the number of low-income housing units in Detroit declined by 26 percent, to 135,000, between 1978 and 1981. The resources for building low-income housing were drastically reduced in the 1980's, and virtually none is now being constructed to meet the increasing demand. While many of the homeless receive some kind of entitlement benefits, consideration should be given to whether the level of benefits is adequate to meet basic needs.

The Detroit HCHP has treated many women and children who were found in shelters because of abusive home situations. Thirty percent of Detroit's HCHP client population is children under nineteen years old. A large number of the women are enrolled in Medicaid but left home hurriedly without their cards. The HCHP had to find a simple way to retrieve these numbers if the program was to get reimbursed for health care services. Further, many women on Medicaid were members of Michigan's Primary Sponsor Plan, a demonstration program in Wayne County which required Medicaid recipients to be enrolled with a single physician or health maintenance organization. In this plan, families had to receive all their health care from a singular provider or obtain authorization from that provider to receive care elsewhere. Since many women feared returning to places where they were known and could be traced by their abuser, they often refused to return to their regular physicians but instead received treatment by the HCHP team physician at the shelter where they were staying. These visit were not eligible for reimbursement.

Of the nineteen RWJF/Pew grant-funded cities, Detroit ranked highest (82 percent) in the percentage of clients known to be receiving some form of entitlement benefit. There are several reasons for this success:

- All shelters in Detroit have case planners on-site. They are responsible for getting clients entitlement benefits.
- Detroit HCHP staff has served as troubleshooters for homeless persons having difficulties obtaining subspeciality medical vouchers.
- Sixty-one percent of Detroit's homeless program clients are women, children, and a small number of elderly, the group with the most potential eligibility for entitlement benefits.

Changes

Many changes in the entitlement picture may be traced to the efforts of the Detroit HCHP and its coalition. Detroit was fortunate in that one of the coalition's early members, Samuel Chambers, Jr., was deputy director of the Wayne County Department of Social Services. His interventions helped modify regulations that previously worked to deny entitled benefits to homeless persons, as follows:

- A permanent address is no longer needed to apply for entitlement benefits. The addresses of shelters or the homeless clinic can be used.
- The Department of Social Services has placed intake workers in two shelters so that applications for benefits can be taken on-site.
- Applications for GA, the primary entitlement for single adults, are now taken under the Emergency Needs Program, only recently applied to help the homeless. Under this program, persons can be certified for GA in eight days, rather than the forty-five days it usually takes.
- Regardless of where in Detroit homeless persons formerly lived, clinic outreach staff now brings them to a single district social services office, where established good relationships help expedite the application process.

Unresolved Questions

An unsettled concern involves homeless persons in the Assertive Community Treatment (ACT) Program. These clients have been hospitalized at Northville Regional Psychiatric Hospital, a major state facility for the mentally ill from Detroit, and then released into the community with intensive support services. DHCH assumed most ACT clients would qualify for SSDI since they had just been released from a psychiatric hospital. This proved not to be true. The majority of this group was hospitalized for treatment of a cocaine-induced psychosis. Because of faulty documentation of past episodes of mental illness, these clients usually do not qualify for GA and food stamps. Without this minimal level of support, it is almost impossible to live and function in the community.

In fact, most of Detroit's homeless receive some form of entitlement benefit. However, the low level of payment, particularly for GA clients, and the lack of affordable low income housing make bare survival a challenge. Thus the Detroit HCHP can enroll the homeless in entitlement programs, even raise the level of benefits, but still fall short of the ultimate goal of placing individuals and families in suitable housing with an opportunity for independent life.

Philadelphia

In Pennsylvania a startling and singularly important reduction in public benefits occurred as a result of the restructuring of the GA program in 1983. Approximately thirty thousand individuals residing in Philadelphia previously eligible for GA cash benefits were restricted to ninety days of benefits in a given twelve-month period.[5] The significance of this event to the homeless of Philadelphia was profound and cannot be overstated.

Entitlements

The Pennsylvania Welfare Reform Act of 1982 divided single individuals ineligible for any other forms of entitlements into two categories, termed chronically needy and transitionally needy. Approximately two-thirds of the homeless receiving GA fall into the latter category, which limits both cash benefits and medical benefits to ninety days per year. The loss of these benefits is, in fact, a precipitating cause of homelessness for many of the individuals and families seen by the Philadelphia HCHP since 1984.

The design of eligibility standards for public entitlement programs in Philadelphia has also presented multiple access barriers to the homeless. Inability to negotiate bureaucracies, such as Social Security and the Department of Public Welfare, and to provide proof of identity and verification of a permanent mailing address and a lack of other income usually results in disallowance of an application.

JM, a chronically mentally ill black man, applied for GA and needed identification. This is the third time he has begun the application process because he either forgot what he was directed to do by the intake worker at the welfare office or cannot obtain the information he needs to apply. Social Security will not accept JM's birth certificate as proof of identity when he tries to replace a lost Social Security card. Confused and discouraged, he gives up and will not be seen again for weeks or months.

In this instance, through considerable support and assistance from a shelter mental health worker and social worker, JM finally received both welfare benefits and SSI.

Small gains occur. For instance, prior to May 1987, homeless individuals living in shelters in Philadelphia were barred from receiving food stamps, ostensibly because meals were provided in the shelters.[6] Through Community Legal Services of the Philadelphia Department of Public Assistance food stamps regulations have been adjusted, and shelter residents are now entitled.[7]

A common problem for homeless persons, perhaps one of the biggest hurdles to overcome in the journey to document one's existence, is the loss of all identification or personal papers. If this difficulty is solved and complete documentation has been accomplished, next may come the arduous task of obtaining a payee so that the SSI-eligible person may receive benefits. Homeless people are often disconnected from their families. The only alternative may be the various public and private agencies as payees. It is often a difficult and even an unpleasant task to accept the responsibility of receiving and managing entitlement benefits for another person. In Philadelphia caseworkers at the Office of Services to Homeless and Adults, Community Legal Services, and some privately run shelters, such as the Bethesda Project, are willing to act as payees for homeless persons.

Veterans' benefits are the easiest to get and maintain once a person has been determined eligible. However, many homeless veterans are not aware that they may be eligible for benefits and are sometimes unwilling or unable to tolerate the application process, although it is relatively simple. Many homeless veterans are alcohol- or drug-dependent and in need of detoxification. Admission to a VA detoxification program may be the first step in gaining benefits. Once in the VA hospital, social work staff is available to complete the necessary benefit application forms. Homeless veterans with little or no income are also entitled to free medical care, an extremely valuable benefit considering the stringency of GA regulations in Pennsylvania.

The VA Medical Center in Philadelphia is also one of thirty-six that received federal funds in 1987 to develop programs specifically for homeless veterans. These are aimed at substance abuse and mental health treatment and housing placement.

Housing

Michael Harrington states that "uprooted" is a far better word than "homeless" when referring to the population we are considering here.[8] And so it is. Affordable housing is almost nonexistent in Philadelphia for this group. Even if homeless persons eventually receive benefits such as welfare and SSI, it is almost impossible to find decent and affordable living quarters. If appropriate housing is somehow found, then additional support services are needed in order to maintain the housing. When such services are not available, it is likely that those just briefly rehoused will once again become "uprooted."

The Philadelphia Housing Voucher Program assists homeless individuals and families in locating suitable living units, pays a portion of the monthly rent, and gives ongoing counseling as well as training in tenants' rights and responsibilities.[9]

Conclusion

Effort and funds will be spent best if entitlement programs are used as a means to achieve long-term benefit, rather than focus on bare survival alone. For instance, a concentration upon training for employment is taking place at shelter sites and in other settings for the homeless across the country. William Wilson[10] has suggested creation of a national labor policy to help the most disadvantaged break the poverty cycle. His agenda lists full employment as the ultimate goal, although he recognizes that jobs alone cannot solve the problems of deep poverty and homelessness. In Wilson's view, a strategy combining a national minimum income, indexed AFDC benefits, child and family allowance, income transfers to supplement low wages, and subsidized child care services is indicated.

This multifactorial approach, worthy of serious discussion, should include as well an affordable national housing strategy. Does anybody have a better idea?

LINDA KEEN SCHARER

IRENE STUART

ADA LINDSEY

MARIA PITARO

BETH ZEEMAN

MARY HENNESSEY

BRENDA PELOFSKY

GAIL SMITHWICK

21

Education and Training

Introduction

The future of health care programs for the poor, including the homeless, depends importantly on attracting the interest of young persons in training. Because much of this work occurs outside a traditional medical setting, it requires cooperation with others and uses skills and techniques rarely observed in a standard well-equipped medical facility. If outreach and an interdisciplinary team approach are proven methods of care for homeless individuals, what are the implications for education and training?

The very nature of this work inhibits an effective response from schools of medicine and nursing and from hospital residency programs. The inpatient service is the preferred site of learning for students and educators. Here patients' physical conditions are often dramatic, the patients are available twenty-four hours a day, and technology for diagnosis and treatment is conveniently at hand. The number of patients for review within the time scheduled for rounds is manageable, and the participants are easily assembled. Furthermore, the teaching function is built into the reimbursement system. In contrast, current methods for teaching ambulatory care, where much of service to the poor occurs, are labor-intensive. Current practice has not surmounted the structural realities of limited clinic hours, the fleeting presence of the individual patient, the large daily volume of work, and the flow of new individuals each day.[1] Reimbursement for teaching functions remains inadequate.[2]

There is, of course, evidence that a change in emphasis in the direction of ambulatory care is occurring.[3] Twenty-five percent of the three years of training in internal medicine must now be spent in an ambulatory care setting.[4] Furthermore, shorter hospital lengths of stay and the economic incentive to perform procedures on an outpatient basis complement this shift in focus.

The ambulatory care setting now envisioned, however, is not the place of contact for the homeless and poor. In fact, the Health Care for the Homeless Program was necessary precisely because these individuals were not going to clinics for care. We now understand that the preferred initial place for treatment is the frontier of the street or outreach clinic. Would any of these locations be approved as valid ambulatory care settings? They are certainly not cited as such.[4] Ambulatory care planning has not yet included these options in an organized manner.

How does one learn to care for human beings in unusual circumstances? We know that an interdisciplinary team approach offers many advantages in working with individuals such as the homeless, who are severely challenged by difficult life situations. Health professional schools are segregated into medicine, social work, and nursing. This separation of disciplines will not easily be altered, yet the ability of individual professionals to sustain work in places such as shelters is easily eroded.

In order to develop young health workers who accept the team concept, emphasis must be placed on the skills of a charismatic, clinically proficient preceptor. This is the individual who engages the students, supervises their work, and acts as an interpreter of the environment. It is a basic requirement that the preceptor work at the site. In this context we should not overlook the value of volunteers in discovering these opportunities. The nurses' clinics in a Nashville shelter, at the Pine Street Inn in Boston, and at the Los Angeles Union Rescue Mission discussed below were outgrowths of volunteer efforts.

This discussion considers the current climate of medical and nursing education with respect to outreach and interdisciplinary care, notes the experiences of students placed at work sites, and provides examples of and guidelines for educational initiatives for health care professionals and patients.

Model Educational Programs for Students in Health Disciplines

Life is short, and the art long, opportunity fleeting, experiment dangerous, and judgment difficult.

　　—Hippocrates, *Aphorisms*

In general, basic sciences form the first two years of the medical school curriculum, followed by clinical rotations that permit a specified number of electives. It is here that the opportunity for training exists.[5,6]

The following comments were made by fourth-year medical students asked to evaluate a community medicine rotation that placed them for one month in shelters and SRO hotels. They suggest that giving students this opportunity may influence their attitudes, if not their career choices.

Learning was mostly by doing. Not much didactics. At this point in med school I liked that. . . . Medicine was not always the center issue with many of the patients, and learning to work with other professionals in a team approach was probably the most valuable lesson I got. . . .

I especially enjoyed working at the Men's Shelter clinic and the Moravian Church. Both allowed exposure to a very different and varied subculture of the New York population. They allowed one to develop, or strengthen a personality of tolerance, humility, and realize what it's like to deal with a much more unfortunate and usually unappreciative population. The problems they face, both medically and psychologically, allowed me to build my academic knowledge—and powers of communication—under almost any circumstances.

From an academic point of view the thing that impressed me was the fact that most of the patients and conditions I saw were first time presentations. This gave me the valuable opportunity of being the first to examine and diagnose the condition. . . . Socially speaking, the experience was equally valuable. The shelters were a humbling and, at times, shocking eye opener to the poverty and destitution that can exist in a wealthy country.

My rotation . . . is best described as interesting. Interesting patients in interesting locations combined to yield a fascinating and educational experience. Working in the SRO clinics and in the shelters could not provide a better grounding in the principles of compassion and care.

This was an interesting experience which shed light on my ignorance. I was not aware of the fact that so many people were lacking primary care either due to a poor financial position or just plain ignorance and sometimes distrust towards medicine. Not only did I learn to deal with someone who may be "different" from an average patient, but my overall knowledge of medicine was expanded since not all the disease forms can be seen in the general population.[7]

The required current information base in the basic sciences and the complexities inherent in teaching acute patient care naturally restrict expansion of the four-year medical school curriculum. However, in at least one medical school—the University of New Mexico—an entire curriculum has been created with a four-year focus on primary care.

Nursing schools have also experimented with curriculum change, allowing students the option to work with the homeless. A noteworthy example took place at the Vanderbilt University School of Nursing in Nashville in 1986. This elective program, although discontinued after one semester as the result of demands for student time by competing courses, stands as a model effort, an important template for other nursing schools interested in this area of work.

In an analysis of the course its creator noted that for nurses there is the possibility of a gap between education and practice. Students, in fact, are often sheltered from the realities of the current health care system. The homeless clinic experience in Nashville gave students a genuinely realistic view of community nursing.

. . . the greatest benefits are derived from the experiences obtained through focusing on the clients' responses to actual or perceived health threats. Students quickly realize that they are on the clients' "turf" and that their clients are not a "captive audience" as they are in acute-care facilities. For their nursing to result in improved health status, students learn not to rely on their technical skills, but to increase the self-care of clients by health promotion activities. They soon learn that merely "telling" the client what to do generally has little, if any, effect upon that client's behavior and they learn to modify their desired client outcomes to reflect more realistically the environmental, developmental and personal characteristics of the clients.[8]

The preceptor for the students already had considerable prior volunteer experience in work with homeless persons before the course began. Therefore, when students were introduced to the clinic, she was able to fulfill well the dual role of faculty adviser and practical role model. "My credibility is increased by 'practicing what I preach.' I admit to the students that at times I am unsure of what to do next with some clients; we then act as co-researchers in attempting to explore both etiological factors and alternative nursing approaches."[8]

The preceptor noted that some students seemed unhappy with their clinical performance, although their work objectively had seemed good. Counseling led to a recognition that they felt ineffectual. Pointing out that the small gains stemming from personal interaction with homeless clients were in themselves of great value proved helpful to students.

A summary of the course experience emphasized that:

Nurses must be involved in the planning of health facilities designed to serve the homeless. There exists an area in the health care for the homeless that is indeed nursing. Nursing is concerned with 1) assisting the individual client or family in maximizing individual health potential by increasing self-care abilities and 2) promoting health of the community itself through advocacy for change concerning environmental conditions, program entitlements, and utilization of existing health care institutions. Nurses are uniquely prepared to assist the client holistically by application of theoretical frameworks from nursing and from other disciplines.[8]

Primary Care Defined: Its Relation to Care of the Homeless

Primary care is health care broadly interpreted, offering health promotion and disease prevention, basic hands-on services for acute and chronic disorders, education, guidance and counseling, and appropriate referrals. It includes:

- Assuring access to care for all
- Comprehensiveness of care
- Coordination and integration of services
- Continuity of care, with emphasis on sustaining long-term relationships between patient and health care staff

How well have the burgeoning primary care training programs in the United States carried out this mission? And have they adapted this definition in real life to the care of homeless persons? Perhaps the best source of information available to answer these questions is the 1987 report on primary care residency training issued by the United States Department of Health and Human Services.[9] Here primary care residency training programs federally funded between 1977 and 1986 were reviewed to determine their degree of success in increasing the number of primary care practitioners (essentially physicians in the fields of general internal medicine, pediatrics, and family practice) and improving access to good-quality care. The results:

- Over the ten-year span the number of resident physicians in primary care fields among the assessed federally funded programs more than doubled.
- Considerably more primary care didactic instruction, clinical experience, and continuity of care were offered than were true of more traditional training programs.
- Graduates of these training programs chose careers in medically underserved areas more frequently than did physicians in traditional programs (perhaps a self-fulfilling prophecy).

However, analysis of the curricula of these and other primary care programs fails to show more than a minimal effort to place physicians in training outside hospital walls and into the field, to those persons difficult to reach, the alienated, the improverished, the homeless.[10] Clearly, although a few sterling attempts have been made to bring resident physicians into health care programs for the homeless, more effort is needed in training primary care doctors to work with these persons.[11]

Among the numerous potential focuses of training interest for primary care-oriented young physicians in major United States cities today are:

- The impact of poverty on disease; questions of access to care and devising means to access; seeking and finding the medically unreached; appropriate tasks for persons in health care fields to address the medical consequences of poverty
- Ethical issues in health care, including as especially pertinent those related to HIV infection; the presence of this and other illnesses in high frequency among minorities, drug users, and the very poor, persons of different social class and with different social values and perspectives from those of most medical students and physicians

"The identification of psychosocial and behavior problems as key elements of a 'new morbidity' adds an important dimension to the care of patients and thus to the training of physicians."[12]

The Training and Education of Nurses: The Los Angeles Initiative

The University of California, Los Angeles (UCLA) School of Nursing has established and maintains a shelter-based nurses' clinic. The history and structure of this program are detailed below.

Background

In March 1983 the UCLA School of Nursing was invited by the administration of the Union Rescue Mission (URM) to participate in providing primary health care to homeless individuals in downtown Los Angeles. The URM, established in 1887, is located in the skid row area. It provides several thousand meals a day and almost seven hundred sleeping accommodations and has a rehabilitation program for job training. In addition, it housed a clinic, in existence for more than twenty years, that was open two afternoons a week, and was staffed by volunteer physicians and nurses.

URM was interested in having assistance in operating its clinic. As a result, the UCLA School of Nursing faculty implemented a nurse-managed clinic at URM with primary health care provided by nurse practitioners. The priorities for faculty involvement in this community-based project were for student education, faculty practice, research, and community service. Since the nurse-managed clinic was to be a clinical experience site for students, faculty began clinical practice there on a volunteer basis. Teachers first developed the philosophy and objectives for this project. They then wrote standardized protocols for the procedures commonly practiced. The protocols served as instructions for the students. Committees were established for development of the patient record, the encounter form, quality assurance, and infection control procedures.

Because of the location of the clinic, the population served, the inadequacy of mechanisms for reimbursement, and many other conditions, it is a most unusual clinical training site for nursing students, yet the distinctive nature of this clinic operation makes it a good learning opportunity for some students.

Current Practice

The nurse-managed clinic is now open five days a week, staffed by full- and part-time nurse practitioners, a licensed practical nurse, and a part-time social worker. One or more physicians are employed part-time. They see patients, serve as consultants, and are always available by phone if a circumstance arises in which the nurse practitioner requires immediate medical consultation. Homeless men who are enrolled in programs at the URM also serve as assistant staff in the clinic. All the health center services are under the management of the director of clinical services, an experienced full-time nurse practitioner.

Because the clinic is small, only a few students can be accommodated at any one time. The faculty believes, however, that if nurses are ever to be attracted to work with the urban underserved population, students should have this type of clinical experience. The majority of students assigned to this site have selected the graduate nurse practitioner specialty. They can practice physical examination and nursing diagnostic skills in this setting. They have the opportunity to evaluate a patient's health status and devise the plan of care based on the problems identified. They must consider the attendant circumstances resulting from homelessness.

In the second year of the educational program, nurse practitioner students focus on health promotion, health maintenance, and disease management. The emphasis in the final clinical course are refinement of their assessment, management, and evaluation skills, family health care, and community health problems. This environment also makes it easier to help students learn about collaboration, cooperation, consultation, referral, and the meaning of follow-up.

Many nurse practitioner students come into the graduate program with work histories in nursing practice ranging from a few months to more than fifteen years. The faculty believes the clinic, where primary health care and social services are provided for homeless individuals, is a good site for these students to begin their transition into nurse practitioners. The faculty also decided that it was essential to integrate overt health-illness, sociocultural, and psychophysical environment considerations into discussions about health care problems.

Observation

When the nurse faculty began this clinic, there was insufficient information available about what types of health problems these homeless individuals were likely to have. There also was little experience reported to suggest that they would even come to a clinic for health care. However, as the clinic and the primary care that was provided became known by the individuals who inhabited the Los Angeles streets, the numbers who sought health care increased. In 1989 almost three thousand individuals were cared for, through more than eight thousand encounters. The School of Nursing has recently received funding to operate a second nurse-managed clinic in downtown Los Angeles, designed especially to give primary health care to children.

The faculty originally began this work because of its primary interest in establishing a clinical training site for graduate student nurse practitioners. The project has evolved into a service that benefits students, faculty, and the underserved urban community of homeless individuals.[13]

The Boston Experience

Educational opportunities for nursing and medical students, and for resident physicians, have perhaps been more thoroughly experienced in Boston than in many other cities with Health Care for the Homeless Programs. The principles, attitudes, spirit, and difficulties of these developments are discussed below. It is important to note that homeless persons at Boston's Pine Street Inn are considered guests of the shelter and are so termed here.

Overview

Since 1977 the Pine Street Inn Shelter has been a clinical placement for nursing students from the University of Massachusetts at Boston.[14] The shelter is the site for the clinical part of a ten-credit course in community mental health nursing. In addition to the clinical hours, students attend four hours of classroom instruction per week. The classroom focus is on theoretical concepts relevant to community mental health nursing, including systems theory, community and family assessment, communication skills, crisis intervention, group therapy, research, and health policy.

Nursing students occasionally elect to go to Pine Street but are more often randomly assigned. A great deal of anger and anxiety is common when assignments become known. Time spent initially in understanding and working through negative reactions has proved invaluable in assisting students to reach their full potential in the shelter.

Orientation

Prior to their first visit to the shelter students meet as a group with the clinical instructor, who fosters a nonjudgmental atmosphere to allow them to express freely their concerns about the placement and to discuss any preconceived notions they may have about homeless persons. Teaching modules, which include games, brainstorming, and role play, help students identify personal feelings and stereotypes and develop a more realistic idea of who the people are who constitute the homeless group. Working in a shelter is a new experience and is for many a difficult adjustment. During orientation students become accustomed to the facility, the guests, the staff, procedures, and policies.

The Clinical Experience

The time commitment is eighteen hours per week for two semesters. Fourteen hours, including one consistent session with the nurses' clinic, are scheduled at the inn. Time is also made available for students to attend self-help meetings such as AA and Al-Anon (attendance at three AA and three Al-Anon meetings is highly encouraged), visit other agencies, and attend professional conferences.

They are oriented to the nurses' clinic by the inn's nursing staff which also provides on-the-spot supervision, consultation and support. Having nursing role models and concrete nursing tasks to perform eases the transition into the shelter.

The majority of students' clinical time is spent among the guests in the inn's lobby. This is a stressful experience. At first the student sees only a mass of homeless faces. Many individuals are vying for their attention. Students may wonder why they are there. How can they possible do nursing and and provide other health care services in this setting? This feeling changes as they mingle with the guests, learn their names, and realize that each person has a unique story to tell.

Students are asked to identify two or three guests as their patients. When possible, therapeutic contracts are made, problem lists written, and goals mutually established. Students often need help in setting realistic goals with, rather than for, the guests. In supervision they are helped to accept the often slow pace of progress and to see the value in small gains. In time, most are able to appreciate the enormous value of the therapeutic relationship itself.

Record Keeping

Students are expected to comply with charting and other documentation requirements of the inn. They must also submit lists of personal goals and how they will measure their own success in achieving these goals. The lists reflect personal objectives for professional growth. They are used in supervision to develop individually meaningful experiences. Each student keeps a journal of clinical activities, a day-to-day record of clinical time, including descriptions of activities, personal reactions, significant thoughts, and learning experiences. Each student also submits a complete data base, problem list, goals, and ongoing notes on the guests being followed. These are reviewed in supervision.

Supervision and Evaluation

An on-site instructor meets with the students in clinical conferences. Supervision is used to help students increase their skill in developing and maintaining therapeutic relationships. Termination issues are stressed in supervision. Students may feel that they are deserting the guests and either want to avoid the issue or say, "I'll probably come back." When termination is mismanaged, guests may have difficulty in trusting nursing students in the future. However, when termination is handled correctly, it is common for a guest to request work with an incoming student.

Long-Term Benefits of the Program

Students have often stated that they reap more benefits from the program than do the guests. They express gratitude to the guests, who have taught them not to take things at face value, who have shown them the fear in suspicion, the hurt in anger, and the strength they manifest in spite of being homeless. The students feel changed by the experience and more accepting of themselves.

The program offers both short- and long-term benefits to the guests. Occasionally a dramatic difference is seen in a guest as the result of a student's intervention. More often the change is slow, resulting from the work of several different students over many semesters.

Students who have worked in the shelter become sensitized to the needs and struggles of homeless persons. Their nursing care plans reflect this. There are now close to two hundred graduates from this program, many staffing area clinics and hospitals.

The Education and Training of Medical Students and Residents

Introducing physicians in training to the established independent nurses' clinics was not easy. Originally, fourth-year medical students were assigned to the Pine Street Inn clinic. There was no on-site preceptor, but a physician was available by telephone for consultation. Unfortunately some of the assigned students had no desire to be at the shelter or to learn about homelessness, and there was no curriculum to facilitate their education. On the basis of this early experience, several guidelines for more fruitful student participation emerged.

First, students must come voluntarily. Secondly, a time commitment is essential for many reasons. Orientation to the shelter and to the clinic is time-consuming but vital to providing care. The clinics have dramatically shown how fostering relationships between guests and providers is a slow but rewarding process that can facilitate medical care. The clinics provide a source of continuity for those whose care is usually fragmented. Students must spend enough time both to benefit from what they can learn in this setting and to give service. Thirdly, there must be adequate supervision, ideally by a physician well informed about care of the homeless. A pitfall to avoid is having the supervising physician devote so much attention to teaching students that the usual interactions of the clinic session are refocused and the physician is less available to the clinic staff and the guests.

The unsuccessful first attempt at placing medical students in Pine Street's clinic was followed by better programs. Harvard Medical School began an Urban Health Project. Students spent ten weeks between their first and second years in shelters, soup kitchens, and prisons. Because they had little clinical experience, they worked in the lobbies, kitchens, and dormitories of the shelters. They spent time sharing meals, playing cards, and escorting guests to appointments. They became significant assets to the shelters and paved the way for further student involvement. They also gathered together once each week to review their experiences with preceptors. Medical students from Boston University had tours of Pine Street Inn included as part of their required curriculum, introducing them to life in the shelters.

Primary care medical residents from Boston City Hospital chose to come to the Pine Street Inn clinic in 1986 after physicians from the HCHP had been there for a year.

The rotation required a one-year commitment to attend one evening clinic each week. A group of clinic staff interviewed interested residents prior to their being selected, to assess motivation and sincerity. The medical residents at first faced reserve but were soon accepted, as their commitment and medical skill became apparent. The success of the program is attested by the fact that two of the first residents who chose the Pine Street clinic are currently working for Boston's HCHP.

A problem inherent in having *medical* students and residents in the shelter clinics is that these units are designed to be independent *nurses'* clinics. Nurses are experts in many areas ignored by traditional medical education. The introduction of physicians is therefore bound to be difficult. This point is well described by Dr. James O'Connell, referring to his first night at Pine Street Inn: "Perhaps I could manage scleroderma or leukemia, but the expertise of these dedicated professionals included maggots, lice and festering feet. There was much for me to learn."[15]

The nurses have come to realize the value of on-site physician support. The ability and ease with which the nurses and physicians are able to learn from each other to the benefit of the guests have become a credit to both and a triumph in a field where traditional rivalries often have impeded patient care.

At first the nurses and clinic staff were protective of the guests, and rightfully so. They had received many offers to do "screening," or to have students come to the clinics to learn without providing any services in return. They experienced firsthand the lack of responsiveness of the medical establishment to their patients and faced daily the end results of impractical therapeutic regiments, which were regularly prescribed when the guests visited the hospital. In addition, they were concerned about having physicians in training "practice" on the guests.[16]

This lack of trust of the existing medical system was eased somewhat by hospital rounds, during which shelter nurses and members of the HCHP team visited hospitalized guests together each week. Here the nurses were able to speak directly with the residents responsible for patient care, and mutual respect grew. The house staff could learn about realistic discharge planning and follow-up, and the nurses offered valuable background information to improve care. The nurses could also see the role and level of responsibility of residents in a teaching hospital and learned that residents were more than "student doctors."

Currently the HCHP in Boston has multiple sites providing a variety of experiences for residents and medical students. Short-term electives in the clinic at St. Francis House, a day shelter, are available. Pine Street's clinic welcomes students who agree to a six- to eight-week commitment. Students and residents also have the opportunity to visit a number of different shelters and their clinics. While on elective, they are invited to the twice-weekly meetings of the HCHP to provide an overview of services available throughout the city, including family services.[17]

Conclusion

In the past it was the unusual young medical or nursing student who was able to break through the traditional in-hospital orientation and to understand in a more than superficial way that the illness of an individual patient was often a result of health problems in the community at large.

Major medical centers and professional schools have generally lagged in finding means to teach about the health care of the homeless. The status of this work has been low, and time in the curriculum carefully guarded. When change has occurred, it has often stemmed from student rather than faculty interest, yet it remains true that "the professional school can serve as the two-way intellectual conduit between the problem as it exists in society and what goes on in the university."[18]

Since teaching of health care providers about the needs of homeless persons is a relatively new field, few models for training and education exist. Several fundamental principles form the basis for developing successful programs.

It must be explicitly taught to all students that *every* patient is to be treated with respect and dignity. Care must be offered in a positive, nonjudgmental manner, recognizing the indignities and humiliations which the homeless regularly endure. Patients have the right to make choices, including unhealthy choices. The role of the provider is to enable patients to make the best possible choices.

Continuity of care is especially important, and emphasis should be placed on developing one-to-one relationships to engender trust.

Homeless persons are usually isolated from the medical system, their care compromised by lack of access to resources and lack of knowledge on the part of hospital providers. Inappropriate follow-up and care plans result.

Finally, the recognition of the central role of nursing and social service must be stressed, especially to physicians. The majority of health-related problems of the homeless are treated outside hospitals. Nurses provide the assessment, personal care, supervision of medications, counseling, and advocacy. Often health care, housing, and food are obtained through the system of federal and state entitlements. It is the social worker and outreach worker who characteristically obtain these benefits. In addition, their counseling and advocacy efforts enhance patient care.

Young people are most likely to be drawn to work in this field if exposed to it at school or during postgraduate training by enthusiastic teachers or peers. The role model is all-important, and this model must include working with teachers and staff who are both talking about and actually delivering care in real life settings.[18]

Teaching about care of the homeless will never be time well spent in a crowded curriculum or service schedule if it is purely didactic. A well-organized, properly supervised clinical experience allows students and young physicians and nurses to overcome stereotyped thinking and obtain a realistic view of life in shelters. Some will recognize the rewards of a career in this field; all will gain a degree of sensitivity and concern for fellow human beings in need.

Acknowledgments: We would like to give special thanks to Marie Gerhardt, M.D., Debra Donovan, and John Noble, M.D., for their help in the planning and preparation of the Boston discussion.

STEPHEN L. WOBIDO

TENA FRANK

BILL MERRITT

SANDRA ORLIN

LARRY PRISCO

MARK ROSNOW

DIANE SONDE

22

Outreach

Introduction

The homeless, whose numbers have grown steadily across the United States, seriously challenge the health and social service systems of this country to respond to what is viewed as a fundamentally new health problem. Outreach has been recommended as one way, among many, to help meet the health needs of these persons. The American Psychiatric Association, for example, has suggested that the reluctance many homeless persons express about having contact with mental health personnel could be overcome by aggressive outreach.[1]

However, the growing interest in outreach as a way of serving homeless persons has introduced conflicting views on the purpose and nature of such programs.[2] As the term is currently applied to a variety of services, outreach may both encompass the activity of engaging people in treatment and service systems and be a form of treatment and therapy itself. It may include various elements of case management, advocacy, community organizing, and political action.[3] In public health, medicine has traditionally been viewed as responsible for providing all those activities in the community that relate to the prevention of illness and suffering, as well as the promotion of health, and to the improvement of the physical and emotional welfare of the people.[4] The history of public health offers several examples of health care that can serve as a basis for examining and understanding those activities we today commonly call outreach to the homeless.

Historical Perspective on Outreach

In the eighteenth and nineteenth centuries the increasingly squalid and over-crowded slums of Europe and the United States produced health conditions viewed as threatening both the public health and the social fabric of Western societies. Controlling, preventing, and treating the diseases that threatened to spill out of the urban slums came to be viewed as essential to maintaining social order and required innovative approaches.

In eighteenth-century Europe one form of such innovation was the development of the concept of "medical police," government workers whose mission was "to apply dietetic and medical principles to the promotion, maintenance and restoration of the public health." The scope and authority of such workers, their proponents argued, must extend beyond the established medical practice of the day to include such areas as nutrition, sanitation, housing conditions, hygiene, accident prevention, epidemic control, and health education.[5]

In late-eighteenth-century England the rising numbers of poor people in London's slums led to the creation of the first institutions designed to provide medical care for the sick poor. The hospital movement and the dispensary movement represented efforts to reach populations not being helped by existing medical practitioners. New public health outreach efforts geared to discovering and *preventing*—as well as treating—the spread of disease were mounted among the urban poor.[6]

Finally, the waves of immigration to the United States in the late nineteenth and early twentieth centuries presented similar health threats to the broader community. One of many responses to meeting such challenges was the development of the first public health nurse programs and the eventual coordination of their efforts along with those of other health activities in the nation's first geographically organized district or community health centers. Assuming responsibility for the entire population within a particular district, such centers spread in New York, Cincinnati, and Boston during the first quarter of this century, offering a broad array of services and reaching out into local communities to find those lacking care.[7]

The principal characteristics of these approaches provide ample foundation for an understanding of the purpose and nature of outreach today. These characteristics include:

Response to need rather than demand alone. Invariably, such efforts have arisen whenever the current medical practice was insensitive or unresponsive to growing health problems, particularly among the poor. Outreach and case-finding efforts are mounted better to define and reach those affected. The approach is proactive rather than reactive and aims to reach the entire population within a given geographic area rather than only those able to demand or seek care.

Greater emphasis on prevention generally characterizes such efforts than is true of the currently institutionalized medical system. The approach goes beyond curative interventions to encompass an often broad array of preventive measures as well as health education and promotion.

An impetus arising from outside medicine, as one component of a broader social change movement. The fate of new public health interventions seems closely related to their ability to maintain their own unique characteristics. When either segregated too sharply from mainstream medicine, or subordinated to it, much of the original approach frequently disappears. When such movements are able to achieve both broad institutional support *and* enduring changes in organized medicine, their contribution seems more lasting.[8]

The Challenge of Outreach Today

Making contact and establishing relationships with homeless persons are the challenge of outreach today.[9] This engagement process begins by nonintrusive offering of basic services (e.g., food, shelter) in the streets and in settings that homeless individuals frequent. Because survival needs are the overwhelming priority for homeless persons, attention to these points is a vital part of gaining initial acceptance. H. Richard Lamb refers to this process as the "opening wedge": developing a climate of trust by meeting an individual's basic priority needs with no strings attached.[10] A. Frances and L. Goldfinger further suggest that only by first providing resources that can meet these primary requirements can health workers establish credibility and differentiate themselves from those in an individual's past who failed to meet such needs.[11] In addition, a provider attempting to engage a person should be flexible, having the ability to respond to each individual's requests and not be locked into a prescribed treatment protocol.[12]

Flexibility means that the approach should be individualized, with respect to both the number and types of services and the manner in which they are provided. Individualized attention involves careful assessment of clients and continued close monitoring and evaluation of service delivery to ensure that needs are being met.[13]

A nonthreatening manner is an integral ingredient of initial and continued involvement with the homeless. This involves a "no questions asked" demeanor. Premature probing for personal background information may be considered intrusive and deter from treatment an individual who is fearful of bureaucracies and possible rehospitalization.

A key characteristic of establishing relationships is emphasis on the voluntary nature of this type of engagement.[14] Treatment and services are considered a choice, and although providers may encourage an individual's participation in a service or specific program, they must respect that person's right to refuse to participate.

Accessibility of services also is a key factor in facilitating participation. The term "assertive availability" refers to services that are accessible even to the most isolated and unmotivated[13] and that maintain involvement with those likely to drop out. It means bringing help to individuals in need rather than waiting for them to come to service sites.[15]

The process of engagement is facilitated by sensitivity to the stigmatizing effects of psychiatric and medical labels. Decreasing the attention to, or eliminating the use of, such labels may help reduce negative reactions.[16]

A key element stressed by S. M. Barrow and A. M. Lovell involves the timing of the mental health referral.[17] Often as many as ten contacts are necessary before mental health services may be offered with the probability of being accepted. A premature offer of mental health treatment, accompanied by probing of the individual's mental health status, may deter an individual from accepting treatment.[17] What appears to be essential before such an offer is made is the development of a climate of trust and the provision of services that mean the most to the client.[11]

Throughout the process, therefore, it is necessary to guard against moving too fast. However, once an individual has initiated contact, it is important to remain responsive and to address progressively that person's more complex and specialized needs for treatment and assistance. Failure to do so could jeopardize the credibility and effectiveness of earlier outreach and engagement efforts.[18]

Defining Outreach

The definition of "outreach" must focus on the essential element of contact with any individual who would otherwise be ignored (or unserved). This avoids hinging the definition on any specific activity. This is important because in actual practice outreach efforts include a number of different services, none of which is necessarily provided by all programs.[3]

There are other common and useful characteristics defining outreach:

- Outreach should bring the point of contact with the service system to the homeless person, no matter where that person is. It should not be limited to a fixed or office-based setting. Thus, while outreach may take place on the street, it can also be accomplished in shelters, drop-in centers, medical and psychiatric emergency rooms, patients' SRO hotel rooms, hospitals, and jails. In addition, some would say that shelters and drop-in facilities are themselves a form of outreach.
- Outreach programs should attempt to engage individuals who are unserved or underserved by existing agencies and service providers.
- Both program administration and outreach staff must have a strong commitment to the team approach to service delivery.
- Chief administrators or program directors must support the outreach team and advocate for their efforts with other service providers in the community.
- Programs should possess a philosophy that aims to restore the dignity of the homeless person, dealing with the client as a person, not as a patient.
- Programs must feature a style of care in which outreach workers are both consistent and persistent in their dealings with clients.[19]

Qualities of an Outreach Worker

A special type of individual is required for working with those who are homeless and out of contact with the health care system and society. Candidates must be genuinely interested in working with severely ill people and prepared for difficulties stemming from such work. In particular, they must possess an expectation of nonresults. They must understand that they will not be able to "cure" or "save," that their clients may be denied access to needed services and programs, and that some may in the end reject them and the help they try to provide.

Thus, programs should seek out individuals who can find other rewards in doing outreach work besides the achievement of clinical improvement in their clients. Such rewards can include those stemming from a religious commitment to helping (as distinct from converting) others, those connected to furthering an academic understanding of illness and poverty, or those that come from simply enjoying work with the underserved.[19]

The process of outreach and engagement can be a lengthy one marked by few obvious accomplishments. It may take numerous contacts, spanning many months or even a year, before an individual accepts help.[17] Outreach workers must have realistic expectations and recognize the limitations as well as the possibilities in a specific situation.[20]

Those working with the homeless must have emotional strength and the capacity to view all individuals positively.[21] In particular, attention to a person's sense of well-being appears to be an important aspect of the provider's role.[22] Stern and Minkoff suggest that staff members can be trapped in a "professional-esteem paradox" in which they are reluctant to participate in activities they believe to be "demeaning" or inconsistent with their professional orientation even if the activities promote the general well-being of the client.[23]

For workers in frequent contact with chemically dependent or mentally ill homeless persons, training in clinical skills and professional supervision are essential. At a minimum, in the nonmental health settings that often serve homeless individuals (e.g., emergency rooms, police stations) service providers should have ready access to skilled guidance.

The ability to assess and address a person's need for care also is important in early outreach contacts. Often staff members are caught in the delicate situation of recognizing a need for help but hesitating to mention treatment out of concern that the individual will flee. Thus, workers—particularly mental health providers—must be able to judge the severity and urgency of the situation and determine whether it warrants immediate attention and treatment or can be postponed until a trusting relationship has developed.[20]

The provider also must have the ability to link the client into the needed community services. This involves knowledge of the services and resources available in the community that may best fit specific needs.[24]

Evaluating Outreach Programs

Evaluations of outreach efforts may be needed for both external and internal reasons.[19] The most common external reason leading to an evaluation is the need to demonstrate program effectiveness to financial supporters. Internal reasons include the staff's desire to answer its own questions about how the program is functioning, understanding and solving operational problems, and determining how work can be more effectively accomplished. The reasons for evaluation determine the types of questions which must be answered and the methods used.

Challenges of Evaluating the Effectiveness
of Outreach Programs

Outreach programs can pose a considerable challenge to evaluators attempting to determine their effectiveness.[19] There are a number of reasons:

- The extreme variability and flexibility in the way services can be delivered among and within any given program
- The mobility of the client population in and out of treatment
- The often subtle effects of the services that are given to clients, making them difficult to measure, and that are manifested only over a lengthy period
- The nature of change in this population, which tends to be cyclical rather than linear in nature (in other words, people with severe mental illnesses do not gradually get better over time; instead they typically experience long-term disabilities characterized by repeated setbacks and recurrences of symptoms)
- The need to measure the impact of outreach services both on individuals and on numerous service systems

In summary, the very factors that contribute to a successful outreach effort (i.e., flexibility, ability to alter service systems) may impede evaluations that strive to measure effectiveness in concrete terms.

Since the effectiveness of outreach programs is determined to a great extent by the availability and quality of other services and programs for homeless individuals in the community, evaluations aimed at measuring the overall function of an outreach program must also focus on the extent to which these other services are available. Similarly, it is important both to evaluate the impact of services on program clients and to determine who is not being served by the program. Is the program meeting the needs of the entire homeless population or just of certain segments?[19]

Use of Quantitative Measures and Scales in Evaluating
Outreach Programs

Outreach programs may also have difficulty in applying to the homeless the scales and measurement tools developed to measure improvement in other populations. Typically, existing scales are not sensitive to improvement in the functioning of the homeless because of the severity of these individuals' symptoms. Improvement in clients is often so subtle that it does not register on typical scales that measure functional improvements in such areas as employment status and higher-level social interaction skills.

These difficulties have led both to the redesign of existing quantitative measures of improvement and the development of alternative designs more relevant to documenting the progress of a homeless person. For example, an existing rating scale for measuring the functional level of mentally ill persons in inpatient and outpatient clinic settings was modified more accurately to reflect the impact of homelessness on client functioning. As another instance, poor personal hygiene was seen both as a possible indicator of poor functional ability and as an indicator of poor access to bathing facilities caused by the client's homelessness.

Alternative measures of improvement in the status of the homeless may also include the number of days per month spent in housing, number of times victimized, level of hygiene, number of contacts with other service providers, and so on. Such measures of success however, reflect the changing nature of the service systems involved as much as they do changes in individual functioning.[19]

Use of Descriptive, Qualitative Measures in Evaluating Outreach Programs

Qualitative evaluation techniques have proved useful for program administrators seeking to answer questions about the functioning of their programs. Some techniques rely on descriptive analyses of program function, often gained from in-depth interviews and observations of staff and clients and other individuals who interact with the program rather than on analyses of numerical measures that may not fully capture essential program and client characteristics.

One qualitative technique helpful to some outreach providers is the questioning of formerly homeless individuals who have been outreach clients to find out which elements in the outreach team's approach were appealing or useful and which were perceived as negative. One way to obtain in-depth, high-quality information on these topics is to include formerly homeless clients in staff training sessions or on staff retreats.[19]

Examples of Outreach

Examples from the Health Care for the Homeless Program show the nature, purpose, characteristics, and principles of professional outreach in action.

Nashville

The Nashville HCHP is based at a fixed-site clinic in the downtown area, within walking distance of the major homeless shelters. Outreach is an essential element in the service provision offered by the clinic, and it includes visits to the riverbank communities, shelters, and soup kitchens.

Much of Nashville's outreach plan was based on knowledge gained from the experience of the city's religious ministries, which had been working for years with the homeless. It was clear that these service providers drew strength from a deeply held spiritual belief that served to motivate and support them over the weeks, months, or years it might take to reach a homeless person. Whether drawn from a spiritual source or from some personally held belief, principle, or ideology, commitment to serving the homeless person was understood to be a basic trait all outreach workers must have in order to sustain themselves and their work. There were no miracles or magic in building trust and support. The first step was often nothing more than a smile and the offer of a cup of coffee.

Milwaukee

The Milwaukee HCHP outreach team has consistently taken the extra step in working with its homeless, as these reports show:

In the case of a homeless man who spent his days drinking, the outreach team found it unproductive to talk with him while he was inebriated. Knowing where he slept on the streets, one of the outreach workers arrived at this spot at sunrise before the man had started his daily drinking routine. While sober, the man viewed the alternatives suggested to him by the outreach worker in a new light, and he eventually agreed to move indoors.

Another example is of the homeless man who had described himself as the "king of the bums." At the time the Milwaukee HCHP outreach team found him, he had been homeless for ten years. Before that he lived in shelters and SRO facilities. When he was moved into his own apartment, the outreach team quickly learned the transition was not going smoothly. One afternoon, when an outreach worker arrived, he heard the man's alarm clock ringing. Asked why the alarm clock was on, the man explained that he feared that if he touched the alarm, the clock would break. Besides teaching him how to set and turn off the alarm clock, the outreach worker also explained to him the importance of not smoking directly under the smoke detector and not placing hot pans on material that would burn.

Successfully managing a household and performing simple daily tasks can be major difficulties for those who have been homeless for an extended period. Assisting this person through his transition from homelessness to renter status made the difference between success and failure. Without guidance of this type, it seemed probable that the man would not have lasted in his new apartment.

San Antonio

The San Antonio HCHP outreach team began its operation by dividing the city into quadrants to be visited on the same day each week. Team members traveled with food, drink, toiletries, and clothing. The dependability of the team in showing up on the same day each week imparted a sense of trust to the homeless in those areas; the giving of basic, usable goods was the beginning of many relationships. While traveling a quadrant, the team members searched out local providers to explain their outreach purpose, enlist their support, and explore ways of mutual assistance in serving the homeless. This activity was the beginning of networking in San Antonio. As the credibility of the outreach team and the HCHP increased, so did the information from the providers and the homeless themselves on how best to accomplish their shared mission. In some instances provider staff or homeless persons accompanied the team to specific locations (camps, safe houses), and the team thereby gained access to places and situations that otherwise would never be noticed by the general public or service community.

The following maps derive from this privileged information and show the routes traveled by the homeless throughout San Antonio. All along these corridors

Map of San Antonio and Bexar County

○ ○ ○ ○ ○ Primary routes
● ● ● ● Secondary routes
★ Campsites

Downtown San Antonio

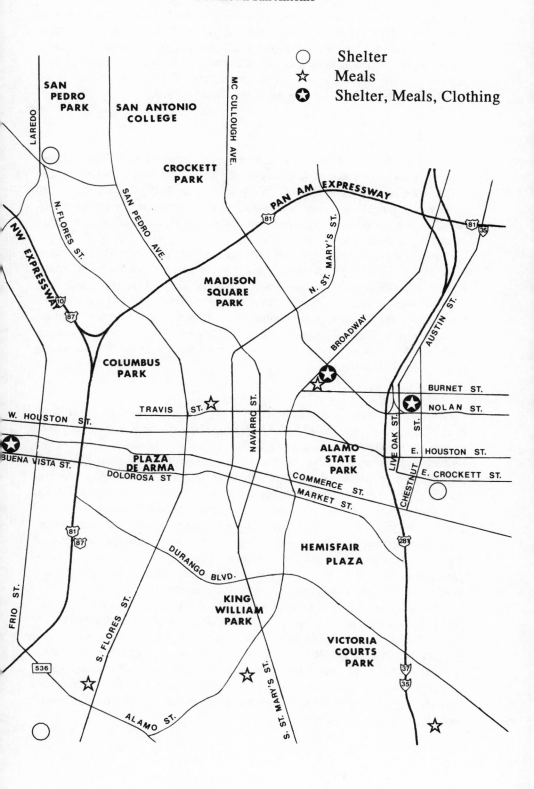

are camps, safe houses, and providers of food, shelter, and clothing. An interesting discovery made by the team was the continuing battle between the homeless, looking for safety and survival, and drug traffickers, attempting to use the same routes. A team member was also shown a map, developed by the homeless community itself, describing desirable campsites and safe houses with names of contact persons who could be relied upon and trusted. Some of the names of the HCHP outreach team were among the listed contact persons.

Philadelphia

In April 1985 a HCHP outreach team began visiting Women of Hope, the low-demand residence for twenty-four chronically mentally ill women who had been living on the streets of Philadelphia for a year or more. The residence was staffed by formerly homeless women with social work supervision. A mental health worker was assigned full-time to assist with treatment plans and engage women in mental health treatment.

Every Tuesday evening the outreach team visited the residence in order to offer health services. The women, who were invited but not forced to accept treatment, retained much of their street life-style. They carried bags and wore layers of infested clothing. Some sat up all night. They shouted or muttered but rarely conversed. They rejected mental health treatment and benefits. Most refused to have their blood pressures checked. They seemed alarmed by the possibility of medical care. However, the nurse practitioner continued the painstaking process of gaining the residents' trust.

Eventually some of the women began to get sick. One woman, named Rose, began to urinate in cups by her bed. The team thought this new behavior might be caused by her hesitance to pass by the raised canes and angry shouts of her roommates. Rose signaled her reluctance to accept health care by telling the nurse practitioner to go to hell. However, she became weaker and, after being unable to get out of bed, agreed to hospitalization. She was discharged on oral medication to control her newly diagnosed diabetes. The team urged the Women of Hope staff to press treatment. Rejecting the "poison," Rose headed for her old street corner, where she remained for several months. On the street Rose became debilitated and eventually returned to the shelter. The director of Women of Hope, a Sister of Mercy who had known Rose for years on the street, said she would rather see Rose inside the shelter in a coma than outside on the street.

The outreach team members felt uncomfortable with Rose's worsening condition. They began encouraging the staff to consider giving her insulin. With time, the staff also grew more alarmed about Rose's health and less worried about injecting her with insulin. When the director of Women of Hope sensed that Rose was too comfortable to return to the street yet too weak to say no, she asked Rose to accept insulin. Rose agreed to insulin, but not to blood tests. Rose's physician from the hospital and the nurse practitioner developed a plan for adjusting insulin doses by urine test results alone.

Over the next three years Rose had only one medical hospitalization, for an infection. She also returned one additional time to the street. This time dense cataracts limited her vision, and she began walking into traffic. This behavior led to Rose's involuntary psychiatric hospitalization. Once Rose was safe in the hospital, options were considered for her care. Negotiations between Rose and the Women of Hope/HCHP staff led to an agreement: Rose agreed to return to Women of Hope; only two staff members would give her insulin. Rose still refused cataract surgery ("They'll cut my eyes out"). She refused psychotropic medication ("poison"). She accepted nail clipping but no other care from the nurse practitioner. Rose usually described her mood as "insulting." She said she disliked Women of Hope, all the staff and residents, yet when two residents died in 1989, Rose barked, "I told them there would be two deaths in the family."

———————

Rose, along with many homeless chronically mentally ill, challenged Philadelphia's outreach team to reconceptualize health care. Through outreach they crossed the lines between health care provider, residential service provider, and support network. The nurse practitioner offered tangible services which the women found helpful. For Rose this meant bringing water to her and cutting her nails.

SUSAN NEIBACHER

23

A Public-Private Partnership in Health Care for the Homeless

Introduction

In times of fiscal restraint, collaboration between public and voluntary agencies is required in order to solve complex problems. The virtues, challenges, and difficulties of developing a partnership that maximizes valuable resources are evident in this description of one city's successful experiment with a coalition, the New York City Coalition for Health Care for the Homeless. The coalition came together as grant applicants for the national Health Care for the Homeless Program and has worked together under four different chairpersons since 1984. It has done this in a city fraught with litigation and in which advocates for the homeless are sometimes pitted against the city government.

Background

In 1984, when the two foundations announced that the fifty-one largest U.S. cities could apply for funds from the national Health Care for the Homeless Program, Mayor Edward I. Koch asked the New York City Human Resources Administration (HRA) to lead in what proved to be a successful grant application on behalf of the city. The HRA is the public welfare agency in New York City responsible for serving homeless families and single adults. The United Hospital

Fund (UHF) of New York was chosen to administer the grant; the UHF, a nonprofit organization that addresses critical issues affecting health care in New York City, has a reputation as a neutral convener of diverse groups around health issues. It could be expected to be objective in the face of contention.

The Johnson / Pew competitive Request for Proposals specified that a coalition must govern the project. There was some concern on the part of some social service agencies that the HRA would assemble a small and unrepresentative coalition, excluding agencies that might be critical of it. Before the first coalition meeting was called, a few agencies, including the Coalition for the Homeless and the Community Service Society, the oldest family service agency in the United States, met and subsequently urged the HRA commissioner to support a broad-based coalition. He agreed, and meeting notices about the coalition were sent to agencies serving homeless people, the federated charities, coordinating and planning councils, and advocacy groups. The notices stated that any agency "related" to homeless issues was welcome.

In 1984, when the foundations announced the national program, New York City already had the nation's most extensive network of services for homeless people. The network included the municipal government, churches and synagogues, and voluntary agencies. Services ranged from soup kitchens, drop-in centers, and mental health outreach programs to traditional missions, large municipal shelters, welfare hotels for families, some health services, and a network of small overnight shelters. Most of these agencies are nonprofit, supported substantially by contracts or grants from city and state agencies, including HRA, the New York City Department of Mental Health, and the New York State Department of Social Services.

Planning Stage

Striving for Inclusiveness

"Leadership of the project will come from a city-wide coalition that includes health professionals and institutions, major voluntary organizations, religious groups dealing with the homeless, and relevant city, county and state agencies, including those related to health and mental health, welfare and housing."[1] Despite this clear mandate for cooperation, the first few months of planning were a genuine test of the consortium's ability to work together. HRA and UHF each assigned a staff member to the coalition during the planning stages, thus demonstrating a major commitment on their part. Other public and voluntary agencies also provided significant leadership. However, although the coalition strove for inclusiveness, there was never any expectation that all organizations would make the same degree of commitment; indeed, this might have created the divisiveness that the coalition wanted to avoid.[2]

What are some of the twenty-five organizations that participated in the coalition and what is their mission in New York City? In addition to HRA and UHF, three other public agencies were active. The New York City Health and Hospitals Corporation, a quasi-governmental corporation established by the city of New York to run the nation's largest municipal hospital system, participated; several of its hospitals were providing health services in municipal shelters. The New York State Office of Mental Health was represented. Active throughout the history of the coalition was the local public health agency, the New York City Department of Health. At the time of the planning stages, the Department of Health was conducting a small homeless initiatives program through which public health nurses screened and referred homeless families in welfare hotels to hospitals and health centers. Significantly, two public agencies were not represented: the New York City Department of Mental Health, Mental Retardation and Alcoholism and the New York State Division of Substance Abuse. Their absence is particularly striking considering the prevalence of alcoholism, drug abuse, and mental illness among homeless persons.

Two coalitions were major players in this new coalition. One was the Coalition for the Homeless, which is known for the class-action suits it files to pressure the city into providing sufficient beds for the homeless and enforcing regulations regarding health and safety codes. The other coalition, the Partnership for the Homeless, was founded in 1982 to assist the religious community in establishing small evening shelters staffed by volunteers. As the partnership's services expanded, it grew from a provider of service to an advocate for homeless persons and a critic of the city.

Another leading organization in the initial coalition was the Community Service Society (CSS). Its staff conducted the seminal urban anthropological research on homeless single adults,[3] and its representative brought substantial knowledge about financing and health care services for indigent persons to the coalition.

The service provider agencies in the coalition were diverse and tended disproportionately to represent services that were targeted to single homeless adults. Project Reachout of the Goddard Riverside Community Center, the oldest mental health outreach program in the country, was represented, as was Columbia University Community Services. This agency is a major training program for volunteers working with the homeless as well as a significant provider of mental health services for single homeless adults. Volunteers of America was represented by the director of its homeless shelter, the city's largest nonprofit shelter for homeless men.

In addition, two health care agencies were actively involved. Betances Health Unit, a freestanding health center located on the Lower East Side of Manhattan, had been providing primary health care services to the homeless and other indigent persons in a specially designed Winnebago van. Betances was licensed by the New York State Department of Health to bill Medicaid for services rendered in the van. The other health care agency, the Visiting Nurse Service of New York, provides services to homeless families.

While a number of the federated charities and planning council agencies attended meetings, the one most actively involved in the planning stages was the Federation of Protestant Welfare Agencies.

Building a Sense of Trust

At the initial coalition meetings, while discussion of issues was usually substantive, there existed an overriding sense of trying to build consensus. At those meetings, and in between, there were informal attempts to build ad hoc alliances supporting different positions.[4] But because HRA sponsored some very large shelters, sometimes described as Dickensian, it was viewed with suspicion by some coalition members. In fact, the Coalition for the Homeless had sued the city over the right to shelter. Naturally, the two agencies were wary of each other. Ironically, at the same time that the coalition was trying to build trust among its members and HRA wanted to show good faith, the coalition's chairperson (from HRA) was called out of a coalition meeting to talk to the city's attorney about one such lawsuit. As a matter of coalition practice, and as a means of avoiding direct conflict, no votes were taken. Discussions became a vehicle for determining whether or not representatives were open to compromise. Issues gradually became clearer and consensus-enhanced. Because it chose to make decisions through consensus, however, the coalition's thinking and planning processes were not as rational and organized as those described by the planning literature.[5] In a coalition with diverse membership, a number of different agendas are played out simultaneously. The following discussion highlights some of the alternatives that demanded consideration both for planning purposes and for building the necessary sense of trust so that these disparate agencies could indeed work together.

Service Model

It was assumed from the beginning that the UHF, which is not a direct provider of health services, would contract for services with other nonprofit facilities. While it was never debated that the delivery of health care to homeless people would require an integration of social services, the coalition did discuss the types of agencies or organizations that would be considered eligible to provide such services. Perhaps one of the least acrimonious discussions was the one about the type of organization with which the UHF should contract. While several of the other cities funded under the national program based their services in social agencies, the thinking in the New York City project from the beginning was that health care should be provided by licensed health facilities. Since the foundations were emphasizing continuity of care and access to the full range of health services, this decision seemed reasonable. An additional incentive was the belief that the only way to sustain the project after the life of the grant was to gain access to the funding stream for indigent health care, Medicaid. Therefore, it was agreed that the contracted agencies had to be licensed by New York State in a manner that qualified them for reimbursement under Medicaid regulations.

Expedited Medicaid Procedure

Related to the coalition's recognition of the need to gain access to the full range of health services was a commitment to finding a way to expedite the Medicaid application procedure. This goal seemed feasible because, for a number of years, hospitals had been using an expedited process to obtain inpatient Medicaid coverage for homeless people. Although homeless single adults are eligible for Medicaid in New York, most do not have all the documents needed to complete the standard application. The coalition agreed to explore the possibility of approaching the New York State Department of Social Services in this regard. The program ultimately became a demonstration project for Alternate Documentation for Medicaid, a procedure in which a program representative may apply for Medicaid on behalf of a homeless person without all the usual documentation, such as birth certificate.

Service Sites and Populations to Be Served

Early in the planning process, HRA made it clear that services would not be delivered at city-run shelters because the city had already accepted this responsibility. Therefore, if New York City were awarded the grant, the services would be provided at nonmunicipal shelters, soup kitchens, and other sites at which homeless persons gather. Those least likely to gain access to health care were targeted for the services. Although it was not always clear whom this group included, the coalition attempted to establish service population boundaries, albeit loose ones.[5] There were, however, some sharp differences of opinion about the type of sites that would be served. Should health services be provided in train and bus terminals like the Pennsylvania Railroad Station, the Port Authority Bus Terminal, and Grand Central Station? After considerable debate the coalition agreed that services would not be provided in these locations because of the lack of privacy for physical examinations and limited possibility for continuity of care.

Mobile Vans

In the course of developing a plan for service delivery, the coalition also debated the use of mobile vans. The group was aware of experiences with vans in New York City, which failed because of frequent breakdowns and the vans' limited mobility in the congested streets. At a later date it was agreed that an equipped mobile van could be tried by one provider at limited sites.

Governance

After resolving some of the service issues, the coalition sought to formalize its role. In order to fulfill its responsibilities, it agreed to take the following actions:
  1. Review the ongoing performance of health services providers
  2. Select new health services providers
  3. Establish annual contractual services along with concomitant budgetary implications
  4. Impose sanctions on existing contractors as applicable
  5. Determine additional sites to receive services as appropriate[2]
The coalition established an executive committee of seven representatives, four from voluntary and three from public sector agencies. Allowance was made for the committee to expand to eleven, with an agreement that there would always be one more voluntary than public agency represented.[1]

New York City Coalition's Search for Providers

After extensive discussions about the population to be served, the type of provider agencies, potential sites, and staffing patterns, the coalition developed a formal Request for Proposals. Only established hospitals and community health centers would be considered appropriate subcontractees. Care was to be provided in a diversity of locations, maximizing overall access to health and social services. Applicants were advised that services would be targeted for "the broadest range of homeless, not just any single category (e.g., youths, alcoholics, or former mental patients)."[1]

In response to the Request for Proposals, eight institutions submitted applications. They were evaluated using the following criteria:

1. Proposed program content
2. Population to be served, understanding of problems and experience in serving homeless populations
3. Geographic area
4. Homeless sites, appropriateness for health service program, compatibility with existing services
5. Scheduling
6. Staffing
7. Health care backup
8. Network of linkages
9. On-site training, education and staff burnout plans
10. Capability for ongoing support beyond the four year grant
11. Budget[2]

While discussions were lengthy and heated, a gradual consensus emerged, and two freestanding health centers and a major teaching hospital were chosen as the providers. Conveniently, these institutions were located in three different boroughs of the city—the Bronx, Brooklyn, and Manhattan—thus assuring that services would be delivered in the areas with the largest concentrations of homeless people. It was agreed that staffing patterns, budgets, sites, and other issues were to be negotiated individually.

Service Delivery Model

All three providers would have interdisciplinary teams with social workers, mid-level practitioners (nurse practitioners or physician's assistants), and supervising physicians. This was an economical and efficient model. The teams would go to selected sites on a prearranged schedule and set up miniclinics in places where the homeless congregated for other services. Sites would include soup kitchens, a traditional mission, small voluntary shelters, and mental health outreach programs. Sites would provide an area close to running water with privacy for physical examinations, but no formal clinic space would be required. In actuality, rest rooms, priest's offices, laundry rooms, and any space with access to water were considered. Teams would provide twenty-four hours of service in the field a week. The rest of the work week would be spent in supervision, team meetings, follow-up on clients, paper work, collaboration with other agencies, and program staff meetings. The two community health center teams would rely on the hospitals with which they were affiliated for backup for inpatient care and speciality services that the center was unable to provide.

Proposal Application

The designated staff members from HRA and UHF developed the proposal that was submitted to the foundations. They combined the three providers' proposals into a cohesive plan; described the population, project governance, budgets, staffing, and potential service sites; developed an organizational chart; and assembled letters of support, including the mayor's endorsement of the coalition. The proposal did not refer to a project director, an omission that later came to light.

An interesting debate arose over the number of homeless people in New York City. City representatives insisted that it was impossible to make an accurate count but were adamant that the estimates provided by advocacy groups were inaccurate and could not be used. Thus, the number of homeless people referred to in the proposal was the actual number "sheltered" by HRA. The leadership of HRA in 1984 did not want to acknowledge the seriousness of the problem; because the city was obligated to house all homeless persons, it may have been concerned that any discrepancy in the numbers of persons sheltered and the approximate number of homeless would make the city look bad.

Site Visit by the Foundations, Advisory Council, and Program Office

New York City was one of the cities selected for a site visit. The foundations' instructions were faithfully followed in planning the agenda. Those preparing for the site visit in the New York City Coalition approached the day with a certain sense of pride that such a diverse group had worked together and had achieved such a high level of coordination and commitment, especially in light of New York's fractious and litigious history on this and other issues. Despite the careful planning, on the day of the visit the chairperson of the site visit team dismissed the group's agenda and proceeded to raise numerous questions about design and governance. In particular, the site visit team questioned the concept of using mid-level practitioners to serve clients, the organization and governance of the coalition, the role and status of the project director, and the role of backup hospitals. It requested the following information be submitted: a short, updated statement of purpose; a more detailed table of organization; a description of the role and status of the project director; an updated and revised description of each team's activities; a proposal for team site long-term financing; letters of support from backup hospitals; descriptions of standard approaches to services; and plans to prevent burn-out.[6] So much time was spent in the meeting that the off-site visit was limited to the provider on the Lower East Side of Manhattan.

It was clear that the site visit team had not been impressed, but its criticism served to strengthen the cohesiveness of the coalition members, who believed that the site visit team did not understand the obstacles surmounted by the coalition. There was now a redoubled and impressive level of commitment by the executive committee members, fueled by the coalition's need to prove its case. It became a running joke that "we'd go broke if we were offered any more money." The HRA and UHF staff members, in consultation with the executive committee and their respective institutions, drafted a "supplement" to the original proposal, a supplement as long as the original proposal itself.

Implementation Stage

On December 18, 1984, the foundations announced that New York City was one of the grantees. Thereupon the coalition faced a whole new set of challenges. The first five months of 1985 were spent formalizing the coalition, clarifying the roles of the coalition and executive committee, hiring a project director, developing contracts for the providers, reviewing budgets and staffing patterns, visiting and selecting sites, and hiring staff. All parties had to have input into each of these concerns.

Governance

It was decided that the executive committee would have responsibility for operational concerns and the coalition itself would set policy. In practice, the executive committee focused on operational concerns and recommended policy to the coalition, which generally approved. The project director, who had been a member of the coalition and the executive committee, administered the program.

The executive committee focused on a range of operational issues. Among the most significant was the need for an expedited procedure for applying for Medicaid. In addition, the committee reviewed the patient data contact forms designed by the University of Massachusetts at Amherst, which Johnson / Pew had contracted to conduct research on the program. The forms were rejected, and the project director advised the program office that the forms were too intrusive and would lead to clients' refusing service.

The coalition now had to decide which sites should be served, and which clients. Should there be a concentration on single adults or homeless families? Which group most needed help? Influencing the decision was the fact that most members of the committee and coalition represented agencies serving single adults. As a result, most of the sites chosen were those serving single adults. The rationale was that homeless families receive AFDC and Medicaid and, therefore, have access to health care through the traditional delivery system.

The coalition considered the creation of committees, including those on finance, health care standards, fund raising, and communications. It established a Health Care Standards Committee to develop reporting forms, protocols, and quality-assurance measures. It designed an audit instrument and later conducted an audit of 10 percent of the medical records of each team. The design for the

other committees fell to the reality that administering a program with three different provider agencies and three different teams at numerous sites in three boroughs
of New York City was so time-consuming that the project director had no time to
staff the other committees.

Service Provision

The project director and a staff member from each of the provider organizations visited potential sites to determine their appropriateness for services. Those
sites that seemed the most appropriate were presented to the executive committee
for review. Two of the providers were actively recruiting staff. The first services
were delivered in June 1985 by the Manhattan provider. The Brooklyn provider
became fully operational in the fall.

The most difficult problem was posed by major administrative changes at the
Bronx provider. The Bronx component was cosponsored by the Department of
Family Medicine and the Home Care Department of Montefiore Medical Center,
so that visits could be billed to Medicaid on a home care rate. However, because
so many administrative changes were taking place at the hospital, including the
departure of its chief executive officer, it was not possible to negotiate the issues
that would lead to employing team members. Program implementation in the
Bronx did not occur until February 1986.

Some Frustration

The executive committee made a significant investment of time and energy
and exemplified the premise that people working together can solve problems
more effectively than one person working alone.[8] However, from the project
director's perspective, there were times of frustration because all decisions were
made by committee. If people were late to meetings or missed them, discussions
were often repeated, and at times decisions were reversed. Those who had the rare
opportunity to be part of the creation of a major new service as complex as this
one were understandably reluctant to let go of the day-to-day operations and
management. Not until there was additional turnover on the executive committee
in the spring and fall of 1986 did operational decision making shift to the project
director.

Middle Phase

Governance

While the new members of the executive committee were deeply committed
to the project, they were not as invested in controlling the decisions as the original
executive committee had been, and they tended to look to the project director for
leadership and direction. The executive committee met monthly to discuss issues
related to the future of the program and the vitality of the sites; it also cosponsored
a major conference. The coalition met quarterly; its sessions tended to be informational since the program was going well and no new policy issues emerged.

Project Administration

It soon became clear that providing services almost exclusively in soup kitchens had drawbacks. Aside from the makeshift aspect of setting up examining rooms in priests' offices, laundry rooms, and rest rooms, most soup kitchens are open for only an hour or two at a time, moving a large number of people through the line as quickly as possible. This arrangement presented several problems: Already impatient clients were especially unprepared to wait, the volunteers who ran the kitchens wanted to "lock up" as soon as possible, and providing services at one site in the middle of the day did not lead to efficiency and worker productivity. Furthermore, some soup kitchens periodically closed to give volunteers a "vacation."

In an effort to find a better balance of sites, the program tried providing services in some new SRO hotels and a new mental health outreach program. The expectation was that the need for services would be high at these new sites and that services could be provided for a larger block of time than in soup kitchens. Unfortunately, for a variety of reasons none of these sites proved fruitful. However, in August 1987 the executive committee agreed to an exception to the policy of not placing the teams in municipal shelters and on a temporary basis the Brooklyn team started providing services at such a shelter. Two soup kitchens had closed, and HRA simultaneously opened a shelter for employed and employable men before it was able to contract health services. By placing staff members of the Brooklyn team at the shelter, the needs of both organizations were met. In fact, the better mix of sites increased both productivity and staff morale.

A computer consultant designed a program to be used by management for determining worker productivity, collecting diagnostic data, clarifying the nature of staff interventions, and developing client profiles. The computer base later proved essential for meeting federal reporting requirements.

Federal Funds

In 1987, through the McKinney Homeless Assistance Act, the New York City program became eligible for federal funding. With federal funds available, a significant amount of thought, discussion, and planning went into deciding whether the program should take a new direction. UHF administrators, staff, and executive committee members discussed alternatives. Serious thought was given to developing several comprehensive, intensive treatment programs that would encompass mental health, education, training, and substance abuse. On balance, however, executive committee members thought that they had a "good thing going" and decided to replicate the existing program. They decided to apply for McKinney funds to expand the program from three teams to seven.

The New York City Coalition believed that the public-private venture had worked so well that there should be one McKinney application for the entire city under the aegis of HRA. However, the Public Health Service decided that it wanted to fund only the coalition's part of the proposal and awarded the UHF a separate grant. Once awarded the significant grant to expand to seven teams, the program returned to writing contracts, reviewing service sites, recruiting staff, and "swapping" sites between providers. Furthermore, the program's information was now computerized. It looked as if with the federal money, the program were here to stay, at least for a while. Foundation funding would be ending, but the federal money would extend the program.

Institutionalized Stage

Governance

The executive committee remained active and decided that the uniqueness of this public-private venture should be further developed. It saw the mission of the coalition as expanding beyond the "programmatic aspects of the Health Care for the Homeless Program by addressing policy issues which affect homeless people."[9] A mission statement was developed (see below), as well as a list of concerns, which included the lack of mental health, substance abuse, and pediatric care resources; the inadequate supply of low-income housing; and the need for infirmary or convalescent care for homeless single adults. Finally, however, the executive committee determined to limit its focus to the specific health care needs of homeless people. It recommended that the coalition concentrate on two areas: infirmary care and pediatric concerns.

NEW YORK CITY COALITION FOR HEALTH CARE FOR
THE HOMELESS PROGRAM MISSION STATEMENT

The New York City Coalition for Health Care for the Homeless was created as a part of the process for receiving funds under the National Health Care for the Homeless Program of the Robert Wood Johnson Foundation and Pew Memorial Trust. The Coalition has met on a regular basis for the past four years to oversee the operation of the program, with a major focus on developing and sustaining the program beyond the life of the Foundation grants. In addition, a number of issues have been identified that impede the treatment of illnesses of homeless people.

While a number of models of health care for homeless people have emerged, there has been no systematic evaluation of the effectiveness of these programs and the problems they face trying to integrate homeless people into the mainstream of the health care delivery system.

Health and social service professionals serving homeless people experience frustration because of difficulties in obtaining a full range of health and social services for homeless people. This is made worse by the fact that homelessness exacerbates illness. The Coalition believes that it is imperative to expand the Coalition's role beyond the programmatic aspects of the Health Care for the Homeless program by addressing policy issues which affect homeless people. In order to make some policy recommendations and advocate for adequate funding of services, a number of issues need to be examined: (i) the availability of the full range of health services including mental health, dental, substance abuse, and optometry, (ii) levels of alternative care for those persons suffering from acute illnesses, (iii) utilization of entitlements, (iv) discharge planning, and (v) continuity of care.

In order to move in the direction of making policy recommendations information and input will be secured from public and private health providers, public and private service organizations, academicians, and governmental agencies. The Coalition, a public-private venture which draws its members from clinical providers, social service providers, and government agencies, is uniquely situated to incorporate these perspectives in analyzing these service and policy issues. The purpose of the analysis is to develop appropriate policy recommendations and to present these recommendations to the parties that are in a position to implement them.

Thus, the Coalition seeks to carry out the analysis, formulate, and advocate for such policy changes as may be deemed necessary as well as to serve in an advisory capacity to the operational aspects of the program.

Committee on Infirmary Care

Over the years of operation of the program it became apparent that there was a need for some type of infirmary or protected place for homeless persons to recuperate from acute illnesses. The Committee on Infirmary Care was established to define the need, examine existing services in other cities, design an appropriate model for New York City, and identify potential resources and sponsorship. The committee worked to quantify the number of individuals who would require such care in a given week and to establish indicators of the length of time needed to convalesce. Committee members included medical personnel, representatives from the New York City Health and Hospitals Corporation, and HRA.

Committee on Pediatric Concerns

The Committee on Pediatric Concerns was created because of the recognition that homeless children were churning through different units of the public welfare system, shelters, welfare hotels, and transitional housing and were seen by many different health providers and often reimmunized and retested. Communication, coordination of services, and continuity of care were limited. HRA's Office of Health Services had played a significant role in linking providers of family health services to the various facilities "housing" the families. However, coordination of the services themselves could occur only if the providers had the opportunity to meet and work out the shared problems. The Committee on Pediatric Concerns comprises representatives of all of the different programs providing health care to homeless families in New York City and such organizations as the New York County Medical Society. This committee selected two areas for immediate action: coordination and tracking of children through the system and into permanent housing, and transportation of families from outreach health services to backup hospitals and health centers for specialty services. The committee established two subcommittees to work on these issues.

The Subcommittee on Coordination and Tracking has recognized that one of the difficulties in coordinating pediatric care for homeless families is the large number of different providers of services. Because of this diversity, the subcommittee is compiling a resource directory, which will serve four distinct purposes. It will:

- Help providers of health care to homeless families obtain health information (e.g., immunization status) from previous health providers

- Facilitate communication among health care providers to homeless families
- Help hospitals that have treated homeless families contact on-site providers when patients need follow-up
- Link families with community providers as they are placed in permanent housing

The Subcommittee on Transportation is concerned with the need to provide homeless patients with assistance in traveling from outreach health programs to clinics for follow-up visits. The subcommittee is currently exploring the feasibility of setting up a transportation network by determining the number of visits that require transportation, the distances to be transported, and possible grouping of families for transportation.

Public-Private Ventures

What does a coalition have to offer in terms of solving a major health and social service problem? Basically it provides the opportunity for a vast array of players to discuss, argue, if need be, but, most important, solve problems constructively. Furthermore, it brings together people and agencies with different experiences, knowledge, and skills.

A coalition can exchange resources for a shared objective, such as more and better health care for homeless people.[2] For instance, social service agencies and providers of service to the homeless know the difficulties of getting health care institutions to respond to their clients, but they don't necessarily understand the stringent regulations and problems that face the health care delivery system. Public welfare agencies mandated to shelter the homeless are overwhelmed by the sheer numbers of those with extensive psychosocial problems and by the general community's lack of commitment to provide sufficient resources or even to welcome shelters in their neighborhoods. Overwhelmed by the depth of human suffering and the whims of a larger society not often committed to social welfare, the agencies often focus on putting out fires, both actually and figuratively. Working together, representatives with different perspectives can design a program that functions.

Another virtue of a coalition is the access it may bring to critical actors who have the power to make certain decisions.[4] For instance, by bringing together the knowledge of those experienced in expediting Medicaid procedure and the "power" of the local public welfare commissioner, the coalition successfully pressed the New York State Department of Social Services to amend Medicaid approval processes for individual homeless single adults.

On the other hand, nurturing the trust necessary for collaboration takes a lot of time. It does not happen simply by putting a diverse set of individuals together in the same room. It demands a willingness and a commitment of key people to work out differences and build sufficient consensus for decision making. It also requires staff support for coordination. At times it may appear that coalition building is inefficient because it drains staff time from programmatic and operational concerns. The process of group decision making takes time that unilateral decisions do not require.

Assembling a coalition requires choosing the agencies that have the necessary resources, expertise, power, or status to commit to the group and to legitimate it. "The central question is whether the potential contribution of a coalition partner, be it symbolic or intense, warrants the organizational investment necessary to secure it."[2]

The New York City Health Care for the Homeless Coalition is a success. It was formed in 1984 to apply for funds from two major foundations. It then moved toward implementing an innovative program that has expanded and is now institutionalized. The coalition itself has begun to address broader social policy issues related to the health care of homeless men, women, and children as public and voluntary agencies work together to solve work on some of the most intractable problems of modern times. The emphasis has been on cooperation rather than on pointing fingers, blaming, and pursuing litigation.

It is fair to say that if people and agencies in the public and private sectors can somehow work together in New York City to create a viable coalition, then the model can probably work anywhere.

BARBARA CONANAN
FRANCISCA RODRIGUEZ
EDWARD CAGAN
PATRICIA DOHERTY
CAMILLE FERDINAND

24

A Twenty-Year Experience in Health Care of the Homeless: The St. Vincent's Hospital (New York) Program

Introduction

For every hour and every moment thousands of men leave life on this earth, and their souls appear before God. And how many of them depart in solitude, unknown, sad, dejected, that no one mourns for them or even knows whether they have lived or not.

—Feodor Dostoyevsky, *The Brothers Karamazov*

ST. VINCENT'S HOSPITAL has been caring for persons at shelters and SRO hotels in New York City since 1969. We have had the opportunity to observe the amazing changes that have occurred during these two decades, changes that include the remarkable growth in numbers of individuals without homes, on the streets, in parks, underground. The use of the word "homeless," in fact, is a product of these changes. This word was not in use to describe the street population in 1969. At that time those we now think as homeless were almost entirely middle-aged alcoholic men on skid row, most of them white. Since then, here in New York City and elsewhere across the country, observers have noted that the homeless are younger, that many more are members of minorities, and that women and children—entire families—have become homeless. Twenty years ago a homeless woman was not to be seen, nor a child.

Measuring the numbers of the homeless has proved to be a daunting task and in our view ultimately unrewarding. For New York City, the Human Resources Administration counts the numbers housed in city shelters and rented hotel rooms. In July 1989[1] this included 12,894 family members in 3,988 families, comprising 5,471 and 7,423 children. In addition, 10,296 single adults were in shelters. The total: 23,190. Further, according to the New York City Police Department runaway unit, there are about 20,000 abandoned kids in the City. Of course, there are uncountable others. The grand total on a typical day may well surpass 60,000 in New York City. Advocacy groups place the numbers higher, and endless disputation results. Yet there is no dispute that large numbers of persons lack regular shelter and need help.

The reasons for homelessness and for these demographic changes have been widely considered both in New York and across the nation and will not be reviewed here. Without question, however, there has been a vast impact on the health status and needs of the homeless as a result of these developments.

Origins of the SRO / Homeless Program at St. Vincent's Hospital

New York City is one of the critical sites in which dynamic change has occurred over the past twenty years in the development of homelessness in our country. Since the St. Vincent's program and its staff have served homeless persons throughout this time, analysis of the program serves as a means of understanding the nature of homelessness in a major city in the late twentieth century and of illustrating how a hospital-based program can survive and thrive over a lengthy period.

The SRO / Homeless Program has amassed a large total experience with homeless persons, allowing an understanding of the nature and extent of illness, their social service needs, and the means of developing relationships that lead to effective involvement. During the twenty years of service reported here, the program has cared for an estimated eighty thousand individuals, and in 1989 alone it saw about seven thousand persons. While this experience is surpassed by several other long-standing agencies in the United States, including the St. Anthony's Clinic in San Francisco and the Pine Street Inn in Boston, it is noteworthy.

1969

In the summer of 1969 a newly fledged intern in the hospital emergency room turned to an attending physician who was passing through and said, "I've been seeing lots of derelicts brought in here by ambulance moribund or DOA [dead on arrival]. What's going on with these men? How come there isn't a system that helps them before it's too late?"[2]

The attending physician had no answers to these questions. The intern then determined to find them on his own. His investigation revealed that within several blocks of St. Vincent's, a large SRO building, the Greenwich Hotel at 160 Bleecker Street, had been taken over by the city government for the housing of men without shelter and that the hospital emergency room was receiving the ambulance referrals.

The hotel building, located in the midst of the entertainment and residential area of Greenwich Village, was constructed in 1893 for poor workingmen without families. Theodore Dreiser, one of its more famous residents, purportedly summarized his experiences there in his novel *Sister Carrie*. Its fourteen hundred rooms, each five by seven feet in size, were considered adequate by the housing standards of that era. No changes had been made in these rooms over the years. Although the hotel operated legally, and structural violations noted by city inspectors were corrected, each space resembled a cage rather than a place to live. Each of the eight floors had a single communal toilet room.

The New York City Department of Social Services used the hotel for referral of destitute homeless men during the clinic's operation. At the maximum, twelve hundred were in residence. Many stayed briefly.

The men could be divided into three general categories: About 200 were elderly, the majority living precariously on Social Security payments, welfare, or salaries from menial jobs; some had lived at the hotel for years, a few for more than two decades. In addition, there were about 450 middle-aged chronic alcoholics, most unemployed and living on welfare. And also present were some 550 young heroin addicts, recently released from prison with no legitimate funds other than welfare payments.

The hotel management attempted to keep these groups separated; but access to all floors was simple, and attempts at segregation were ineffective. Consequently, the younger, more aggressive men freely abused the others. At night the hotel became a jungle in which the aged and disabled barricaded themselves in their rooms or were subject to assault. The number of visits to the clinic for treatment of trauma reflected this problem. Nevertheless, men remained at the hotel because there was no better place to go.

Efforts were started to bring health services to the men at the hotel. In partnership with nurses from the Visiting Nurse Association of New York, residents and attending physicians from the hospital conducted a free clinic in three rooms donated by management. The clinic functioned for eighteen months from 1969 to 1971.[3]

The unit met four afternoons per week. Costs of salaries were borne by the Visiting Nurse Service and St. Vincent's Hospital; both organizations donated equipment. Some medications were stocked. Others were supplied by Medicaid prescriptions, for which virtually all the men were eligible. It was not possible to bill Medicaid for visits because the clinic site was not approved by the state government.

To make the unit as attractive as possible, no fee was accepted, and no registration procedure took place, although records were kept of all visits. Men who desired medical help simply appeared at the clinic or were referred by workers from the Department of Social Services who shared the space. The nurse or physician obtained a history if possible. Physical examination was performed, and advice or treatment, or both, was given. For more extensive services, St. Vincent's Hospital stood ready to receive the patients.

When the nurses were not occupied in the clinic, they toured the hotel, looking for disabled men who could not leave their rooms. Needed medical help was occasionally provided in this way, sometimes against great resistance.

Experience included care for men who would not permit themselves to be properly treated and for whom disability seemed to be preferable to good health.

———————

Patient AB, a sixty-five-year-old man, was found in his room and induced to come for treatment of a massive leg ulcer caused by venous stasis, trauma, and neglect. The ulcer involved the entire anterior and lateral surface of the left leg below the knee. Exuberant granulation tissue made the circumference three times that of the right leg. When the patient was first seen, purulent, foul-smelling drainage was marked. Maggots were found in the lesion.

Treatment lasted for ten months and consisted of warm antiseptic soaks (up to five times per week), sterile dressings, and oral antibiotics. Although the patient was persuaded to visit the clinic daily, he often refused soaks and antibiotics. When reepithelialization was almost complete and drainage minimal, the patient refused to leave his room and would not return to the clinic. On visits to the room by physicians and nurses the patient would not discuss his leg, which was seen to be reinfected: The newly formed skin had been destroyed, and gross purulent drainage was present.

At a final visit the patient was semicomatose on the floor. The leg was gangrenous. He was removed to the hospital.

———————

Maintaining professional standards of care in working with manipulative patients was an early challenge.

———————

Patient LE, a thirty-eight-year-old alcoholic man, was seen in the clinic seventeen times over a period of eight months. Initially he requested medication because of insomnia, anxiety, and depression. Thioridazine and glutethimide were prescribed in quantities sufficient for two weeks. Three days later the patient returned and requested more medication. When this was refused, he became extremely agitated. He was eventually given a two-week supply of ethchlorvynol for sleep. Three days later the patient returned and requested paraldehyde, but this was refused. Six days later he insistently demanded more medication and was given meprobamate and chloral hydrate, on condition that he accept referral to the Psychiatric Clinic at St. Vincent's Hospital. He visited the Psychiatric Out-Patient Department on several occasions and received a variety of psychopharmaceuticals from that unit as well.

The patient continued his near-violent approach to obtaining tranquilizers and hypnotics. Finally it was necessary to tell him that we were no longer allowed to write such prescriptions at the clinic.

Subsequently he began to complain of pruritus. He succeeded in eliciting a prescription for diphenhydramine hydrochloride, a soporific antihistamine. When renewals of medication were refused, the patient began to complain of a cough, for which he received elixir of terpin hydrate with codein (a narcotic).

This patient succeeded in manipulating clinic personnel despite major efforts to counsel him and to place him in a more appropriate program for treatment of his emotional disorder, alcoholism, and drug dependence. Our contact ceased when he left the hotel to move to Washington, D.C.

———————

Appreciating irony is essential to survival in this kind of work, as the fate of the clinic shows.

Since there was virtually no place in the hotel for recreation, the men spent their time loitering in front of the building and wandering in the community streets and park. The reaction of the community members to the hotel as a residence for destitute persons, and to the men themselves, was vigorous. These men were easily distinguished from most community residents by their inebriated or "high" appearances. Local businesspeople believed that the SRO residents created a negative effect on their trade. Burglaries, muggings, and purse snatchings in the area were generally attributed to hotel residents. Local pressure was placed on the mayor's office and the Department of Social Services to end referral of new welfare clients to the hotel. This took effect in May 1971. Subsequently a mobile task force from the Department of Social Services was brought to the hotel, and many of the men were moved to flophouses on the Bowery, while others drifted away. When the men left, community interest abated. In October 1971 the clinic closed because of insufficient demand for medical service. The building itself was taken over by Manhattan real estate interests, refurbished internally, and reopened two years later as an expensive condominium called The Atrium.[4]

At about the same time as the program began work at the Greenwich Hotel, St. Vincent's was contracted by the New York City Human Resources Administration to staff a clinic at the Municipal Men's Shelter on the Bowery, New York's skid row. This building serves as the clearing center for most of the other shelters in the city and places about six thousand men each night. Our clinic, now in its twenty-first year, is open forty hours per week and is staffed by a physician, a nurse, and corpsmen. From the start it has seen about twelve hundred individuals through about five thousand visits each year. To date more than twenty thousand records have been gathered.

Clinical Evaluation

The most prominent health concerns for the 309 men seen at the Greenwich Hotel clinic were alcohol abuse (about half of those seen), psychoses (15 percent), heroine use (20 percent), and trauma (20 percent). Heralding the future, 5 men were seen with active tuberculosis. Cocaine was not an issue, nor, of course, was HIV disease. Since then a comprehensive, decade-spanning review of clinical disorders in persons seen at a variety of sites in the SRO / Homeless Program from 1969 to 1984 has been conducted by James Wright and associates.[5]

The project data consist of information derived from clinical charts of homeless persons who received medical services at one or more of the program's clinics. Each contact in these clinics between a homeless individual and our health care team generates a note or an entry in that person's clinic chart related to medical symptoms, conditions, diseases, and social background.

The records from which data were derived were not kept for research intent, but rather for medical and clinical purposes. The data available for analysis were therefore a filtered subset of the actual behaviors, conditions, and diseases of the study population. Wright's analysis noted that the clinical records gave good information on medical condition, diseases, and presenting symptomatology—"far more detailed and extensive information than has hitherto been assembled for this population." Data on topics other than the strictly medical were spotty: Age, race, and sex were recorded in almost all instances, but other information of a social nature was available for only a very small number.

An effort was made to extract information from every chart (both active and inactive) in every clinic operated through the St. Vincent's program. In one case (the Men's Shelter), the sheer number of charts made a compete census impractical, and a 10 percent sample was used instead.

The principal study conclusions of 6,415 records are as follows:

- The demography of homelessness in New York City changed substantially between 1969 and 1984. "In the past, the homeless were predominantly old, white, broken down alcoholic men. Today, the population is much younger on the average, better educated, dominated by blacks and Hispanics, and less substance abusive; and a sizable fraction are women."
- Although alcoholism appears to be declining, abuse as a whole remains a prime health problem. Fully 30 percent of the records reveal chronic substance abuse. Illnesses known to follow substance abuse are common.
- Trauma is the next most common problem, followed in order by acute upper respiratory disorders, chronic lung disease, diseases and disorders of the extremities, mental impairments, skin ailments, and hypertension.
- Comparisons with the National Ambulatory Medical Care Survey[6] confirm that the homeless are at much higher risk from most diseases. "The largest difference is in the rate of substance abuse and, correlatively, in the rate of diseases and disorders linked to substance abuse. Disorders resulting from environmental exposure are also much more widespread."
- Subgroups among the homeless who are at particularly high risk of disease include the old, heavy smokers, chronic alcoholics, drug users, and homosexuals.

In the fifteen years of the analysis Wright estimated that the average age of homeless men declined by eight years and that the percentage of whites fell from about 50 to 15. The incidence of most age-linked diseases also fell over the fifteen years. These included neurological disorders, eye and ear, heart, and chronic lung diseases. The rate of substance abuse decreased from 49 percent in 1969 to 28 percent in 1984.

Most of the disease trends reflect the falling age of the population and the apparently sharp decline in substance abuse, particularly chronic alcoholism. In the earlier years half the men treated at the Men's Shelter were chronic substance abusers; in 1984 the figure fell to about a quarter. "The significance of this pattern is probably more social than medical: 10 or 15 years ago, the road to homelessness was apparently paved with substance abuse; today, many alternate routes seem to have been opened."[5]

The SRO / Homeless Program in 1990

A Leap to Today

The program, a unit of the Department of Community Medicine, has gradually evolved since its first steps into a hotel and shelter in 1969. St. Vincent's founding mission is care of the sick poor. Since homelessness is the ultimate in poverty, this work is seen by the hospital as a highly appropriate means of fulfilling its abiding mission. Thus, when opportunity for increases in services have been recognized, either by staff or through requests from community or city agencies, these have been grasped whenever possible.

The program now serves in twenty-five locations throughout Manhattan, ranging from the Keener Men's Shelter on Wards Island in the East River to the Beaver Street Drop-In Center in the Wall Street area. These sites include two shelters, three drop-in centers, one agency for homeless female substance abusers, and nineteen SRO hotels, three of which house homeless families. (See map on page 361.)

Program Goals and Objectives

Our goal is to seek and find homeless persons and bring them into effective relationships with health care services to help obtain entitlements. We give direct hands-on care to the homeless, emphasize the forming of relationships with families and with the elderly, and serve those with HIV disease. We strive for effective coordination with other community agencies.

Our objectives are to:

- Treat clinical disorders on the spot
- Reduce the frequency of acute medical crises
- Decrease fragmented and episodic care
- Encourage independent use of the health care system through counseling and education
- Encourage independent living through learning resources and utilizing networks
- Provide dignity and humanity to health care services

Staff Attitudes and Approaches

The program evolved and has developed to address specific needs and concerns of the homeless in general, but we pride ourselves on remaining aware that each person is an individual with strengths and weaknesses, abilities and disabilities. Our approach is person-centered and is based on that individual's needs. We

MANHATTAN

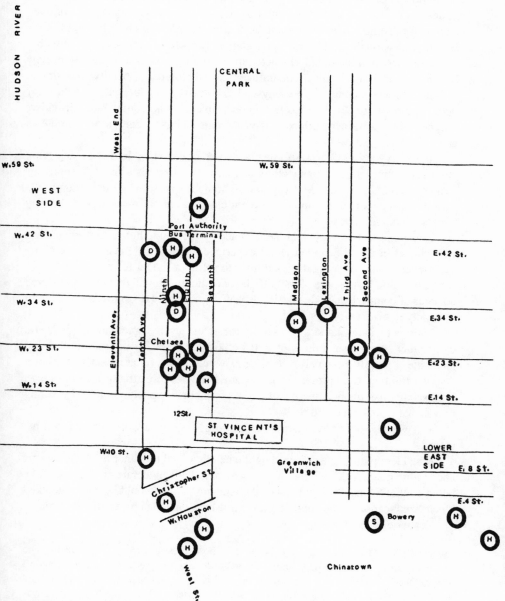

Ward's Island (S)

HUDSON RIVER

CENTRAL PARK

West End

W. 59 St.   W. 59 St.

WEST SIDE

Port Authority Bus Terminal

W. 42 St.   E. 42 St.

Madison   Lexington   Third Ave   Second Ave

Ninth   Eighth   Seventh

W. 34 St.   E. 34 St.

Eleventh Ave.   Tenth Ave.

Chelsea

W. 23 St.   E. 23 St.

W. 14 St.   E. 14 St.

12 St.

ST VINCENT'S HOSPITAL

LOWER EAST SIDE

W. 10 St.   E. 8 St.

Greenwich Village

Christopher St.

E. 4 St.

W. Houston

(S) Bowery

West St.

Chinatown

City Hall

(D) Drop-in Center
(H) Hotel
(S) Shelter

(D) Wall St.

have identified and work with all the subgroups of the homeless and SRO population: the mentally ill, substance abusers, runaway or throwaway kids, veterans, the unemployed and unemployable, the elderly, and mothers with children.

Attitudes of the staff clearly can make or break a program and be supportive or destructive for patients.[7] Recognition and prevention of generalizations derived from class distinction are important. A distinct middle-class bias is the norm for health professionals. Health care providers may prefer middle-class patients because of their mutual social characteristics. There often is a tendency to view lower-class patients in terms of unfavorable stereotypes. Socially undesirable patients include alcoholics, the physically dirty, the uneducated, and the very poor. The poor are perceived to lack cooperativeness and compliance. Providers may reveal negative perceptions of their patients' status by derogatory comments and indicative gestures.[8]

As Al Elvy points out,[7] staff must be aware, or be helped into awareness, that body and facial language, as well as words, can impart distaste or disapproval. "There is probably no quicker way to lose homeless persons' participation in the treatment process than to indicate to them that you are not pleased with the way they conduct their lives."

This point is clarified in comments made by the young house staff physicians who shared in the Greenwich Hotel experience. One had hoped that the clinic experience would be a good opportunity to set up a model for private practice, where he could learn some of the pitfalls. He quickly learned that the unit offered no areas of comparison with a desirable private practice. He continued largely out of loyalty to his co-workers.

Another resident stated: "Working at the hotel was like practicing medicine on the frontier—or worse. I think of it as outpost medicine, as opposed to hospital medicine. Possibly an experience like this would be useful at an early stage of a doctor's training, but I prefer to work where I can be more effective, even though I did accomplish the heading off of a few cases of early pneumonitis. My feeling now is that I'm down on bums."

This was the only physician in the group who stopped work before the clinic closed.

A resident planning a career in public health joined to gather firsthand experience in his field. Although the project was of at least moderate effectiveness, he believed that the health problems of the men at the hotel could be better attacked by early education of the pubic in preventive medicine than by a walk-in clinic.

Yet another said:

I originally went to work at the hotel because of moral pressure. My senior resident, who had worked there, was leaving, and I was asked to take his place. I felt that I couldn't refuse. Once I started work I began to see myself as the great healer bringing enlightened medicine to the dregs of the earth. After some experience, I realized how little I was accomplishing. This brought on despair. I stayed on until the clinic closed because there was no one to take my place, and someone had to care for the men.

One of the leaders in the founding of the clinic was a resident physician, an idealist, who had dealt in college and medical school with disadvantaged people.

I went to the hotel simply to see what it was all about. In medical school we get little or no awareness of the social problems contributing to the common illnesses which flood our wards. The futility of treating this group of men is common knowledge. They often refuse to come to us until they are carried into the emergency room in extremis.

In my work at the hotel I had to lower my professional standards. I began dispensing medication more freely in an attempt to effect a therapeutic trial in patients whom I knew would never consent to hospital diagnostic procedures.

I've learned a lot about why these men don't seek out health care at institutions. They have short attention spans, an antiestablishment orientation, a low level of tolerance for standing in lines, and they are turned off by the regimentation of a hospital.[3]

A Three-Tier Approach

Our program's doctor-nurse-social worker teams regularly visit the temporary living sites of the homeless and SRO residents. Consistent yet gentle persistence eventually can penetrate the homeless person's world. Team members must create a favorable milieu so that a trusting relationship is established. Such an atmosphere of acceptance helps the shelter or hotel residents take the first step toward a health care system that is nonthreatening, accessible, and their own. In order to provide comprehensive health care, a three-tier approach is needed. Outreach workers (Tier 1) need the backup resources of shelter health stations and satellite clinics (Tier 2) and hospital backup for ambulatory care and inpatient services (Tier 3).

First Tier: Outreach

. . . Act of reaching or stretching out as if to grasp someone. Hence, power of seizing, obtaining, touching or affecting something. Power of stretching out or extending action, development of influence or the like. Power of attainment; striving after something.[9]

If you turn the word "outreach" around, you are "reaching out." Staff must go to the people if they do not come forward. Through the mental health movement, "outreach evolved from a growing social concern and sense of responsibility for those community members in need of health care but unable to use the established, central hospital system."[10] Outreach describes the intent of health workers to maintain extra-institutional contact with community members who are actually or potentially at risk, for the purpose of therapeutic intervention.

If staff must reach out, it implies that the homeless have certain characteristics that require this approach, particularly in regard to health care. Many are disaffiliated, lonely, alienated, angry, mistrustful, distrustful, and paranoid; they live disorganized lives and have poor judgments because of substance abuse or mental illness; many have had previous negative experiences with health institutions and have become passive with regard to their own health or lack the ability to use traditional systems. The objective of outreach is to engage them to *themselves* and the health care institution. Staff can accomplish this by going to the homeless where they congregate, on a regular, consistent basis, thereby becoming a factor in their lives. By going to their territory, staff members develop a relationship built on equality instead of on an authority-subservient role of oppressor to the oppressed. Care is offered, not forced. Clients have control over the medical intervention. The equality posture sets up the dynamics to build trust that can develop into a relationship. It is the relationship with the team members that opens the homeless to the health care system. The process is labor-intensive and time-consuming and offers no guarantee of tangible positive results. Outreach workers may be rejected, tested, and scorned and more often than not must prove that they can give concrete services before they are accepted. Staff members must be confident, self-assured, have good senses of humor, and be able to deal with numerous stimuli and contradictions. They must possess the three *P*'s—persistence, patience, and perseverance—and the three *C*'s—creativity, consistency, and caring.

Outreach in SROs, compared with congregate settings such as shelters and drop-in centers, has its own particular qualities. SROs tend to be housing sites for the elderly or handicapped homeless, substance abusers, and families. Each SRO possesses its own distinct character and personality.

To find cases, health providers need to know the hotel system and how it works. In performing outreach in the hotel, staff must work with the manager, obtain rosters, consult with HRA workers on-site, knock on doors, pass out flyers, become familiar with gatekeepers, and develop tricks of the trade to get inside doors. "Sometimes you never knew what's on the other side—you take a chance."[11] The pervasive use of crack has created a volatile mood in hotels, with erratic, potentially explosive behavior, particularly in families. In 1988 the program terminated services at a hotel for single adults and temporarily halted services at a family hotel for six months because of fear for staff safety.

Other characteristics of staff outreach in SROs include:

- Becoming known by mingling or hanging out in the lobby, listening, and assessing.
- Speaking to other residents and other service providers who could indicate those with immediate needs.
- Aggressively reaching out by knocking on doors to introduce oneself, explaining the purpose of the visit, and, if clients are not available, leaving a note informing them of the team visit and the next time the team will return.
- Providing concrete services. If something is promised, the promise must be kept.

These characteristics are revealed in the way staff relates to homeless families in SROs. An outreach team describes its function:

Because of our open and informal approach, families find it's easy to relate to the team. The initial visit usually takes 3 to 5 minutes. The team does not wish to overwhelm them or invade their privacy needlessly. If a family requests that the team not visit them, that wish is respected. We let them know that if an emergency should arise, they can still feel free to contact us. We always leave them our brochure.

By the third visit, new families become accustomed to the routine and the relationship often starts to flourish. By this time, families ask the team to make appointments for their children as well as for themselves, consulting us about symptoms and other medical data or social service problems.

The families who function well tend to get involved immediately with our clinics and use the services we offer. Some families whose children are enrolled in another clinic eventually change to our clinic also because we are very accessible in case they need consultation.

The less functional tend to wait until a crisis arises and end up as emergency room walk-ins. In these families, many of the mothers have a history of substance abuse and usually show poor compliance.

For the most part, families are not inhibited in discussing their problems with the team as a whole but occasionally a family member will request to speak to a particular member of the team alone. This wish is honored.[12]

The SRO environment has its own special appeal, used by successful outreach workers:

We were visited by state auditors responding to a grant proposal. These were two men both over six feet tall. They were appalled at the environment in the Barbour Hotel. The building was dilapidated, the paint was peeling off the lobby walls. Both visitors seemed uncomfortable but accompanied the team on its rounds through the hotel. Half-an-hour into the visit, we heard harrowing screams and doors slamming. Our social worker suggested the visitors remain on the ground floor with the nurse while he investigated. Within five minutes, he returned assuring everyone that all was under control. Within two weeks, we received notice of funding, with the feedback that "if the team was crazy enough to go to the hotel, let's give them the money."[12]

Second Tier: Shelter Health Stations

Bringing doctors, nurses, and social workers into shelters to establish clinics is the critical next step. In early years of the program many shelter sites were analogous to frontline aid stations. At first staff was able to give only basic rudimentary services. Physicians relied on visual and listening skills. Our motto was "High Touch—Low Tech." As funding improved, so did quality and comprehensiveness. The word "clinic" became appropriate, a location where a host of services could be offered, such as laboratory studies, electrocardiograms, and Pap test, everything except X rays.

Today all shelters, all drop-in centers, and some hotels have identified examining rooms with table, sink, and basic equipment. At the hotels, if a room is unavailable, assessment and treatment occur at any place. At all locations our staff is able to perform the following: outreach, case finding, physical and psychosocial assessment, acute and long-term medical care, health screening, health education, crisis intervention, concrete social services, individual and group counseling, referral and treatment, monitoring of appointments and medications, and case management.

Tier 2 services in family SROs are less definable than in shelters and drop-in centers. When our interdisciplinary teams of physicians, nurses, and social workers visit the family hotels, each team member is introduced by name and function. This helps the family members easily identify the staff at subsequent visits and allows them to direct their questions to the appropriate team member. The approach is informal and nonthreatening, creating a favorable milieu for establishment of a relationship. When the team meets a family for the first time, it is told about the team's services. The staff assesses needs, collects basic data, and informs families when the team plans to return to the hotel.

In the family hotels Tier 1 and Tier 2 functions tend to combine, because few of these SROs contain examining areas. Family hotel care is outreach—plus. If during initial contact an immediate health problem is evident, action is necessary. Making a future clinic appointment misses the point.

Third Tier: Hospital-Based Clinics

The hospital-based clinics are the third tier of care. Providing primary care to a nontraditional population in a traditional setting can be a daunting task. Creating a clinic compatible with the needs of the recalcitrant, the mentally ill, and substance abusers takes motivation, commitment, and an understanding of their viewpoint. As a homeless woman recently told one of our staff, "I just came here for the doctor to look at my eyes. What does that have to do with where I was born or my mother's name before she got married?"[7]

Slow nurture and guidance are necessary to equip each person with skills necessary to navigate the system and to learn to use the clinic for follow-up and ongoing care. A hospital clinic is an intimidating, bureaucratic maze and a major barrier to care.

There is a wide chasm between the homeless and their access to traditional medicine and social services. The hospital clinic staff must be made sensitive to the problems and needs of this group of patients. Arrangements can be made, for instance, to take clinic staff (physicians, nurses, unit clerks, security guards) for an educational visit to the outreach sites.

We insist that every homeless person brought to the hospital clinic must have a referral form. This serves two purposes: First, it identifies the client as the program's patient and permits entry to the St. Vincent's Hospital system without the complications that ordinarily ensue from insufficient identification or insurance coverage; secondly, it provides the receiving medical team with pertinent information that should avoid the duplication of a second examination and reduces repetitive questioning. The form also allows the tracking of our patients through subspecialty clinics.

One of our objectives is to teach clients to use the health care system appropriately. We will teach some of them how to register. For those unable or unwilling to register, the team social worker obtains the required information or whatever portion the client is willing to provide, and it is recorded on the appropriate registration forms.

At the hospital we conduct clinic sessions for our own referrals. The SRO/Homeless Primary Care clinic has evolved to meet our clients' needs and promote continuity of care. This clinic meets twice a week. Primary care resident physicians are assigned to patients, and the attending physicians who work at outreach sites supervise them and examine the patients as well. This design serves two purposes: Clients become accustomed to other physicians, and the site's attending physicians become educators and mentors for younger doctors. It is valuable for medical residents to be exposed to the homeless in their training.

The SRO/Primary Care clinic sessions are anxiety-provoking for both staff and patients. Clients' anxieties run the gamut. They are frightened and intimidated by the institution, staff, policies, and fear of invasive procedures. Unlike the clinics at shelters, where patients dictate time and pace, in the hospital-based SRO/Homeless clinic sessions, a range of services must be given in a limited period of time without alienating or losing the client. The first clinic visit is important. The staff strives to make it comprehensive without making it overwhelming. It is necessary to interact with many other departments, such as X ray and laboratory, that do not make special arrangements for the homeless.

Pre- and postclinic conferences are important in promoting continuity, ensuring that treatment plans are realistic, and identifying who is responsible for following through. For example, if a patient needs daily dressing changes, who will do it and where; or if medication is ordered, who will get and pay for it? For those who break their clinic appointments, charts are reviewed, and the appropriate staff is notified in order for follow-up at the outreach site to take place.

Medication and problem lists and profile cards are completed on each patient, documenting all necessary medication information, lab test results, and clinic appointments. The purpose of the profile card is to summarize important data about every client who comes to the clinic.

Health Education and Preventive Medicine

Trying to convey or carry out an abstract concept such as good health and teaching good health care practices in the midst of daily chaos and chronic crisis may seem an insurmountable task. People in crisis become disorganized and immobilized. Therefore, the team members must deal first with the issues at hand, the acute problems. Only later can education about health maintenance and disease prevention take place. We should be wary of a presumption of control over life which many homeless people do not have. Yet despite chaos, health education can be accomplished, and it appears to be most effective on an individual basis.[13]

Health education is translated into reality through disease prevention strategies, such as immunization campaigns. Each November we launch a massive effort to provide flu shots and Pneumovax for those in risk groups. Teams equipped with acetaminophen, epinephrine, and the vaccines go to the shelters, SRO hotels, soup kitchens, and street corners. Pneumovax is given once in a lifetime. Patients should be so instructed. Careful records documenting immunizations are maintained.

Many homeless persons are aware of the impact of even a minor illness on daily survival. The program finds many takers for immunizations. Tetanus-diphtheria shots are also offered as indicated, including a booster every ten years.

All portable immunization stations should include equipment for safe needle transport back to the hospital or office base. Needles should never be recapped because of the risk of HIV and hepatitis transmission from needle stick injuries.

Shelter employees also need education from the medical outreach team. Emergencies often arise when the team is not on the premises. Shelter staff members can be taught how to intervene in crisis situations, such as seizure disorders, poisoning, and drug overdose. In addition, they are a resource to help identify those needing medical intervention. Therefore, they should learn to recognize common illnesses and problems among the homeless and the importance of anti-tuberculosis or antihypertensive medication being taken. There is a definite need to discuss patients with shelter staff to enhance the quality and comprehensiveness of care. To meet this need, a formal bimonthly meeting with shelter, hotel, and drop-in staffs has been established both to discuss concerns related to patients and to give educational sessions.

Clinical Issues

Through this program, initiatives in understanding tuberculosis, diabetes mellitus, HIV disease, hypertension, and nutritional disorders have been launched,[14-19] and genuine progress has been made in working with clinical issues that at first seemed intractable. However, the widespread disorder of alcoholism remains a tough challenge for staff and for many patients. Both motivation and treatment resources are often in short supply, although an occasional success occurs. The following instance illustrates the difficulties:

DY is a sixty-four-year-old, white, fragile man living in one of the infamous SROs in the garment district. We met him in the spring of 1982. He has a history of alcoholism, chronic obstructive pulmonary disease (COPD), and hypertension. His drinking maintained an elevated blood pressure and exacerbated his COPD, which necessitated frequent hospitalizations. His SRO room was cluttered with beer cans and infested with fleas. His cat aggravated his COPD and added a distinct odor to the room. He could not walk without help and therefore paid "runners" to purchase alcohol for him. He denied abusing alcohol even though beer cans and vodka bottles were sprawled throughout the room. He used to say, "I'm bored, so I drink," but expressed no interest in relocating. After several months of counseling and being offered options, he entered a three-week detoxification and rehabilitation program. We developed a treatment plan to promote sobriety including registering him with a senior citizen center, AA, and meals on wheels, with a long-term goal of relocating him to supportive housing. Two days out of the rehabilitation unit he began drinking again.

It is a struggle for a middle-class alcoholic to maintain sobriety, even with family support and an understanding employer. If a disaffiliated alcoholic is discharged from detoxification or rehabilitation back to the shelters or an SRO without support, one can predict he will resume drinking, even though warned of the consequences.

Abstinence is hard. The following letter was sent to one of the program social workers:

Hi Grace:

How are you and all the rest there? I'm happy but a little shaky. I'm leaving Camp LaGuardia this week. I'm going to the Salvation Army Rehab in Poukeepsie [sic]. After that I don't know what I'll do. I have to find a job up there with room and board and save some money before I come back to New York City. I'll keep going to AA meetings. I promise you that Grace. This is the hardest job I ever had to face in my life. I hope I can do it but believe me Grace I'm still a little scared. After I make enough money to live, I'll come back and start all over. I'll get back to you and tell you what's what. I'll follow up with AA too. I always have a good job with the Market Diner. I hope Jesse is okay. Please keep an eye on him for me. He's a good guy but he won't stop till he kills himself. I don't want to see that. I know him for 15 years. I love Jesse like he's my own brother. Grace, I lost a lot of my life and I don't want to lose him. So Grace, I'm leaving here Wednesday, June 14th. Now lets see what's happening. Thank you for all your help.

Love
JJ

SROs are also a haven for seriously mentally ill persons. These individuals challenge the ingenuity of staff, as the following case history extracted from an SRO / Homeless Program chart illustrates:

The patient, a forty-seven-year-old man, gives a history which is unclear. He apparently has been in a state mental hospital and also has been seen in a local emergency room or clinic.

We find him living in an eight- by ten-foot room in the Hotel Earle. Numerous ashtrays are piled high with cigarette stubs. The patient is unwashed and is thin but appears to be in basically good health, based on the superficial physical exam permitted. He says that a clinic doctor told him that he could not let water touch him for one year from the date of visit. He couldn't have an erection for three and a half years from that date either. The patient says he was told at a clinic last year that the six or seven packs of cigarettes he smokes per day were inadequate to sustain his blood pressure and that the should be smoking one carton daily. However, he cannot afford the cigarettes, or food either, for that matter, because he is not able to make the thirty-five dollars per day to which he is entitled through begging. By law every person he accosts on the street through panhandling is required to give him twenty-five cents. Since most of them don't, he is legally permitted to call them lice, finks, and perverts, as he does, loudly.

Because he has no money for food, he is equally entitled to receive free meals in any restaurant. The restaurants do not cooperate, even though by law they are required to set aside 21 percent of their money to feed people like him.

The patient says he is a member of the government of Greenwich Village, but he remains a very unpopular person, he says, because he speaks explicitly to people on the street who do not give him the money to which he is entitled.

Our psychiatrist consultant felt that the patient should be hospitalized. He refused, moved from the Hotel Earle, and has been lost to contact.

Staffing and Financing

Twenty-six part- or full-time salaried staff members serve in our program. These include eleven physicians (both internists and pediatricians), nine nurses, one nurse practitioner and one nurse-health educator, four social workers, one substance abuse counselor, two drivers, two corpsmen, two outreach workers, a program coordinator, two secretaries, and the program manager. In addition, volunteer psychiatrists and an ophthalmologist share in the work.

The total salary cost of the program is about $1.6 million. An additional sum in the range of $100,000 is used for rent, transportation, and supplies. These costs are met through contracts with the New York City Human Resources Administration, a federal grant through the McKinney Act, and a grant from the New York State Department of Health, Comic Relief, foundation grants, private philanthropy, and hospital support.

Conclusion

We have served in many capacities in our goal of providing primary care to homeless persons. For many, we become their significant other: surrogate family, parents, siblings, grandparents, aunts, teachers, or whatever role is suitable to meet the need. Several patients when admitted to the hospital record a staff member's name as the next of kin. We become their supporters and guide them through an impersonal system. We comfort, care, help, heal, and sometimes provide a glimmer of hope.

In an article evoking the memory of a homeless man,[20] a St. Vincent's staff physician observes that "a health care team at any . . . homeless shelter must construct a biography for tens of . . . individuals each month." The life story is written as a medical document of historical facts and symptoms, old records, physical signs, and conjecture. We listen; we measure; we ponder; we advise. Our work is this: We testify that in this location and at this time a person who had no place to live, who had no place, a *placeless* person sought and accepted care from others. In this way we record our common humanity.

RITA ALTAMORE

MAUREEN MITCHELL

CAROL MARTINEZ WEBER

25

Assuring Good-Quality Care

Introduction and Overview

Simply *providing* health and human services to homeless persons might seem enough of a challenge. Most service providers and program managers, however, want to do more than simply count visits; they want to be sure that good-quality care is being provided. This discussion uses experiences drawn from three health care for the homeless (HCH) projects to highlight some of the issues confronting those who undertake to assess and assure high-quality care.

Talking About Quality of Care

What is good-quality care? It's easy to think that you know it when you see it, but it's often hard to define and measure. Many authors have offered definitions of "quality," ranging from the adherence to established standards of performance to the achievement of good results.[1-3] The Congressional Office of Technology Assessment defines "quality of medical care" as "the degree to which the process of care increases the probability of outcomes desired by patients and reduces the probability of undesired outcomes, given the state of medical knowledge."[4] We will not attempt to define quality. Those organizing, providing, receiving, and paying for care should discuss and compare their own definitions.

The literature on quality of care has often been divided into two general areas. Quality *assessment* deals with the methods by which quality is measured.[1-4]

Quality *assurance* deals with the ways in which a system can be organized to make sure that an appropriate quality of care is being provided.[5,6,7] In both quality assessment and quality assurance there are choices to be made.

Choices in Quality Assessment

Structure, process, or outcome? One can choose measures from any or all of these categories. "Structure" is defined as the resources and organizational arrangements that are in place to deliver care. Structure includes providers and their credentials, facilities, supplies, and equipment, the presence of which allows good-quality care to be provided.[8] One measure of quality might be whether or not an otoscope is available; if it is not, it is impossible to examine the ears of a child with a suspected ear infection. "Process" is defined as the actual care provided, the activities of physicians, nurses, and others involved in providing services. The process of care has both technical and interpersonal components. One aspect of process which can be examined is its appropriateness in a given clinical situation.[9–12] Was the appropriate history obtained and the physical exam done? If an ear infection was diagnosed, was the appropriate antibiotic prescribed? Were the appropriate instructions given? Was the documentation complete? "Outcome" is defined as the results of care, including changes in health status and patient satisfaction.[13–18] Did the symptoms improve? Were the ears normal on recheck? Were the parents happy with the way they and the child were treated?

The link between outcome and process is key. If an outcome is not related to some aspect of care, then how can a provider or system of care be held accountable? The best outcome measures are those that have the strongest association with the process of care; the best process measures are those that have been shown to affect outcome.[19,20]

Explicit or implicit criteria? Explicit criteria most often take the form of lists of very clearly defined elements whose presence in a specific case is agreed to represent good care (for example, temperature taken, medication allergies documented, antibiotic prescribed). Providers use implicit criteria when they review the care provided and use their best professional judgment on whether or not it is good.

From whose perspective? The individuals receiving care, their families, the professional(s) providing the care, the organizations delivering the care, the payers, and the society at large may have very different ideas of what constitutes good-quality care.[21–24] Any choice of measures incorporates the views and values of at least one of these groups; those doing quality assessment should consider whose views ought to be represented.

What scope of care? Health care for the homeless requires attention to physical, social, and psychological needs. How well can quality be assessed if the method does not attend to all the elements of care provided?

Where do the data come from?[25,26] Many quality assessment methods use data collected for other purposes, most often on a billing or encounter form. Use of such secondary data usually reduces cost but may limit the information available.

For example, how often are important outcomes such as client satisfaction or functional status recorded on a billing form?[27] Even the medical record is often a poor source of such information. However, use of secondary data can still yield important insights into process and outcome and may help focus more intensive review.[28]

Choices in Quality Assurance

Once choices have been made about what definition of quality is to be used and what methods of assessment are to be employed, a variety of possible approaches exist for "closing the loop," for looking at the quality provided and, if problems are found, making sure they are addressed.[29] The key in quality assurance is that it is a cycle; problem identification, problem analysis, intervention, and reevaluation all are vital steps. A variety of strategies has been used to try to change provider behavior, with varying success.[30] There is considerable evidence that education alone has limited and often short-term effects.[31,32] More effective may be changes in the system, such as reminders of necessary care which are available to the provider while the client is being seen.[33]

Medical Care Evaluations: These include traditional chart audits and many group peer review activities. The old "every month an audit" approach, using a randomly selected medical problem, such as urinary tract infection, has not been shown to have a high enough yield to warrant the time and cost to perform. It is recommended that audits be focused by choosing to review high-volume, high-risk, and problem-prone diagnoses, procedures, or services.[34–36]

Monitoring of Indicators: In addition to focusing on a specific problem or case for review, there is a trend in the quality assurance field toward the use of indicators, routinely collected data that allow performance to be monitored on a regular basis.[37–38] Indicators are chosen because they can be shown or are believed to reflect quality of care. For example, the number of homeless clients admitted to the hospital each month might be followed because an increase might reflect some problems in primary care. Indicators serve as screening tools; once a change in an indicator points to a problem, further investigation is usually necessary to identify the cause and appropriate interventions. In the example cited, is *access* to primary care the problem, or are there problems in the primary care actually provided?[39–42]

Continuous Quality Improvement: In the last few years quality assurance in health care has begun to adopt some of methods of industrial quality control. Fundamental to this approach is the continuous effort to improve quality; all persons involved in providing care are encouraged to examine their own work and are provided support for doing so.[43] They are rewarded for identifying opportunities for improvement; the underlying belief is that most people are doing the best that they can and that 80 percent or more of problems in quality are the result of difficulties in the system, not problems of individuals. Although still new in health care, this approach may be of particular relevance in health care for the homeless, where factors outside the control of providers profoundly affect what they are able to do.

Making Choices

There are many models for quality assessment and assurance in traditional hospital and ambulatory care settings, as well as in nursing homes, hospices, mental health centers, psychiatric hospitals, and rehabilitation facilities.[44] Many accreditation agencies and quality assurance (QA) practitioners are moving away from reliance primarily on structural measures to the incorporation of some combination of process and outcomes and from periodic audits to routine monitoring of indicators. Doing quality assessment and assurance takes time and money,[45] including the scarce commodity of provider time; however, the costs of poor quality and its effects may be even greater. Unfortunately there is as yet little evidence that will allow a choice of methods based on effectiveness. A critical look at one's own program and its goals may be the best way currently available to identify the structural, process, and outcome measures that are believed to be a reflection of quality and the most cost-effective approach to quality assurance.[46,47] Three different HCH programs with three different service delivery models have answered these questions somewhat differently, as the following case studies show.

Case in Depth: Nursing Care Audit in Seattle

The Model

The Seattle HCH project is based on a model of nursing care provided in shelters, together with mental health, social work, and substance abuse counseling services. Seattle has a strong community health care network; a major goal of the project is to provide homeless clients access to those resources. Most of the contacts in the project are with registered nurses.

In the Seattle project, practitioners, the project director, and governing council members worked together to develop a QA plan which incorporated several standard elements:

- Requirements for supervision and backup of practitioners
- Development and maintenance of protocols for clinical care
- Requirements for peer review and team conferences
- Chart reviews and audits of selected common, important, and high-risk problems
- Review of selected indicators
- Periodic surveys of client satisfaction and of provider satisfaction
- Incident reporting
- Requirements for quality assurance of contracted services

The group agreed that these elements would provide a reasonable assessment of quality at a cost, in time and money, that could be borne.

One of the most successful quality assurance activities undertaken was an audit by project nurses of their compliance with their own protocols regarding follow-up of priority referrals. This activity was part of a larger comprehensive nursing quality assurance process in which project nurses worked together to develop a statement of purpose and philosophy, as well as standards of nursing practice. Each practice standard was accompanied by a rationale and by structural, process, and outcome criteria that could be measured to assess compliance with the standard.

Priority referrals were chosen for audit because of their importance; one goal of the Seattle project is to connect clients to existing resources. It is important to know whether appropriate referrals are being made and successfully completed, especially for clients with "priority" problems, such as acute illness and injury, communicable disease, or suspected child abuse. The audit began with a review of the existing protocols and the development of a checklist of explicit criteria based on the protocol. For each nurse, the records of ten clients with priority problems were reviewed, using the criteria, and the findings compiled and reviewed. Problems in the referral process were discussed, and new log systems instituted in several sites. Six months later the records of all patients with priority problems who were seen within a two-week period were reviewed. The results were encouraging: There was a rise from 62 percent compliance with the criteria to 100 percent on the repeat audit.

The audit was a major project, requiring substantial practitioner involvement, some of it on their own time. One important lesson learned was that the time was well spent. Not only were the nurses able to point with pride to evidence of their own good quality of care, but the process itself was valuable in building team spirit and morale. The protocol review and criteria development process allowed nurses to share their experiences and problems and to focus on their goals for care and the processes they thought most important in achieving those goals.

Unfortunately not all the quality assurance activities have proceeded quite so smoothly. The review of indicators has proved to be one of the most difficult elements to maintain because of the continuous data collection and analysis required. In Seattle all project services are provided through contracts with existing health agencies; the project itself has no direct access to client charts, only to encounter forms. Therefore, the project office cannot conduct chart reviews and must rely on activities within the contracting agencies. It remains difficult to ensure that services to homeless clients are included in the routine quality assurance activities at the contracting agencies and even more difficult to obtain results of such reviews specific to HCH clients.[48]

Case in Depth: Physician Protocols in Cleveland

The Model

In keeping with the Patient's Bill of Rights, the Cleveland Health Care for the Homeless Program aspired to develop a quality assurance program that safeguarded the delivery of health care that respects and advocates for the human dignity of this patient population. The Cleveland project evolved and developed as a result of a collaborative effort between the City of Cleveland Health Department and the MetroHealth System, the county hospital system, both agencies that serve an indigent population. The comprehensive health care delivery model incorporates nursing and medical care, alcohol and substance abuse counseling and referral, social work counseling for employment and housing placement, and shelter outreach nursing and health education, screening, and referral for women, children, and men.

Barriers to Quality Assurance

Merging two bureaucratic agencies, each with its own health care policies, procedures, and transient physician staff, proved to be one of the project's greatest challenges in developing a standardized quality assurance program. Further complicating the goal of delivering good-quality care was the fact that medical services are delivered at two nontraditional clinic sites geographically removed from the city's health centers and the country's hospital system. One Westside makeshift clinic, operated by the city, is housed in an agency providing meals and transient shelter for the homeless. A freestanding homeless social service and counseling drop-in center, which evolved from the Health Care for the Homeless Program, is the Near Eastside site of the county's clinic. There are few full-time health care staff members, with medical care given by staff members who have full-time responsibilities within the city and county systems. The Cleveland project uses physicians rather than nurse practitioners to deliver medical care.

Impetus for the Development of a Quality Assurance Program

The project operates without benefit of a computer information system. However, during monthly meetings the medical staff met and reviewed patient records targeted at specific health alterations. It became evident that the variability between the city and county health policies and procedures made a quality assurance program untenable without major revisions in the program's health care delivery practices. The project's community governing council selected the director of nursing for the Cleveland Health Department to develop health care protocols for the program with the ultimate aim of designing and implementing a quality assurance program. The challenge would eventually incorporate an interdisciplinary approach. The first step to realizing this goal was to develop protocols for physicians.

Protocols Addressing Major Health Alterations

The project's medical director expressed the desire that the program not rewrite textbooks for internal medicine when it developed physician protocols. Taking this concern into consideration, the director of nursing targeted major health concerns common to the homeless population which include the alterations found in Table 25.1. Protocols involving specific disciplines (i.e., nursing, substance abuse and mental health counseling, nutrition, and social work) were developed by discipline-specific personnel. Discipline volunteers from each system

Table 25.1 MAJOR HEALTH ALTERATIONS REQUIRING
QUALITY ASSURANCE MEDICAL PROTOCOLS FOR
HEALTH CARE FOR THE HOMELESS

Hypertension	Malnutrition secondary to hepatic disorders
Upper respiratory tract infection	
Influenza; immunization program	Immunizations
Minor skin trauma	TB screening and treatment
Dermatitis	Basic orthopedic problems
Substance and physical abuse; management / referral	Gastrointestinal disorders; ulcers
	Infestations
Sexually transmitted disease; treatment / referral	Peripheral vascular disease
	Urinary tract infections
HIV testing; counseling and referral	Pregnancy testing; gyn referrals
Nutrition counseling for patients on special diets	Seizure disorders; management / follow-up
	Hepatic disorders; hepatitis / cirrhosis
Eating at hunger centers	

were solicited to develop protocols if these disciplines were not represented on the project's staff.

Since the project uses the pharmacy and the clinical diagnostic laboratory in both systems, protocols had to consider the availability of medications and laboratory tests specific to each system. For cost containment purposes, medications and tests available within each system are the first choice in the care of the patient. Quality assurance standards and practices inherent in each system for the pharmacy and laboratory are ongoing and incorporated within the Cleveland project.

Getting the Quality Assurance Program Started

It was decided to target the five most frequently seen health alterations for standard of care development: upper respiratory tract infection, malnutrition, alcohol and substance addiction, dermatitis, and hypertension. The project initiated protocols that highlighted the major standards of care for these alterations. Table 25.2 identifies the basic performance criteria items included in each protocol.

Referring to protocol guidelines when delivering patient care was a new concept for the staff of this project. The staff believed that if a choice had to be made between seeing patients and documenting for quality assurance purposes, the priority would be patient care. The staff is committed to providing accessible health care for the homeless in Cleveland. The time spent in quality assurance meetings and protocol evaluation is a constraint that takes the staff away from direct patient care. However, in an effort to ensure that the homeless receive care comparable in quality with that for others, the good intentions of providing care needed to be backed by a structure that supports this aim.

Sensitivity to the staff's concerns regarding the bureaucracy involved in qual-

Table 25.2 PROTOCOL PERFORMANCE CRITERIA ITEMS

Name of health alteration

A. Assessment criteria
    1. Subjective criteria (listed)
    2. Objective criteria (listed)

B. Diagnostic criteria
    1. Noninvasive tests available in clinic
    2. Invasive tests: in-house and referred
        a) Standard tests (listed)
        b) Nonstandard tests (M.D. rationale needed)
    3. Preliminary diagnosis without invasive test results
    4. Confirmatory diagnosis with invasive test results

C. Treatment plan
    1. Medication (drug of choice; specify rationale for other; consider in-house availability)
    2. Interdisciplinary considerations
        a) Management of patient's human response to illness; nursing diagnosis and interventions
        b) Patient education; materials given to patient
        c) Medication administration options; return to clinic for daily administration; specify other
        d) Diet management specific to diagnosis and available meal options
    3. Referral to outside agency
        a) Transportation arranged
        b) Report from agency for future clinic follow-up

D. Evaluation of health care
    1. Patient returns to clinic for evaluation
    2. Objective/subjective symptoms managed
    3. Need for alternate treatment: Specify medication/referral/further diagnostic testing
    4. Repeat Steps B–D

ity assurance programs was essential if the program was to be successful. For want of an information system, a uniform color-coded sticker system was to be used to tag patient records according to the patient's primary diagnosis. This feature would enable quick retrieval of patient records for audit purposes. It was decided to keep the QA program simple and "user-friendly" since the project has many inherent barriers to developing a workable program.

Quality Assurance: Safeguarding Continuing Health Care Services

Quality assurance can also be used to document the need for continued health care service, as was the case in the Cleveland project. The project was focused on determining ways to extend its financial resources. One proposal was to eliminate

care delivered by physicians at the Westside clinic, substituting nurse practitioners. It was believed that many patients came to the Westside clinic for social
purposes or repeated minor health problems. An audit which included surveying
patients' primary diagnosis, frequency of visits, and on-site observations over a
period of months revealed that this patient population presented with complex,
unstable multisystem health alterations, complicated by compromised socioeconomic factors. Patients who visited the clinic more than once each week did so to
enhance their own compliance with medication therapy for seizures and hypertension. With the intervention of the nurse and social worker, patients whose primary
diagnoses were complicated by substance abuse or psychiatric disorder returned
for frequent follow-up evaluation, medication, and nursing care.

Because the audit revealed the complexity of health alterations and the need
for an interdisciplinary approach, medical care delivered by physicians remained
an integral part of the clinic operation. Although the clinic was shortened by one
hour on each of the three clinic days, a comprehensive interdisciplinary approach
remains. In this instance a quality assurance mechanism helped health care professionals to continue to deliver accessible, free health care to a segment of society
that is homeless not by choice but by circumstance.

Case in Depth: St. Vincent's Hospital
(New York) Experience

QA of the performance of an interdisciplinary team of health care providers
requires evaluation of both the group and the individuals. In the St. Vincent's
Hospital SRO / Homeless Program QA responsibility is shared among all staff
members, one of whom also serves to oversee QA coordination. Outcome assessment integrates and evaluates the work of the team as a whole. This can be done
with case conferences, chart reviews, and prospective monitoring of designated
outcomes. Chart reviews also provide a format for assessing an individual's performance within the team.

Formal case conferences are scheduled quarterly and consist of in-depth analysis of one case by the entire staff. Cases are chosen through an informal consensus
process among program staff. Generally a particularly challenging case is selected
to provide the team with new input that may crystallize a workable management
plan. Each team member gives a brief presentation. Then one team member
reviews the team's goals, its understanding of the client's goals, and the perceived
problem areas. Occasionally the client will be asked to attend all or some part of
the conference to provide a "consumer's perspective." Routinely, however, only
staff attends. Client input comes primarily from interactions with the team at the
site. The outlining of team behaviors and monitoring of outcomes are key to the
presentation. Program staff members respond with comments and suggestions
based on personal experience and insight, thus providing mutual support and
guidance. Divergent aims among team members are addressed, and various means
of resolution discussed. A common example of differing goals would be a client's
desire for symptomatic relief (e.g., of cough and fever) and a health care provider's desire for long-term cure (e.g., of active pulmonary tuberculosis). Conflicting

goals among the health care providers appear much less often, but when they do occur, expeditious resolution is essential for good patient care.

Formal case conferences as well as informal discussions among team members on-site identify goals and create a workable plan for achievement. The case conference format serves many functions beyond QA. It is a vital technique for review of a team's work as well as a forum for supervisors to observe the group dynamic.

Chart reviews and concurrent monitoring of outcomes are two other modalities for assessing the efficacy of the health care team. For instance, the staff screened a large series of clients for tuberculosis exposure by skin test reactivity to purified protein derivative. Few candidates for isoniazid prophylaxis actually cooperated with a full course of therapy, and it was decided that the limited personnel resources could be spent more efficaciously in primary case finding. However, the current rise in active tuberculosis among HIV-infected individuals has provoked renewed efforts at implementing programs for prophylaxis. Thus, information from chart reviews can guide the selection of future QA indicators as well as yield invaluable data about patterns of illness for use in needs assessment.

Detailed individual chart review provides another mechanism for assessing compliance with good standards of care. The physician staff members in the St. Vincent's program review a medical chart monthly for one hour. The clinical reviewer in conjunction with the program director and the QA coordinator chooses the chart for its educational value. All seek cases that lead to numerous "teachable moments" on various aspects of health care. First the purely structural aspects of the chart and then the skills and performance of individual providers are analyzed. All the outreach charts are organized in a standard format. When a provider must go to an unfamiliar site to cover for an ill or vacationing colleague, the uniformity of the chart structure eases the transition and facilitates organization and tidiness. The reviewer looks for the following components: compliance with standard chart format, proper labeling of each page, legible notes and signature, dating and coherent organization of individual provider notes. The reviewer then breaks the team down into its staff components and sees how the chart reflects its work. The reviewer is most often the QA coordinator, but at times another care provider may assume this role. Key questions include:

- Are the problem lists current? Are diabetes and hypertension flow sheets used when indicated?
- Are historical and demographic data recorded or noted as unobtainable or unreliable (e.g., "poor historian" or "refuses to answer")?
- Is the physical examination appropriate and documented in sufficient detail to address the client's chief complaint? Is the reason for a limited examination documented (e.g., "patient refuses to undress" or "room too noisy for accurate cardiac auscultation")?
- Does the clinical impression grow from the chief complaint, history and physical? Is it a reasoned process, not just a problem list?
- Does the plan of management grow from the chief complaint, history, and physical exam? Is it reasonable on the basis of the client's resources and abilities?

Judgment of a plan's "reasonability" can be reassessed retrospectively because the outcome of early plans is reflected in later progress notes in the chart.

To complete this sort of detailed chart review in one hour requires lengthy preparation. The structural aspects are scrutinized beforehand by the reviewer, and the general pattern is briefly announced as a reminder to all staff. Most of the hour is spent discussing the "impressions" and "plans." In contrast with case conference meetings that focus on outcome and team interaction, these sessions focus on process and individual physician performance. Minididactic sessions are woven into the discussion, and a packet of relevant journal articles is distributed. Although the educational aspects of the case are emphasized and the tone is kept nonpejorative, such problems as errors in judgments, careless documentation, or inadequate provider follow-up are noticed. As one of the physicians has stated, these sessions "are not for the faint at heart." Yet presented in the spirit of team-work and self-improvement, they have usually been well received. Individual commitment to excellence and a sense of collegiality have been essential to the implementation of this project. Without the staff's cooperation and enthusiasm this format for peer review cannot be undertaken.

Implicit in the involvement of all staff is the philosophy that all team members are of equal stature. All bring the special insights of their own professional disciplines and integrate them into the group process of provision of holistic health care. However, review of the technical process of care of a member of a professional discipline is best done by others of that discipline. It is not appropriate for the social work staff to review a physician's antibiotic choice, nor should a physician be reviewing the thoroughness of a social work intake note. For these purposes nurses, social workers, and team extenders meet quarterly with colleagues of their own profession. The monthly in-depth chart review serves this function for the physicians. Additionally, all staff members meet at least annually with their supervisors for a formal evaluation, the results of which are kept in employee files.

Certain intangibles of humanistic, holistic health care provision cannot be assessed by chart review alone. However, many vital aspects of care *are* easily defined and quantified and should be improved through in-depth chart reviews linked with education and follow-up. Most simply, shortcomings in care (missed immunizations, overlooked abnormal laboratory values, for example) can be corrected. Improvement in the quality of care given by individual providers has not yet been examined in St. Vincent's program but is an expected result.

Quality assurance of the system is another ongoing function of the health care teams and the QA coordinator. For instance, in St. Vincent's program nonradiological laboratory reports appear on computer printouts. All results are reviewed daily by a designated physician (a rotating task), and any significantly abnormal value leads to notification of the primary physician. How can an abnormal laboratory value pass unseen? What safeguards can be created to minimize this possibility?

All these review processes are time- and energy-consuming. Staffing and time constraints must be overcome in initiating a team-centered QA program. Preparation for case conferences and in-depth chart reviews are divided among the staff on a voluntary basis. The QA coordinator has office time designated for this function alone and thus plays a larger role in the chart review and didactic functions than other workers of the team. However, as with other aspects of this approach to health care provision for homeless populations, QA work is above all a team effort, and all staff are encouraged to participate.

Summary

Quality of Care for the Homeless: Should It Be the Same as for Everyone Else?

Some may argue that the standards applied to care in traditional settings cannot be the same for homeless persons because the challenges are so different. Providing even routine care is made difficult by limited program resources and by the fact that clients have disrupted lives and poor or absent social support and may have substance abuse or mental health problems. Their physical health problems may be more complex or severe than those who are housed.[49]

The use of mortality rates as a measure of hospital quality presents similar problems. How can the figures be adjusted to reflect the fact that some hospitals take care of sicker patients?[50] The development of severity-adjusted measures of outcome is a current focus of intense interest by providers, accrediting bodies, and payers.[51,52] It is a challenge to develop systems that are reliable and valid measures of the severity of *physical* illness; few systems under development take into account the psychosocial factors that are so important in care for homeless persons.

Those who would assess care for homeless persons must decide if standards for process and outcome should be adjusted. For example, in a traditional clinic the standard may be that 95 percent of children should have evidence of having received a complete OPV series (less than 100 percent to account for those patients whose parents object on religious grounds or who have medical contraindications). Should the same standard be 75 percent in a clinic which cares for homeless children (according to the argument that the mobility of homeless families makes completion of an immunization series unlikely)? Should it be 50 percent? In a traditional clinic the standard may be that 90 percent of children with uncomplicated cases of otitis media should show no evidence of acute infection at a three-week recheck. Should the standard be 70 percent for homeless children (again according to the argument that it is unlikely that parents will be able to comply with the antibiotic regimen?)

We believe that the expectations for quality should be no different for the care of homeless persons from that of others. This does not necessarily mean that the process of care should be identical. Indeed, to treat homeless clients the same as others may indicate *poor*-quality care, if, for example, an antihypertensive medication that must be taken four times a day is prescribed when one that can be taken once daily would be equally safe and effective. To ignore the realities of homelessness is as potentially serious a cause of poor-quality care as to fail to offer the same opportunities for treatment to clients simply because they are homeless and therefore *assumed* unable to understand instructions or adhere to a regimen.

Quality Assurance in Health Care for the Homeless

Quality assessment and assurance are important parts of the delivery of health care. In addition to responding to the requirements of accrediting and licensing agencies, they embody the providers' commitment to give the best care possible. Quality assurance can also provide data that are useful in the fight for continued support, as demonstrated by the Cleveland experience.

For quality assurance to be accepted, however, its benefits must be seen as equal to, or exceeding, its costs. As each of the case studies makes clear, quality assurance activities inevitably take precious provider time, while the benefits may be intangible. It is the responsibility of those who administer the quality assurance process to choose strategies that appear in their setting to offer the best yield for the effort required.

The individuals involved in quality assurance for HCH are not alone in health care in needing better information with which to make these choices. There needs to be better evidence about medical efficacy, so that quality assurance activities can focus on those interventions proved to make a difference.[53] There needs to be better information on what constitutes effective care for specific health problems among the homeless in order to be able to make appropriate adjustments in "standard" care protocols. Quality assurance activities can provide data that will help link process and outcome in specific client groups. Examining our own experience is essential, even though it cannot substitute completely for more rigorous and formal research activities.

Is there any bottom line to quality assurance? The literature on continuous quality improvement suggests, and the experiences in many HCH projects corroborate, the following precepts:

- Make quality the heart of the project's mission.
- Hire leader-managers dedicated to good quality.
- Organize the system in support of the staff's desire to deliver good-quality care.
- Reward staff for identifying opportunities for improvement.
- Provide a structure for the creative search for solutions to identified problems.
- Keep doing it![54]

ANDREW R. GREENE

PHYLLIS B. WOLFE

FREDA MITCHEM

HOPE BURNESS GLEICHER

RON BURRIS

BOB ZMUDA

DENNIS ALBAUGH

26

Program Sustainment

Introduction

Is there life after foundation funding? An excellent measure of success and value for programs supported by philanthropy is their ability to achieve financial independence when demonstration dollars run out. The nineteen HCHPs supported by Johnson/Pew during the period 1985–88 are worthy of study in this regard.

It was a prerequisite of each grant proposal submitted to the foundations that a discussion of plans for long-term sustainment be included. While guessing about details of funding sources four years into the future was in fact unrealistic, it distinctly forced attention of all parties in the national program on 1989 as the year when financial independence was expected or programs would die.

Foundation staff viewed philanthropic monies as start-up funds for the development and the initial services for each of the HCHP projects. It was never the intent to fund the sites permanently. The objective was rather to help the projects build on the strength that would ultimately enable them to become self-sustaining programs, leveraging and substituting other funds.

Foundation Funding

In the launching of a program of this type it was important at the outset to think about and deal with what happens after the grant funding is fully utilized. The issue of program sustainment was considered at the time the HCHP was in the design stage. The maximum figure of a $1.4 million grant per site was agreed to after a number of pro forma budgets were examined. The four-year term was also arrived at after considerable discussion at the foundation level. The amount and duration were finally deemed sufficient to allow a health care operation for homeless persons to start up, achieve steady state, and procure future funding. Included in the total grant was up to $50,000 per year to support specific activities of a citywide coalition and project governing body for planning and, in large part, for project continuance after the grant.

Each site was faced with the dilemma of where to find its ultimate home after foundation support was concluded. Should it attempt to stay at the institution that originally sponsored the project, operate as a freestanding organization, or become folded into an existing public agency such as the local health department? The decisions rested on financial and ideological considerations. For example, would a local health department be able adequately to support site efforts in treating homeless persons, or would the program be swallowed by the bureaucracy and lose its identify, become vulnerable to periodic cutbacks, or even become extinct? In the Washington, D.C. program the matter of survival was dealt with aggressively from the beginning:

Over the life of the demonstration project, each time a new key individual took office within the DHS [Department of Human Services], the Executive Director, in concert with the Board Chair and other key board members, met to orient the new administrator. Of paramount importance was their understanding of the nature of the public / private partnership that had developed, the key role that it played in providing health care to the homeless and to solicit their support in making sure that the program continued to grow and thrive. Ultimately their support was required for resources that would be necessary to maintain service delivery in January, 1989 after the Johnson-Pew funding terminated.[1]

Since private foundations can be more flexible than some public funding sources, the sites were told that foundation funds unexpended at the end of the four-year grant could be used for an extension period. Thus, each site was encouraged from the start to obtain other funding and substitute those funds for line items in their approved foundation budget.

A characteristic of dealing with an RWJF/Pew grant is the strict view of budget negotiating and financial reporting of all grantees. In this program all sites were observed carefully by the foundations' Financial Monitoring Office. Each line item in each year was required to fit into the overall objective of the HCHP site's proposal and its goal, or it was disallowed. If a grantee can demonstrate that it can handle its internal operations well, the thinking goes, then other funders, public and private, will be more apt to support.

The foundation reinforced this point by requiring the site to submit quarterly financial reports before the next payment was made. In this way, the project director would be familiar with and be able to respond to questions about the budget from any forum—i.e., media, funder, potential funder, or public official.

An example of the benefits of close monitoring is shown in this statement issued by the Washington, D.C. program:

As a new non-profit corporation, we are faced with the challenge of obtaining funding for FY '90 at a time when the city faces an enormous budget deficit. We will have to make sure that our service delivery is properly quantified. In 1988, we saw over 7,000 individuals with over 19,000 patient visits at an approximate cost of $62.00 per patient visit. This kind of data along with the referral and diagnostic information that we are retrieving with our computer system allows us to statistically show the impact of our service delivery. This is important not only for seeking continued funding from the district government, but also important as we move to continue generating resources from the private sector.[2]

The San Antonio Story

Embezzlement

Another, more dramatic example of the need for financial monitoring occurred in San Antonio, one of the Pew-supported sites. In late February 1987 the new program director of the HCHP in San Antonio, Ron Burris, had a problem. The approved budget showed that there were more than enough funds to reimburse him for the trip he had taken to a meeting. He called the foundation and confirmed that there were funds budgeted for this purpose. This was in contradiction to advice from the chief fiscal officer of the sponsoring organization, the San Antonio Urban Council, that there were no funds left in that line item. Where was the money?

The financial problems of the Urban Council then began to emerge. In December 1986 all programs operating under the council began to note problems with cash flow. Soon thereafter it was discovered that council funds had been commingled, and in January 1987 it became apparent that approximately seventy thousand dollars were missing from funds given to support the HCHP. In addition, Social Security payments had not been made for several quarters, increasing the total shortfall to about ninety-four thousand dollars.

When board members attempted to review the financial records, which were computerized, they learned that the financial tapes had been erased. Quickly thereafter the chief fiscal officer resigned and disappeared from San Antonio.

The program would not be able to meet its payroll. A due payment of sixty-five thousand dollars was stopped by Pew because of the instability. On March 10, 1987, Pew informed the program director and the Urban Council that while the foundation staff would remain as supportive as possible, the financial situation demanded that Pew withhold future payments to the program until the Urban Council fully documented the events leading to the deficit and reinstated the missing funds. It was clear that this process might take several months and that depending on the findings, continuing grant payments to the council might or might not be possible because by that time the HCHP might have folded.

This was the only responsible action that Pew could take with regard to missing funds. However, it raised the difficult matter of what would happen to the program until mid-April. What actions would or could the program director and the program advisory board enact that could keep the staff together and continue services?

At this point Ron Burris began discussions with the United Way of San Antonio. It was willing to be helpful but was not totally sure of how to help. It is interesting to note that the United Way was a key factor in the long-term sustainment strategy outlined in the original proposal from San Antonio. Therefore, the groups were aware of and on friendly terms with each other before the crisis.

Desperation Demands a Response

On March 12, 1987, the RWJF vice-president for financial monitoring undertook a last-ditch site visit to see if the project could be saved. The visit was made to ascertain the following:

- Since funding from Pew had been stopped, was there sufficient evidence that the program was continuing to meet its objectives despite the grantee's problems?
- To what extent, and in what manner, was the money funding this program from Pew missing?
- Could short-term funding be found from other organizations in San Antonio to sustain the program while efforts were made to deal with longer-term issues of support?
- Could an appropriate nonprofit organization be found to satisfy Pew so that funding could begin again with sufficient knowledge that a reputable organization was handling the financial transactions of the program? Pew had $624,311 in unexpended funds earmarked for San Antonio.

The financial officer met with key participants. Members of the HCHP Advisory Board in San Antonio gathered on short notice and ratified the viewpoint that the spirit of the program remained vigorous and that the ills plaguing the Urban Council had not daunted them. The paid staff of the program noted a sense of unity produced by the crisis. A visit to the two shelter clinics hinted at the viability of the situation, tenuous as it was. Both were staffed and busy, seeing homeless clients with a wide range of health problems. In fact, cumulative data revealed that more visits took place at these sites in February and March 1987 than in other typical winter months. The staff attitude, and evidence that services continued unabated, proved essential to later positive developments.

A meeting took place the next day with the United Way. The objective, from the viewpoint of the foundation site visitor, was to obtain a guarantee of interim financial support while a suitable grantee could be sought for Pew funds. The request to the United Way board included cash support for the program through mid-April, at which point Pew might be able to resume payments. The United Way immediately offerred thirty-thousand dollars in temporary payroll funds and expressed its willingness to consider longer-term help.

The process of seeking a grantee organization then was accelerated. A long list of potential organizations was considered. Finally, when no appropriate agency seemed available, the United Way decided to take an innovative step and accept the direct management of the project itself. This was a significant shift for the United Way, from being only a funding source and into direct services. The United Way had the necessary virtues of

- Having a willing board
- Having impeccable financial position and fiscal controls
- Not being a governmental organization, barred from serving in a grantee capacity

The San Antonio program was salvaged by the willingness of the salaried staff to persevere under stress, by the ability and desire of major local organizations, such as the United Way and St. Philip's of Jesus Clinic (the principal subcontractor for health services to the project from its beginning, which had gone many weeks without contract payments), to risk their money for a good cause, and by the energy and catalytic quality of a foundation officer who would not allow the program to fold.

And what of the embezzler? Several months after these events a man was heard bragging in a Milwaukee bar about how he had ripped off a do-good program in San Antonio. Milwaukee was the site of another homeless program, and many individuals in Milwaukee were aware of the theft. The police were called, the man was arrested and convicted, and he is now serving time. None of the stolen money was recovered.

Considering Sources of Long-Term Support
Medicaid

During the second and third years of the program there was a concerted effort to obtain Medicaid and other public entitlement funds for program support. Each site was encouraged to help clients obtain Medicaid coverage. Intuitively many of the program directors doubted that public programs for society at large would make much of a difference for homeless persons or programs.

Medicaid is a joint federal and state program that reimburses the cost of medical services for persons with little or no income and assets. It is a voluntary program for physicians, pharmacists, and other providers of health services.

In most states recipients of general assistance (GA) or Aid to Families with Dependent Children are automatically eligible for medical assistance. In others, income and assets are considered in the determination of eligibility. Eligibility is usually established for limited periods, such as three or six months. An estimated 90 percent of all homeless clients are theoretically eligible for medical assistance. The more clients with an active medical assistance status, the more income the program could derive from it.

The experience in Baltimore illustrates the results of a yearlong effort to bring homeless people onto Medicaid:

In strictly financial terms, the value of Medical Assistance to the program might be computed as income earned less expenses. In 1988, with 30–35% of our clients having active Medical Assistance at the time they received service, the program earned approximately $35,000. This represents less than 3% of total revenue. Consider this in light of the $21,000 in administrative and casework expenses related to billing Medical Assistance, and the real income earned is $14,000 or 1% of total revenue. Because a far greater percentage of clients are eligible for Medical Assistance than actually receive this benefit, it would, in theory, be possible to devote resources to the certification of clients and recovery of expenses.

However, the return on such an investment, especially in light of existing barriers, may militate against such a solution.[3]

Many barriers and disincentives inhibit the homeless from obtaining medical assistance. A voluminous application must be completed at each redetermination. Also, a personal interview and possibly a physical examination are necessary. This additional step may prove impossible for persons with no access to transportation. Lack of a permanent address or frequent changes of address make it difficult for homeless clients to receive such mail as a medical assistance card. For those who should be eligible automatically by virtue of their GA or AFDC status, clients report that department of social services workers often either neglect to inform them of their entitlement to medical assistance or do not complete the necessary forms. Also, compared with other pressing needs such as shelter, food, and transportation, medical assistance satisfies a relatively intangible need. Unless homeless persons are experiencing an acute medical problem, such as a severe toothache or sore throat, they may not perceive medical assistance as a valuable benefit or at least not worth the hassle and red tape. Furthermore, experience in the nineteen cities shows that approximately half the clients visit homeless clinics only once. This visit often does not afford the opportunity to convince clients to apply for medical assistance and to help them negotiate the application procedure.

On the other hand, the program must consider the political value of participating in Medicaid. The demonstration of a willingness to utilize the system designed to assure access to health services is significant. It reinforces the nation's commitment to offer medical care for all persons within the existing system. Additionally, there is a value for the client: An individual armed with a Medicaid card is greatly empowered with the ability to choose a provider.

Medicaid has not helped significantly with cash-flow needs of most programs. However, lessons learned in attempting to fight for Medicaid dollars gave programs important experience with the city, county, and state agencies involved in the funding of health care for the poor in their jurisdiction. These early interactions between programs and public agencies proved to be a significant element in long-term funding strategies. More than 50 percent of the program sites ultimately received direct state, county, or city aid to continue their work.

The state of Maryland appropriated six hundred thousand dollars in postfoundation support, and Massachusetts granted one million dollars for the program in Boston. Each was able to show that cost-effective, good-quality health care was being delivered. Programs in Chicago, Albuquerque, Detroit, and San Francisco received specific categorical funds from their states. The majority of the categorical funding went toward mental health services at the street level.

City and county governments also contributed when foundation funding stopped. Baltimore, Chicago, Los Angeles, Maricopa County (Phoenix), San Francisco, and Seattle all helped in meaningful ways, largely for categorical programs.

Comic Relief

In 1985 RWJF was contacted by members of a group that called itself Comic Relief (CR). The idea for Comic Relief originated with Bob Zmuda, a comedy writer and producer who believed that humor, long a source of relief for the stress and burdens of everyday life, could be tapped to help the growing homeless population in the United States. His confidence in the tremendous fund-raising potential inherent in a mobilized comedy community was supported by Chris Albrecht, senior vice-president for Home Box Office (HBO). This union would result in the live, televised Comic Relief benefits on HBO, the nation's largest subscription-television network, along with a host of ancillary fund-raising activities.

Faced with the task of selecting the most direct and cost-effective means of processing funds directly into local areas was Comic Relief Vice-President Dennis Albaugh. Albaugh worked with the Comic Relief Organizing Committee and Board of Directors to determine the means of distribution. Rather than set up a new bureaucracy to handle these monies, the national RWJF/Pew HCHP was the designated recipient, a move unique to celebrity fund-raising endeavors. With the machinery already in place, Comic Relief avoided significant costs and delays associated with developing new systems, and donors could be assured that all monies would be put to practical use as quickly as possible.

March 29, 1986, marked the first gathering of the country's top comedic talent for the benefit concert presentation of "Comic Relief." Hosted by Billy Crystal, Whoopi Goldberg, and Robin Williams, the sellout performance was telecast live on HBO from Los Angeles's Universal Amphitheater. The event proved a spectacular success in raising both funds and awareness for the telecast, with "Comic Relief '87" again bringing together the nation's comedy stars. The program has continued its commitment to the cause of aiding the homeless, and the "Comic Relief III" and "Comic Relief IV" presentations, held on March 18, 1989, and May 12, 1990, respectively again played to sold-out crowds and large television audiences.

Within five months of the original event, an audit was completed, and more than $2.5 million was allocated for services at project sites across the nation; "Comic Relief '87" reaped $2.3 million, "Comic Relief III" raised a record-breaking $5 million in pledges, and "Comic Relief IV" will probably prove even more successful. HBO's multimillion-dollar commitment to cover all production costs and operating expenses has made it possible to channel all pledged and realized dollars directly into services for the homeless. Further, HBO unscrambled its signal during each show's broadcast to allow those with cable in their homes to tune in and assist in the fund-raising efforts via toll-free pledge lines.

While the annual "Comic Relief" benefit concerts serve as the core of the organization's efforts, the commitment for both celebrity spokesmen and CR staff continues year-round. City-by-city fund-raising efforts have established strong relationships across the United States, creating a viable impact that can indeed be felt on the streets. The Cleveland, Albuquerque, Milwaukee, and Boston projects have used CR monies to purchases vans, making staff and client transportation possible in outreach programs. In Nashville, San Antonio, Baltimore, and Boston, funds are used to equip and renovate existing facilities so that medical, dental, and counseling services are made available. CR monies were used to purchase a fully equipped mobile clinic, and Los Angeles, Baltimore, and Cleveland hired homeless persons to work at their project sites, thereby facilitating their mainstream reentry. In Denver, CR funds are responsible for opening the new Homeless/Stout Street Clinic, and across the nation these dollars are at work expanding such services as shelter, shower and laundry facilities, food vouchers, and assistance with security deposits and emergency medicine, as well as other enhanced care services in each location.

CR efforts have fostered a network of regional fund-raising venues through the involvement of comedy clubs in cities across America. This sustained effort can be seen in the strong support for comedy-themed benefits on both a national and a local level, which has created a coalition of entertainers eager to raise funds and awareness for the homeless. Local project directors have now developed ongoing relationships with cable companies, radio stations, and entertainment organizations through which events are produced to broaden the base of support. These relationships were developed via CR involvement and are key to the program's longevity.

Stretching Foundation Dollars

The amount of time and effort used to achieve program sustainment began to take on more intensity in early 1987. It became clear that considering all of the best efforts on obtaining future support, not all the projects might be able to continue existing programs, let alone expand into other areas of need. Even the programs that had been merged into existing public agencies faced cuts. While CR was an important contributor, it was not originally designed or thought of as funder of "core" services or personnel.

It became evident that the nineteen programs were spending the foundation dollars at a rate actually lower than their approved budgets. All the projects were attempting to conserve these funds in order to have them available for extensions after the original end date of the grant, December 31, 1988, was reached. In fact, every program sequestered funds sufficient to cover some program services for at least twelve additional months with foundation money.

The foundations supported this action and, in addition, implemented an unusual action. Pew allowed programs to retain interest monies on funds advanced and not deduct the interest from grant payments. RWJF made prepayment advances that averaged five hundred thousand dollars to allow programs to show their local communities that the major funder had faith in their efforts. Many of the sites were able to leverage the advances into challenge grants in their cities and earn extra interest on those funds as well.

The Stewart B. McKinney Homeless Assistance Act

A FEDERAL RESPONSE

In early 1987 word was obtained about possible federal action to support health care for the homeless programs. Prior to this, federal participation had been minimal, limited to small amounts of agency categorical funding mostly through the Department of Housing and Urban Development in a few locations.

The Stewart B. McKinney Homeless Assistance Act (P.L. 100–77) was passed by Congress and signed by President Reagan in July 1987. The act was a response to the growing problems of homelessness in the United States. It provided for supplemental funding to help provider agencies spanning fifteen different programs operated by six federal agencies to be coordinated by the Interagency Council on the Homeless. In fiscal years 1987–89 approximately seventy-five million dollars was appropriated for health care services. In fiscal year 1990, the figure is about forty-six million dollars, including twelve million dollars in fiscal year 1991 advance funding.

FIRST-YEAR ACCOMPLISHMENTS

The first-year accomplishments of the McKinney-funded HCHP projects were notable. As many as 109 projects served 230,000 homeless persons, compared with a projected goal of 200,000 even though most projects were actually in operation only six to nine months of the first year as the result of the phasing in of activities. More than 783,000 patient encounters, or an average of 3.4 encounters per patient, were recorded, indicating that care provided on the average was more than one-time episodic care. The projects served homeless persons approximately in proportion to the changing demographics of the homeless population. About 40 percent were children and their parent(s) living as a family unit, and homeless/runaway youth. Approximately 60 percent were minorities. Of those served, 56 percent received no public benefits despite their extreme poverty, while 21 percent were reported to receive or be eligible for Medicaid—similar to the percentage found to be eligible for Medicaid by the RWJF/Pew projects. In addition, 6 percent received unemployment compensation, indicating that they had recently been in the job market.

The health needs identified by the McKinney-funded projects in their first year of operation are similar to those identified by the RWJF/Pew projects.

Originally, the McKinney Act was authorized only for 1987 and 1988. However, in recognition of the need and of the burden that homelessness created in urban areas of the country, the Stewart B. McKinney Homeless Assistance Amendments Act of 1988 (P.L. 100–628) was approved by Congress in November 1988. This served to extend the authorization for health care programs for three more years (1989–91).

It is widely known and understood that the model for this federal program was the national HCHP. For the health care portion of the act, the text was drawn from the original RWJF-Pew Request for Proposals of 1984. The nineteen program sites were well prepared by experience and background to apply for McKinney Act grants, and all were successful.

Most McKinney Act programs provided supplemental funding for ongoing federal initiatives for the indigent to enable them to accelerate or upgrade their delivery of services to homeless persons. The act also created a new section (340) of the Public Health Service (PHS) Act for the Primary Health Care and Substance Abuse (Health Services for the Homeless) Program. Responsibility for implementing the program was assigned to the Health Resources and Services Administration's Bureau of Health Care Delivery and Assistance (BHCDA), the same bureau that is responsible for administering the Migrant and Community Health

Centers Program funded under Sections 329 and 330 of the PHS Act. These sections of the PHS Act provide federal support for community-based primary health care centers for the indigent and uninsured, migrant and seasonal farm workers, and rural and urban communities underserved by primary health care providers.

BHCDA's response to the new McKinney indigent health care initiative was swift by bureaucratic standards. The McKinney Act was signed into law in July 1987. Notices of grant awards had been issued to most grantees by January 1, 1988. Approximately 146 organizations requested $83 million in funding to implement health programs for the homeless in their communities. Of the $46 million appropriated by Congress in FY 1987, $44.5 million was awarded to 109 applicants, and the balance utilized for a variety of capacity-building purposes, including training, evaluation, and administration.

Community health centers, the nineteen RWJF/Pew pilot projects, and inner-city hospitals and local pubic health departments succeeded in securing funding to launch new or strengthen their current health care and substance abuse efforts for the homeless. In this first competitive cycle, projects were funded in forty-three states, excluding only Alaska, Arkansas, Delaware, Maine, Montana, Nevada, North Dakota, and Wyoming.

Fifty-seven community health centers served as lead grantee agencies, and another forty-eight served as subcontracting providers for health services to the homeless. By and large, only one grantee was funded in each community, with the exception of New York City, which, because of its size and complexity, received multiple grants. As a result, applications from most areas represented communitywide coalition efforts, with a lead applicant agency and multiple service providers designated to play a role in caring for the homeless in their neighborhoods or in their fields of specialty. In all, 533 health and human services organizations participated in the original 109 McKinney-funded communities, an average of almost 5 providers per community. The participating community health centers represented the single largest provider type as both lead agency and subcontracting providers, but because of the comprehensive, interdisciplinary nature of services required under the McKinney legislation, mental health, substance abuse, and social services organizations usually were also part of the McKinney-funded HCHP provider networks. The RWJF/Pew projects generally assumed the responsibility of lead agency role for McKinney funds in their communities.

ROLE OF THE NATIONAL ASSOCIATION OF COMMUNITY HEALTH CENTERS

Implementation of the McKinney HCHP was facilitated by the role played by the National Association of Community Health Centers (NACHC), a Washington-based membership association founded in 1970 to promote comprehensive, high-quality health care for the indigent. NACHC recognized that a large number of its community health center members would receive funding through the McKinney Act to extend or enhance their primary health care and substance abuse services for the homeless. NACHC also realized that although its members were experienced primary health care providers, the centers would need orientation to the requirements of the McKinney Act, training around the issues involved in the substantial amount of subcontracting to be involved, and exposure to the most effective models for staffing and delivery of care to the homeless.

In addition to training, NACHC played a leadership role in attempting to develop a strong national network of HCHP providers. The objective here was to have input into federal administrative policies affecting the programs and to provide feedback from the field to Congress on the health problems of the homeless and needed changes in legislation.

FUTURE LEGISLATIVE PROSPECTS

A McKinney Act reauthorization bill was passed in November 1988, extending the HCHP for three more years (1989–91) at increased authorization levels and incorporating needed revisions. Furthermore, the program's prospects received a boost when the Bush administration budget requested Congress in January 1989 to provide full funding for all of the McKinney Act programs, including $63.6 million for FY 1990 for health services. Support from the incoming Bush administration for homeless assistance programs represented a significant reversal of the Reagan administration's position on the McKinney programs. The Reagan administration had requested only $15 million in FY 1990 appropriations for the HCHP, a funding level that would have resulted in dismantling two-thirds of the 109 HCHP projects established in 1988 and termination of health services to the more than 165,000 homeless patients who had just gained access to health care. While the new administration's support for the HCHP was a positive sign, the FY 1990 budget request at the same time called for an overall $21 billion reduction in nondefense spending, without specifying exactly which domestic programs would be reduced. As a result, even through the McKinney HCHP received administration support, it would still have to compete in FY 1990 in a very tight budget climate for reduced appropriations for domestic programs. Thus, considering the federal budget deficit problem, the struggle for sufficient appropriations in FY 1990 to stabilize funding for the HCHP would prove to be difficult despite the administration's support. As of May 1990, this projection remained accurate.

Conclusion

The burden of obtaining long-term financial support has been the responsibility of project directors and their board members. That all nineteen RWJF/Pew programs succeeded in graduating from dependence on foundation demonstration funds is noteworthy. It is clear that the programs are perceived as conducting valuable services within their own communities and as legitimate, honest (past experiences in San Antonio noted) recipients of government and philanthropic funds.

Lessons may be learned from this broad experience. Each program in its own way managed to handle local concerns, develop a legitimacy, carry out needed functions under the intense scrutiny of neighboring citizens and agencies, and capture political support. Each proved as well to be an effective demonstration of

Table 26.1 FUTURE SUSTAINMENT RESOURCES: HEALTH CARE FOR THE HOMELESS PROGRAM

(December 31, 1988)

CITY	MCKINNEY	COMIC RELIEF	FOUNDA-TION ROLLOVER	UNITED WAY	STATE REVENUES	LOCAL REVENUES	MEDICAID BILLING	FUND RAISING	GRANTS	OTHER
Albuquerque	yes	yes	yes	?	?	?	no	yes	yes	
Baltimore	yes	yes	yes	no	yes	no	yes	yes	yes	
Birmingham	yes	yes	yes	yes	no	yes	no	yes	yes	
Boston	yes	yes	yes	?	yes	no	?	yes	yes	*
Chicago	yes	yes	yes	no	?	no	no	yes	yes	
Cleveland	yes	yes	yes	no	yes	no	no	yes	yes	
Denver	yes	yes	yes	no	no	no	no	yes	yes	
Detroit	yes	yes	yes	no	yes	no	yes	no	yes	†
Los Angeles	yes	yes	yes	no	no	no	no	yes	yes	
Milwaukee	yes	yes	yes	no	yes	?	no	yes	yes	
Nashville	yes	yes	no	yes	yes	yes	yes	yes	yes	
New York City	yes	yes	no	?	no	no	yes	yes	yes	
Newark	yes	yes	yes	no	no	no	yes	yes	yes	
Philadelphia	yes	yes	yes	no	no	no	no	yes	yes	
Phoenix	yes	yes	yes	no	yes	no	yes	yes	yes	‡
San Antonio	yes	yes	yes	yes	no	no	no	yes	yes	
San Francisco	yes	yes	yes	no	no	yes	no	yes	yes	
Seattle	yes	yes	yes	no	no	yes	no	yes	yes	
Washington, D.C.	yes	yes	yes	no	no	yes	yes	yes	yes	

* Corporate sponsors.

† Federal community health center funds.

‡ ACHHS (Medicaid).

service and probity which made outside funders comfortable in providing support. Perhaps the ultimate evidence of the program's standing is its enshrinement in federal legislation through the McKinney Act.

Table 26.1, drawn up at the end of December 1988, when the original four years of foundation funding ceased, summarizes the state of long-term stability of the nineteen projects. The diversity of support is of particular interest.

The programs must remain ever-vigilant to secure funding, use it well, and account for it, but the initial objective of a secure advance into postfoundation life and self-sustainment has been achieved by all.

Notes

1. Health Care for Homeless Persons:
Creation and Implementation of a Program

1. J. B. Reuler, "Health Care for the Homeless in a National Health Program," *American Journal of Public Health* 79, no. 8 (August 1989): 1033–35.
2. F. Earls, L. N. Robins, A. R. Stiffman, and J. Powell, "Comprehensive Health Care for High-Risk Adolescents: An Evaluation Study," *American Journal of Public Health* 79, no. 8 (August 1989): 999–1005.
3. C. Martinez-Weber, "The Homeless Person with Diabetes: A Diagnostic and Therapeutic Challenge," *Postgraduate Medicine* 81, no. 1 (January 1987): 289–93, 296, 298.
4. Council on Scientific Affairs, "Health Care Needs of Homeless and Runaway Youths," *Journal of the American Medical Association* 262, no. 10 (September 8, 1989): 1358–61.
5. E. Luder, E. Boey, B. Buchalter, and C. Martinez-Weber, "Assessment of the Nutritional Status of Urban Homeless Adults," *Public Health Reports* 104, no. 5 (September–October 1989): 451–57.
6. L. Gelberg and L. S. Linn, "Assessing the Physical Health of Homeless Adults," *Journal of the American Medical Association* 262, no. 14 (October 13, 1989): 1973–79.
7. P. W. Brickner, B. C. Scanlan, B. Conanan, A. Elvy, J. McAdam, L. K. Scharer, and W. J. Vicic, "Homeless Persons and Health Care," *Annals of Internal Medicine* 104 (1986): 405–9.
8. W. R. Breakey, P. J. Fischer, M. Kramer, G. Nestadt, A. J. Romanoski, A. Ross, R. M. Royall, and O. C. Stine, "Health and Mental Health Problems of Homeless Men and Women in Baltimore," *Journal of the American Medical Association* 262, no. 10 (September 8, 1989): 1352–57.
9. R. H. Ropers and R. Boyer, "Perceived Health Status Among the New Urban Homeless," *Social Science Medicine* 24, no. 8 (1987): 669–78.
10. National Ambulatory Medical Care Survey, United States, 1979 Summary. Public Health Service, National Center for Health Statistics, Hyattsville, Md., 1982, series 13, no. 66.
11. P. W. Brickner, "Health Issues in the Care of the Homeless," in *Health Care of Homeless People,* ed. P. W. Brickner, L. K. Sharer, B. Conanan, A. Elvy, and M. Savarese (New York: Springer, 1985).
12. J. D. Wright and E. Weber, *Homelessness and Health* (Washington, D.C.: McGraw-Hill, 1987).
13. J. D. Wright, *Address Unknown: The Homeless in America* (New York: Aldine de Gruyter, 1989).
14. T. L. Savitt, "Slave Health," in *Disease and*

Distinctiveness in the American South, ed. T. L. Savitt and J. H. Young (Knoxville: University of Tennessee Press, 1988).

15. M. Morgan, *Skid Road: An Informal Portrait of Seattle* (New York: Viking Press, 1962).

16. J. D. Wright et al., "Health and Homelessness in New York City," Research report to the Robert Wood Johnson Foundation, January 1985. SADRI, University of Massachusetts, Amherst 01003.

17. L. U. Blumberg, T. E. Shipley, Jr., and J. D. Moor, Jr., "The Skid Row Man and the Skid Row Status Community," *Quarterly Journal of Studies in Alcoholism* 32 (1971): 909–41.

18. J. Erickson and C. Wilhelm, "Introduction," in *Housing the Homeless,* ed. J. Erickson and C. Wilhelm (New Brunswick: Center for Urban Policy Research, Rutgers University, 1986): xix–xxxvii.

19. R. Reich and L. Siegel, "The Emergence of the Bowery as a Psychiatric Dumping Ground," *Psychiatric Quarterly* 50, no. 3 (1973): 191–201.

20. J. D. Wright, P. H. Rossi, J. W. Knight, et al., "Health and Homelessness." Amherst, University of Massachusetts, 1985, 1–97.

21. S. J. J. Freeman, A. Formo, A. G. Alampur, and A. F. Sommers, "Psychiatric Disorders in a Skid-Row Mission Population," *Comprehensive Psychiatry* 20, no. 5 (1979): 454–62.

22. H. R. Lamb, "Deinstitutionalization and the Homeless Mentally Ill," in *The Homeless Mentally Ill,* ed. H. R. Lamb (Washington, D.C.: American Psychiatric Association, 1984): 55–74.

23. H. H. Goldman and J. P. Morrissey, "The Alchemy of Mental Health Policy: Homelessness and the Fourth Cycle of Reform," *American Journal of Public Health* 75, no. 7 (1985): 727–31.

24. S. P. Segal and U. Aviram, *The Mentally Ill in Community-Based Sheltered Care: A Study of Community Care and Social Integration* (New York: John Wiley, 1978).

25. E. Baxter and K. Hopper, *Private Lives / Public Spaces: Homeless Adults on the Streets of New York City* (New York: Community Service Society, 1981).

26. R. W. Redick and M. J. Witkin, *State and County Mental Hospitals, United States, 1979–80 and 1980–81.* Mental Health Statistical Note No. 165 (Rockville, Md.: National Institute of Mental Health, August 1983).

27. H. H. Goldman, N. H. Adams, and C. A. Taube, "Deinstitutionalization: The Data Demythologized," *Hospital and Community Psychiatry* 34 (1983): 129–32.

28. A. A. Arce and M. J. Vergare, "Homelessness, the Chronic Mentally Ill and Community Mental Health Centers," *Community Mental Health Journal* 23 (1987): 242–49.

29. Reports to the Robert Wood Johnson Foundation from Health Care for the Homeless Program sites.

30. E. Baxter and K. Hopper, "The New Mendicancy: Homeless in New York City," *American Journal of Orthopsychiatry* 52, no. 3 (July 1982): 393–408.

31. C. Marwick, "The 'Sizable' Homeless Population: A Growing Challenge for Medicine," *Journal of the American Medical Association* 253, no. 22 (1985): 3217–25.

32. D. Lamm and L. Reyes, eds., "Health Care for the Homeless: A 40-City Review." Washington, D.C., United States Conference of Mayors, April 1985.

33. R. Pear, "Economic Recovery Is Seen as Bypassing at Least 10 Million," *New York Times,* March 16, 1986.

34. L. Uchitelle, "Recession Fears Are Growing," *New York Times,* July 7, 1989: B1.

35. Z. Kolbert, "Single-Room-Occupancy Housing May Be Demolished, Court Rules," *New York Times,* July 7, 1989: B1.

36. S. Crystal, "The Homeless Elderly," Department of Community and Family Medicine, School of Medicine, UCSD, M-022, La Jolla, CA 92093, June 1986.

37. National Network for Runaway and Homeless Youth, Washington, D.C.

38. Council on Scientific Affairs, American Medical Association, "Health Care Needs of Homeless and Runaway Youth," *Journal of the American Medical Association* 262, no. 10 (September 8, 1989): 1358–661; and J. C. Barden, "Strife in Families Swells Tide of Homeless Youth," *New York Times,* February 5, 1990: A1 and B8.

39. S. Crystal, "Psychosocial Rehabilitation of Homeless Youth," Department of Community and Family Medicine, School of Medicine, UCSD, M-022, La Jolla, CA 92093, January 1986.

40. J. Kelly, personal communication, October 1983.

41. K. McBride and R. J. Mulcare, "Peripheral Vascular Disease in the Homeless," in *Health Care of Homeless People* loc. cit.: 121–28.

42. Allerton Hotel data, available from the Department of Community Medicine, St. Vincent's Hospital and Medical Center, New York City.

43. E. A. Kutza, "A Study of Undomiciled Elderly Persons in Chicago: A Final Report," School of Social Service Administration, University of Chicago, October 1987.

44. L. K. Scharer, A. Berson, and P. W. Brickner, "Lack of Housing and Its Impact on Human Health: A Service Perspective," *Bulletin of the New York Academy of Medicine* (in press).

45. A. Elvy, "Access to Care," in *Health Care of Homeless People,* loc. cit.

46. L. K. Scharer and B. Price, "Working with Hospitals," in ibid.

47. D. Hilfiker, "Are We Comfortable with Homelessness?" *Journal of the American Medical Association* 262, no. 10 (September 8, 1989): 1375–76.

48. C. I. Cohen and J. Sokolovsky, "Old Men of the Bowery," *Strategies for Survival Among the Homeless* (New York: Guilford Press, 1989).

2. The Health of Homeless People: Evidence from the National Health Care for the Homeless Program

1. J. D. Wright, "The 'Health Care for the Homeless' Program: Evaluation Design and Preliminary Results," presented at American Public Health Association meetings, 1985.

2. J. D. Wright and E. Weber, *Homelessness and Health* (Washington, D.C.: McGraw-Hill, 1987).

3. Committee on Health Care for Homeless People, *Homelessness, Health, and Human Needs* (Washington, D.C.: National Academy Press, 1988).

4. P. W. Brickner, L. K. Scharer, B. Conanan, A. Elvy, and M. Savarese, eds., *Health Care of Homeless People* (New York: Springer, 1985).

5. J. D. Wright, P. H. Rossi, J. W. Knight, et al., "Homelessness and Health: Effects of Lifestyle on Physical Well-being Among Homeless People in New York City," in *Research in Social Problems and Public Policy*, vol. 4, ed. M. Lewis and J. Miller (Greenwich, Ct.: JAI Press, 1987): 41–72.

6. P. H. Rossi, J. D. Wright, G. Fisher, and G. Willis, "The Urban Homeless: Estimating Composition and Size," *Science* 235 (1987): 1336–41.

7. P. H. Rossi and J. D. Wright, "The Determinants of Homelessness," *Health Affairs* 6 (1987): 19–32.

8. P. H. Rossi and J. D. Wright, "The Urban Homeless: A Portrait of Urban Dislocation," *Annals of the American Academy of Political and Social Science* 501 (1989): 132–42.

9. J. D. Wright, J. W. Knight, E. Weber, and J. Lam, "Ailments and Alcohol: Health Status Among the Drinking Homeless," *Alcohol Health and Research World* 11 (1987): 22–27.

10. J. D. Wright and J. W. Knight, "Alcohol Abuse in the National 'Health Care for the Homeless' Client Population," Washington, D.C.: National Institute on Alcohol Abuse and Alcoholism, 1987.

11. V. Mulkern and R. Spence, "Alcohol Abuse / Alcoholism Among Homeless Persons: A Review of the Literature," Washington, D.C.: National Institute on Alcohol Abuse and Alcoholism, 1984.

12. P. Archard, *Vagrancy, Alcoholism and Social Control* (London: Macmillan, 1979).

13. P. Koegel and A. Burnam, "Traditional and Non-traditional Homeless Alcoholics," *Alcohol Health and Research World* 11 (1987): 28–34.

14. J. D. Wright, "The Mentally Ill Homeless: What Is Myth and What Is Fact?" *Social Problems* 35 (1988): 182–91.

15. L. Bachrach, *The Homeless Mentally Ill & Mental Health Services: An Analytical Review of the Literature*. Alcohol, Drug Abuse and Mental Health Administration, U.S. Department of Health and Human Services, 1984.

16. L. Bachrach, "Interpreting Research on the Homeless Mentally Ill: Some Caveats," *Hospital and Community Psychiatry* 35 (1984): 914–16.

17. J. F. L. Ball and B. E. Havassy, "A Survey of the Problems and Needs of Homeless Consumers of Acute Psychiatric Services," *Hospital and Community Psychiatry* 35 (1984): 917–21.

18. E. Bassuk, "The Homeless Problem," *Scientific American* 215 (1984): 40–45.

19. N. Cohen, J. Putnam, and A. Sullivan, "The Mentally Ill Homeless: Isolation and Adaptation," *Hospital and Community Psychiatry* 35 (1984): 922–24.

20. H. R. Lamb, "Deinstitutionalization and the Homeless Mentally Ill," *Hospital and Community Psychiatry* 35 (1984): 899–907.

21. S. Segal, J. Baumohl, and E. Johnson, "Falling Through the Cracks: Mental Disorders and Social Margin in a Young Vagrant Population," *Social Problems* (1977): 387–400.

22. S. Crystal and M. Goldstein, *Correlates of Shelter Utilization: One-Day Study* (New York: Human Resources Administration, 1984).

23. R. Ropers, M. Robertson, and R. Boyer, *The Homeless of Los Angeles County: An Empirical Evaluation* (Los Angeles: UCLA, Basic Research Project, Document No. 4, 1985).

24. C. Marwick, "The 'Sizable' Homeless Population: A Growing Challenge for Medicine," *Journal of the American Medical Association* 253 (1985): 3217–25.

25. D. Lamm and L. Reyes, eds., "Health Care for the Homeless: A 40-City Review," Washington, D.C.: United States Conference of Mayors, 1985.

26. J. Wright and P. W. Brickner, "The Health Status of the Homeless: Diverse People, Diverse Problems, Diverse Needs," presented at the American Public Health Association meeting, 1985.

27. A. Elvy, "Access to Care," in *Health Care of Homeless People*, loc. cit.: 223–31.

28. H. Freeman, R. Blendon, L. Aiken, S. Sudman, C. Mullinix, and C. Corey, "Americans Report on Their Access to Health Care," *Health Affairs* 6 (1987): 6–18.

29. J. D. Wright, "The Worthy and Unworthy Homeless," *Society* 25 (1988): 64–69.

30. J. W. Knight and J. Lam, *Homelessness and Health: A Review of the Literature* (Amherst, MA: SADRI, 1986).

31. J. Lam, "Homeless Women in America: Their Social and Health Characteristics," Ph.D. thesis, University of Massachusetts, 1987.

32. F. S. Redburn and T. F. Buss, *Responding to America's Homeless* (New York: Praeger, 1986).

33. M. Stoner, "The Plight of Homeless Women," *Social Service Review* (1983): 565–81.

34. J. D. Wright and E. Weber, "Determinants of Benefit-Program Participation Among the Urban Homeless: Results from a 16-City

Study," *Evaluation Review* 12 (1988): 376–95.

35. R. Moore and F. Malitz, "Underdiagnosis of Alcoholism by Residents in an Ambulatory Medical Practice," *Journal of Medical Education* 61 (1986): 46–52.

36. N. Fisk, "Epidemiology of Alcohol Abuse and Alcoholism," *Alcohol Health and Research World* 9 (1984): 4–7.

37. M. Shepherd et al., *Psychiatric Illness in General Practice* (London: Oxford, 1966).

38. N. Briggs, "Mental Health and Homelessness," Ph.D. thesis, University of Massachusetts, 1988.

39. J. D. Wright, *Selected Topics in the Health Status of America's Homeless* (Washington, D.C.: Institute of Medicine, National Academy of Science, 1987).

40. National Ambulatory Medical Care Survey, United States, 1979 Summary. Public Health Service, National Center for Health Statistics. Hyattsville, Md., 1982, series 13, no. 66.

41. F. R. Kellogg, O. Piantieri, B. Conanan, P. Doherty, W. J. Vicic, and P. W. Brickner, "Hypertension: A Screening and Treatment Program for the Homeless," in *Health Care of Homeless People,* loc. cit.: 109–19.

42. K. McBride and R. Mulcare, "Peripheral Vascular Disease Among the Homeless," ibid.: 121–29.

43. J. Wright, "Homelessness Is Not Healthy for Children and Other Living Things," *Journal of Children and Youth Services* (forthcoming).

44. J. W. Curran, H. W. Jaffe, A. M. Hardy, W. M. Morgan, R. M. Selik, and T. J. Don-

dero, "Epidemiology of HIV Infection and AIDS in the United States," *Science* 239 (1988): 610–16.

45. Centers for Disease Control, *Morbidity and Mortality Weekly Report* 36 (1987): 524–25.

46. C. Norman, "Sex and Needles, Not Insects and Pigs, Spread AIDS in Florida Town," *Science* 234 (1986): 415–17.

47. Centers for Disease Control, *Morbidity and Mortality Weekly Report* 34 (1984): 299–305.

48. J. McAdam, P. W. Brickner, R. Glicksman, D. Edwards, B. Fallon, and P. Yanowitch, "Tuberculosis in the SRO/Homeless Population," in *Health Care of Homeless People,* loc. cit.: 155–75.

49. Centers for Disease Control, *Morbidity and Mortality Weekly Report* 34 (1985).

50. Centers for Disease Control, *Morbidity and Mortality Weekly Report* 34 (1985): 40.

51. T. P. Gross and M. L. Rosenberg, "Shelters for Battered Women and Their Children: An Under-recognized Source of Communicable Disease Transmission," *American Journal of Public Health* 77 (1987): 1198–201.

52. "Tracking the Homeless," *Focus* 10 (1987): 20–24.

53. P. H. Rossi, *Without Shelter: Homelessness in the 1980s* (New York: Priority, 1989).

54. J. D. Wright, "Poverty, Homelessness, Health, Nutrition, and Children," presented at National Conference on Homeless Children and Youth, Washington, 1989.

55. D. Altman, E. L. Bassuk, W. R. Breakey, et al., "Health Care for the Homeless," *Society* 26 (1989): 4–5.

3. Overcoming Troubled Relationships Between Programs and the Community

1. R. Meister, personal communication.
2. *Nashville Banner,* July 17, 1987: 1.
3. Nashville Mayor Bill Boner, letter to members of the Metropolitan Council, *Tennessean,* April 1, 1988.

4. Slouching Toward Chaos: American Health Policy and the Homeless

1. Committee on Health Care for Homeless People, Institute of Medicine, *Homelessness, Health, and Human Needs* (Washington, D.C.: National Academy Press, 1988).

2. Boston Foundation, *Homelessness: Critical Issues for Policy and Practice* (Boston: Boston Foundation, 1987).

3. J. D. Wright and E. Weber, *Homelessness and Health* (Washington, D. C.: McGraw-Hill, 1987).

4. T. S. Kuhn, *The Structure of Scientific Revolutions,* 2d. ed., enlarged (Chicago; University of Chicago Press, 1970).

5. A. Koestler, *The Ghost in the Machine* (Chicago: Henry Regnery, 1967).

6. B. Ehrenreich and J. Ehrenreich, *The American Health Empire: Power, Profits, and Politics* (New York: Random House, 1970).

7. K. J. Mueller, "The Role of Policy Analysis in Agenda Setting: Applications to the Problem of Indigent Health Care in the United States," *Policy Studies Journal* 16 (1988): 441–53.

8. J. Morris, *Searching for a Cure* National Health Policy Reconsidered (Washington, D.C.: Berkley Morgan, 1984).

9. J. L. Locher, ed., *The World of M. C. Escher* (New York: Abrams, 1984).

10. P. A. Butler, *Too Poor to Be Sick: Access to Medical Care for the Uninsured* (Washington, D.C.: American Public Health Association, 1988).

11. M. B. Sulvetta and K. Swartz, *The Uninsured and Uncompensated Care: A Chartbook* (Washington, D.C.: National Health Policy Forum, 1986).

12. Task Force on Health Care of the Poor, *No Room in the Marketplace: The Health Care of the Poor* (St. Louis: Catholic Health Association, 1986).

13. C. E. Rosenberg, *The Care of Strangers: The Rise of America's Hospital System* (New York: Basic Books, 1987).

14. M. Foucault, *The Birth of the Clinic: An Archeology of Medical Perception* (New York: Pantheon, 1982).

15. J. Hadley, *More Medical Care, Better Health?: An Economic Analysis of Mortality Rates* (Washington, D.C.: Urban Institute, 1982).

16. K. R. Levit and M. S. Freeland, "National Medical Care Spending," *Health Affairs (Millwood)* 7 (1988): 124–36.

17. I. Frazer, T. A. Granatis, and E. A. Pryga, *Medical Indigence: Definitions, Scope, and Consequences of the Problem* (Washington, D.C.: American Hospital Association, 1985).

18. S. Mulstein, "The Uninsured and the Financing of Uncompensated Care: Scope, Costs, and Policy Options," *Inquiry* 21 (1984): 214–29.

19. J. Feder, J. Hadley, and R. Mullner, "Falling Through the Cracks: Poverty Insurance Coverage and Hospital Care for the Poor, 1980 and 1982," *Millbank Memorial Fund Quarterly* 62 (1982): 544–66.

20. G. R. Wilensky, "Solving Uncompensated Hospital Care," *Health Affairs (Millwood)* 3 (1984): 50–62.

21. Robert Wood Johnson Foundation, *Access to Medical Care in the United States: Results of a 1986 Survey* (Princeton, N.J.: Robert Wood Johnson Foundation, 1987).

22. H. E. Freeman, R. J. Blendon, L. H. Aiken, S. Sudman, C. F. Mullinex, and C. R. Corey, "Americans Report on Their Access to Care," *Health Affairs (Millwood)* 6 (1987): 6–18.

23. G. D. Lundberg and L. Bodine, "Fifty Hours for the Poor," *Journal of the American Medical Association* 258 (1987): 3157.

24. K. Davis and D. Rowland, "Uninsured and Underserved: Inequities in Health Care in the United States," *Millbank Memorial Fund Quarterly* 6 (1983): 149–76.

25. G. Bazzoli, "Health Care for the Indigent: Overview of Critical Issues," *Health Services Research* 21 (1986): 353–93.

26. D. L. Patrick, J. Stein, M. Porta, C. Q. Porter, and T. C. Ricketts, "Poverty, Health Services, and Health Status in Rural America," *Millbank Memorial Fund Quarterly* 66 (1986): 105–36.

27. M. E. Moyer, "A Revised Look at the Number of Uninsured Americans," *Health Affairs (Millwood)* 8 (1989): 102–10.

28. P. J. Farley, "Who Are the Underinsured?" *Millbank Memorial Fund Quarterly* 63 (1985): 476–503.

29. M. C. Berc and G. R. Wilensky, *Health Care of the Working Poor* (Anaheim, CA: American Public Health Association, November 13, 1984).

30. M. E. Guy, J. Alexander, J. Bronstein, C. Hale, J. Roseman, and G. Stowers, *Why Employers Choose Not to Offer Health In-* *surance* (Portland: American Society for Public Administration, April 17, 1988).

31. National Health Care Campaign, *Facing Facts: A Statistical Profile of Health Care in the United States* (Washington, D.C.: National Health Care Campaign, 1986).

32. R. J. Blendon, L. H. Aiken, H. E. Freeman, and C. R. Corey, "Access to Medical Care for Black and White Americans: A Matter of Growing Concern," *Journal of the American Medical Association* 261 (1989): 278–81.

33. M. O. Mundinger, "Health Service Funding Cuts and the Declining Health of the Poor," *New England Journal of Medicine* 312 (1985): 44–46.

34. N. Lurie, N. B. Ward, M. F. Shapiro, C. Gallego, R. Vaghaiwalla, and R. H. Brook, "Termination of Medi-Cal: Does It Affect Health?" *New England Journal of Medicine* 311 (1984): 480–84.

35. N. Lurie, N. B. Ward, M. F. Shapiro, and R. H. Brook, "Termination of Medi-Cal Benefits: A Follow-up Study One Year Later," *New England Journal of Medicine* 314 (1986): 1266–68.

36. C. C. Korenbrot, "Risk Reduction in Pregnancies of Low-Income Women," *Mobius* 1 (1984): 36–43.

37. A. Castaner, B. E. Simmons, M. Mar, and R. Cooper, "Myocardial Infarction Among Black Patients: Poor Prognosis After Hospital Discharge," *Annals of Internal Medicine* 109 (1988): 33–35.

38. S. Woolhandler and D. U. Himmelstein, "Reverse Targeting of Preventive Care Due to Lack of Health Insurance," *Journal of American Medical Association* 259 (1989): 2872–75.

39. B. V. Aiken, L. Rucker, F. A. Hubbell, R. W. Cugan, and H. Waitzkin, "Access to Medical Care in a Medically Indigent Population," *Journal of General Internal Medicine* 4 (1989): 216–20.

40. I. Shapiro and R. Greenstein, *Holes in the Safety Nets: Poverty Programs and Policies in the States* (Washington, D.C.: Center on Budget and Policy Priorities, 1988).

41. American Hospital Association, *Promoting Health Insurance in the Workplace: State and Local Initiatives to Increase Private Coverage* (Chicago: American Hospital Association, 1988).

42. *Access to Health Care: The New Jersey Uncompensated Care Trust Fund*. New Jersey Department of Health, 1988.

43. R. Desonia and K. M. King, *State Programs of Assistance to the Medically Indigent* (Washington, D.C.: George Washington University, Intergovernmental Health Policy Project, 1985).

44. D. J. Lipson, "The Massachusetts Health Security Act Draws Reaction from Across the Nation," *State Health Notes* no. 82 (1988): 4–5.

45. C. M. McCarthy, "Financing Indigent Care: Short- and Long-range Strategies," *Journal of the American Medical Association* 259 (1988): 75.

46. J. Wolfson, P. J. Levin, and W. J. Brock,

"Linking Health Care to the Poor to Health Care for Profit," *Health Affairs (Millwood)* 6 (1987): 129–35.

47. G. R. Wilensky, "Public, Private Options to Cover Uninsured Workers," *Business and Health* (January 1987): 42–43.

48. S. A. Freedman, B. R. Klepper, R. P. Duncan, and S. P. Bell, "Coverage of the Uninsured and Underinsured: A Proposal for School Enrollment-Based Family Health Insurance." *New England Journal of Medicine* 318 (1988): 843–47.

49. A. S. Relman, "Universal Health Insurance: Its Time Has Come," *New England Journal of Medicine* 320 (1989): 117–18.

50. S. Woolhandler and D. U. Himmelstein, "Resolving the Cost / Access Problem: The Case for a National Health Program," *Journal of General Internal Medicine* 4 (1989): 54–60.

51. President's Commission for the Study of Ethical Problems in Medical and Biomedical and Behavioral Research, *Securing Access to Health Care: A Report on the Ethical Implications of Differences in the Availability of Health Services,* vol. 1 (Washington, D.C.: Government Printing Office, 1983).

52. D. Mechanic, "Health Care for the Poor: Some Policy Alternatives," *Journal of Family Practice* 22 (1986): 282–89.

53. V. W. Sidel and R. Sidel, *A Healthy State: An International Perspective on the Crisis in United States Medical Care* (New York: Pantheon Books, 1983).

54. H. Waitzkin, *The Second Sickness: Contradictions of Capitalist Health Care* (New York: Free Press, 1983).

55. A. L. Schorr, *Common Decency: Domestic Policies After Reagan* (New Haven: Yale University Press, 1986).

56. Ad Hoc Committee on Medicaid, *The Final Report of the Ad Hoc Committee on Medicaid. Including the Poor* (Chicago: American Medical Association, 1989).

57. S. Woolhandler and D. U. Himmelstein, "Free Care: A Quantitative Analysis of Health and Costs Effects of a National Health Program for the United States," *International Journal of Health Science* 18 (1988): 393–400.

58. U. E. Reinhardt, "Health Insurance for the Nation's Poor," *Health Affairs (Millwood)* 6 (1987): 101–12.

59. F. Mullan, "Poor People, Poor Policy," *Health Affairs (Millwood)* 6 (1987): 113–17.

60. G. R. Wilensky, "Viable Strategies for Dealing with the Uninsured," *Health Affairs (Millwood)* 6 (1987): 33–46.

61. D. U. Himmelstein and S. Woolhandler, "A National Health Program for the United States: A Physicians' Proposal," *New England Journal of Medicine* 320 (1989): 102–8.

62. H. M. Stevenson, A. P. Williams, and E. Vayda, "Medical Politics and Canadian Medicare: Professional Response to the Canadian Health Act," *Millbank Memorial Fund Quarterly* 66 (1988): 65–104.

63. A. Enthoven and R. Kronick, "A Consumers-Choice Health Plan for the 1990's," *New England Journal of Medicine* 320 (1988): 29–37, 94–101.

64. National Leadership Commission on Health Care, *For the Health of a Nation: A Shared Responsibility* (Ann Arbor: Health Administration Press, 1989).

65. Committee for National Health Insurance, *The Health Security Partnership: An Equitable and Universal National Health Plan* (Washington, D.C.: Health Security Action Council, 1989).

66. V. Navarro, "The Rediscovery of the National Health Programs by the Democratic Party of the United States: A Chronicle of the Jesse Jackson 1988 Campaign," *International Journal of Health Services* 19 (1989): 1–18.

67. National Association for Public Health Policy, *A Progressive Proposal for a National Health Care System* (Burlington, VT: National Association for Public Health Policy, 1989).

68. Vanderbilt Institute for Public Policy Studies, *Covering the Uninsured: How Much Would It Cost?* (Nashville: Vanderbilt University, 1986).

69. K. E. Thorpe, J. E. Siegel, and T. Dailey, "Including the Poor: The Fiscal Impacts of Medicaid Expansion," *Journal of the American Medical Association* 261 (1989): 1003–7.

70. P. W. Brickner, L. K. Scharer, B. Conanan, A. Elvy, and M. Savarese, eds., *Health Care of Homeless People* (New York: Springer, 1985).

71. J. K. Ingelhart, "Medical Care of the Poor: A Growing Problem" *New England Journal of Medicine* 313 (1985): 59–63.

72. E. Ginsberg, "Medical Care for the Poor: No Magic Bullets," *Journal of the American Medical Association* 259 (1988): 3309–11.

73. R. H. Brook, "Practice Guidelines and Practicing Medicine," *Journal of the American Medical Association* 262 (1989): 3027–30.

5. Creation and Evolution of a National Health Care for the Homeless Program

1. Robert Wood Johnson Foundation / Pew Memorial Trust Health Care for the Homeless Program, "Request for Proposals," 1984.

2. United States Conference of Mayors, "The Continued Growth of Hunger, Homelessness and Poverty in America's Cities: 1986" (Washington, D.C.: December 1986).

3. United States Conference of Mayors, "The Continued Growth of Hunger, Homelessness and Poverty in America's Cities: 1987" (Washington, D.C.: December 1987).

4. United States Conference of Mayors, "A Status Report on the Stewart B. McKinney Homeless Assistance Act of 1987" (Washington, D.C.: June 1988).

5. United States Conference of Mayors, "A Sta-

tus Report on Hunger and Homelessness in America's Cities: 1988" (Washington, D.C.: January 1989).
6. L. Corcoran, "Report Prepared for the Albuquerque Health Care for the Homeless Program," 1985.
7. City of Denver grant application to the Robert

Wood Johnson Foundation, 1984.
8. Nashville Metropolitan Government grant application to the Robert Wood Johnson Foundation, 1984.
9. City of San Antonio grant application to the Robert Wood Johnson Foundation, 1984.

6. Clinical Concerns in the Care of Homeless Persons

1. E. Baxter and K. Hopper, "The New Mendicancy: Homeless in New York City," *American Journal of Orthopsychiatry* 52, no. 3 (1982): 393–408.
2. J. D. Wright, "Homelessness Is Not Healthy for Children and Other Living Things," *Journal of Children and Youth Services* (forthcoming).
3. J. D. Wright and E. Weber, *Homelessness and Health* (Washington, D.C.: McGraw-Hill, 1987).
4. J. D. Wright, P. H. Rossi, J. W. Knight, E. Weber-Burdin, R. C. Tessler, C. E. Stewart, M. Geronimo, and J. Lam, *Health and Homelessness* (Amherst, MA: SADRI, 1985): 1–97.
5. J. D. Wright, *An Analysis of the Health Status of a Sample of Homeless People Receiving Care Through the Department of Community Medicine, St. Vincent's Hospital and Medical Center of New York City: 1969–1984* (Amherst, MA: SADRI, 1985).
6. J. T. Kelly, "Trauma: With the Example of San Francisco's Shelter Programs," in *Health Care of Homeless People,* ed. P. W. Brickner, L. K. Scharer, B. Conanan, A. Elvy, and M. Savarese (New York: Springer, 1985).
7. See Chapter 16.
8. C. H. Alstrom, R. Lindelius, and I. Salum, "Mortality Among Homeless Men," *British Journal of Addiction* 70 (1975): 245–52.
9. P. W. Brickner, D. Greenbaum, A. Kaufman, F. O'Donnell, J. T. O'Brian, R. Scalice, J. Scandizzo, and T. Sullivan, "A Clinic for Male Derelicts: A Welfare Hotel Project," *Annals of Internal Medicine* 77 (1972): 565–69.
10. K. McBride and R. J. Mulcare, "Peripheral

Vascular Disease in the Homeless," in *Health Care of Homeless People,* loc. cit.: 121–29.
11. See Chapter 26.
12. P. Webb, "Disorders Due to Heat and Cold," in *Cecil Textbook of Medicine,* 15th ed., P. B. Beeson, W. McDermott, and J. B. Wyngarden, eds., (Philadelphia: W. B. Saunders, 1979): 84–86.
13. L. R. Goldfrank, "Exposure: Thermoregulatory Disorders in the Homeless Patient," in *Health Care of Homeless People,* loc. cit.: 57–73.
14. C. Martinez-Weber, "The Homeless Person with Diabetes," *Postgraduate Medicine* 81 (1987): 289–97.
15. Centers for Disease Control, "Revision of the CDC Surveillance Case Definition for Acquired Immune Deficiency Syndrome," *Morbidity and Mortality Weekly Report* 36, supplement 15 (1987).
16. *Morbidity and Mortality Weekly Report* 37 (1988): 54–52, 547–49.
17. *Morbidity and Mortality Weekly Report* 37 (1988): 1–22.
18. R. Reich and L. Siegel, "The Emergence of the Bowery as a Psychiatric Dumping Ground" *Pscyhiatric Quarterly* 50, no. 3 (1973): 191–201.
19. A. A. Arce, M. Tadlock, M. J. Vergare, and S. H. Shapiro, "A Psychiatric Profile of Street People Admitted to an Emergency Shelter," *Hospital and Community Psychiatry* 34 (1983): 812–17.
20. F. R. Lipton, A. Sabatini, and S. E. Katz, "Down and Out in the City: The Homeless Mentally Ill," *Hospital and Community Psychiatry* 34 (1983): 818–21.

7. Health Care for Familyless, Runaway Street Kids

1. R. C. Hermann, "Center Provides Approach to Major Social Ill: Homeless Urban Runaways, 'Throwaways,' " *Journal of the American Medical Association* 260 (1988): 311–12.
2. B. Tyler, "Teenage Throwaways: How Many?" letter, *Journal of the American Medical Association* 260, no. 21 (1988): 3132.
3. C. L. M. Caton, "The Homeless Experience in Adolescent Years," in *The Mental Health Needs of Homeless Persons,* ed. E. L. Bassuk (San Francisco: Jossey-Bass, 1986).
4. G. R. Adams, T. Gullotta, and M. A. Clancy, "Homeless Adolescents: A Descriptive Study of the Similarities and Differences Between

Runaways and Throwaways," *Adolescence* 20, no. 79 (1985): 715–24.
5. J. Bucy, executive director, National Network of Runaway and Youth Services, Washington, D.C., personal communication, July 1989.
6. "Runaway and Homeless Youth: National Program Inspection," U.S. Department of Health and Human Services, Office of the Inspector General, Region X, October 1983.
7. American Academy of Pediatrics Committee on Community Health Services, "American Academy of Pediatrics: Health Needs of Homeless Children," *Pediatrics* 82, no. 6 (1988): 938–40. See also United States Con-

ference of Mayors, unpublished data, December 1987.

8. Federal Bureau of Investigation, National Crime Information Center, Washington, D.C. 20535.

9. "Plight of the 'Boarder Orphans,'" *Newsweek* (July 24, 1989).

10. B. Ritter, "Abuse of the Adolescent," *New York State Journal of Medicine* 89 (1989): 156–58.

11. D. Griffin, associate director, National Network for Runaway and Youth Services, personal communication September 1989.

12. N. Brozan, "Van is Hope for Bronx 'Throwaways,'" *New York Times*, October 6, 1989.

13. P. H. Rossi, J. D. Wright, G. A. Fisher, and G. Willis, "The Urban Homeless: Estimating Composition and Size," *Science* 235, no. 4794 (1987): 1336–41.

14. D. Freeman, *Techniques of Family Therapy* (New York: Jason Aronson, Inc., 1981).

15. K. Kufeldt and M. Nimmo, "Youth on the Street: Abuse and Neglect in the Eighties," *Childhood Abuse and Neglect* 11, no. 4 (1987): 531–43.

16. M. Twain, *The Adventures of Tom Sawyer* (New York and London: Harper & Brothers, 1917).

17. J. Haley, *Uncommon Therapy: The Psychiatric Techniques of Milton Erickson* (New York: Norton, 1973).

18. M. D. Janus, A. W. Burgess, and A. McCormack, "Histories of Sexual Abuse in Adolescent Male Runaways," *Adolescence* 22, no. 86 (1987): 405–17.

19. E. D. Farber, C. Kinast, W. F. McCoard, and D. Falkner, "Violence in Families of Adolescent Runaways," *Childhood Abuse and Neglect* 8, no. 3 (1984): 295–99.

20. D. M. Paperny and R. W. Deisher, "Maltreatment of Adolescents: The Relationship to a Predisposition Toward Violent Behavior and Delinquency," *Adolescence* 18, no. 71 (1983): 499–506.

21. E. Farber and J. Joseph, "The Maltreated Adolescent: Patterns of Physical Abuse," *Childhood Abuse and Neglect* 9 (1987): 201–6.

22. E. Bassuk and L. Rubin, "Homeless Children: A Neglected Population," *American Journal of Orthopsychiatry* 57, no. 2 (1987): 279–86.

23. E. Bassuk, L. Rubin, and A. S. Lauriat, "Characteristics of Sheltered Homeless Families," *American Journal of Public Health* 76, no. 9 (1986): 1097–101.

24. D. Shaffer and C. L. M. Caton, "Runaway and Homeless Youth in New York City," report to the Ittleson Foundation, New York, 1984.

25. W. G. Kearon, "Abuse of Runaway and Homeless Children on the Streets," letter, *Childhood Abuse and Neglect* 11, no. 4 (1987): 587.

26. J. M. Robertson, "Homeless Adolescents: A Hidden Crisis," *Hospitals and Community Psychiatry* 39, no. 5 (1988): 475.

27. M. Beyer, "Psychosocial Problems of Adolescent Runaways," Ph.D. dissertation, Yale University, 74–25718 35/05-B:2420, 1974.

28. S. Wolk and J. Brandon, "Runaway Adolescents' Perceptions of Parents and Self," *Adolescence* 12 (1977): 175–88.

29. American College of Physicians, "Health Care Needs of the Adolescent," *Annals of Internal Medicine* 110, no. 11 (1989): 930–35.

30. S. K. Schonberg, "Adolescents and AIDS," *Journal of Adolescent Health Care* 10, no. 3 (1989): suppl.: 4S.

31. E. Bassuk, W. R. Breakey, A. A. Fischer, C. R. Halpern, G. Smith, L. Stark, N. Stark, B. Vladeck, and P. Wolfe, "Supplementary Statement on Health Care for Homeless People," *Homelessness, Health, and Human Needs* (Washington, D.C.: National Academy Press, 1988).

32. S. D. Proctor, "To the Rescue: A National Youth Academy," *New York Times*, September 16, 1989.

33. H. Dow, "Forty-eight Hours on Runaway Street," CBS Television, March 10, 1989.

34. Council on Scientific Affairs of the American Medical Association, "Health Care Needs of Homeless and Runaway Youths," *Journal of the American Medical Association* 262, no. 10 (1989): 1358–61.

35. A. Manov and L. Lowther, "A Health Care Approach for Hard-to-Reach Adolescent Runaways," *Nurses Clinics of North America* 18 (1983): 333–42.

36. K. Johnson, "Building Health Programs for Teens," Adolescent Pregnancy Clearinghouse Report (Washington, D.C.: Children's Defense Fund, May 1986).

37. S. Davis, "Pregnancy in Adolescents," *Pediatric Clinics of North America* 36, no. 36 (1989): 665–80.

38. C. R. Hayman and J. C. Probst, "Health Status of Disadvantaged Adolescents Entering the Job Corps Program," *Public Health Reports* 98, no. 4 (1983): 369–75.

39. G. Alperstein and E. Arnstein, "Homeless Children—A Challenge for Pediatricians," *Pediatric Clinics of North America* 35, no. 6 (1988): 1413–25.

40. American Academy of Pediatrics, Committee on Community Health Services, "Health Needs of Homeless Children," *Pediatrics* 82, no. 6 (1988): 938–40.

41. G. Alperstein, C. Rappaport, and J. M. Flanigan, "Health Needs of Homeless Children in New York City," *American Journal of Public Health* 78, no. 9 (1988): 1232–33.

42. S. H. Vermund, R. Belmar, and E. Drucker, "Homeless in New York: The Youngest Victims," *New York State Journal of Medicine* 87, no. 1 (1987): 3–5.

43. D. S. Miller and E. H. Lin, "Children in Sheltered Homeless Families: Reported Health Status and Use of Health Services," *Pediatrics* 81, no. 5 (1988): 668–73.

44. S. Fitzpatrick, J. Johnson, P. Shragg, and M. E. Felice, "Health Care Needs of Indochinese Refugee Teenagers," *Pediatrics* 79, no. 1 (1987): 118–24.

45. G. Yates, R. MacKenzie, J. Pennbridge, and E. Cohen, "A Risk Profile Comparison of Runaway and Non-runaway Youth," *American Journal of Public Health* 78, no. 7 (1988): 820–21.

46. Select Committee on Children, Youth, and Families, *Down These Mean Streets: Violence By and Against America's Children* (Washington, D.C.: Government Printing Office, 1989).

47. D. M. Paperny and R. W. Deisher, "Maltreatment of Adolescents: The Relationship to a Predisposition Toward Violent Behavior and Delinquency," *Adolescence* 18, no. 71 (1983): 499–506.

48. C. Newell-Withrow, "Observations of Children, Youth, and Violence," *Journal of Pediatric Health Care* 1 (1987): 77–84.

49. S. Rimer, "The Short Life of a Former Foster Child," *New York Times,* November 11, 1987.

50. T. J. Flanagan and E. F. McGarrell, eds., *Sourcebook of Criminal Justice Statistics 1985,* U.S. Department of Justice, Bureau of Justice Statistics, 1986.

51. A. F. Schiff, "A Statistical Evaluation of Rape," *Forensic Science* 2 (1973): 339–49.

52. American Academy of Pediatrics Committee on Adolescence, "American Academy of Pediatrics Committee Statements: Rape and the Adolescent," *Pediatrics* 81, no. 4 (1988): 595–97.

53. A. G. Getts, "Diagnosing Chlamydia Trachomatis Urethritis by First Catch Urine Enzyme Immunoassay in Adolescent Males," *Journal of Adolescent Health Care* 10 (1989): 209–11.

54. P. H. Hardy, J. B. Hardy, E. E. Nell, D. A. Graham, M. R. Spence, and R. C. Rosenbaum, "Prevalence of Six Sexually Transmitted Disease Agents Among Pregnant Inner-City Adolescents and Pregnancy Outcome," *Lancet* 2, no. 8398 (1984): 333–37.

55. New York City Department of Health, "Congenital Syphilis," *City Health Information* 8, no. 6 (1989): 1–2.

56. J. Kennedy, unpublished data.

57. J. J. Fraser, P. J. Rettig, and D. W. Kaplan, "Prevalence of Cervical Chlamydia Trachomatis and Neisseria Gonorrhea in Female Adolescents," *Pediatrics* 71 (1983): 333–36.

58. H. H. Handsfield, R. J. Rice, M. C. Roberts, and K. K. Holmes, "Localized Outbreak of Penicillinase-Producing Neisseria Gonorrhoeae: Paradigm for Introduction and Spread of Gonorrhea in a Community," *Journal of the American Medical Association* 261, no. 16 (1989): 2357–61.

59. "Syphilis and Gonorrhea Are Spreading Among Urban Teens," *Medical World News* (May 22, 1989).

60. F. N. Judson, "Management of Antibiotic-Resistant Neisseria Gonorrhoeae," *New England Journal of Medicine* 110, no. 1 (1989): 5–7.

61. C. D. Berry, T. M. Hooton, and S. A. Lukehart, "Medical Intelligence: Neurologic Relapse After Benzathine Penicillin Therapy for Secondary Syphilis in a Patient with HIV Infection," *New England Journal of Medicine* 316, no. 25 (1987): 1587–89.

62. State of New York, Department of Health Memorandum, "Recommendations for Diagnosing and Treating Syphilis in Human Immunodeficiency Virus Infected Patients," Series 89–65, August 23, 1989.

63. "White Paper on Adolescent Health" (Chicago, Ill.: American Medical Association, 1986).

64. R. Deisher, G. Robinson, and D. Boyer, "The Adolescent Female and Male Prostitute," *Pediatric Annals* 11 (1982): 819–25.

65. F. T. Weber, D. S. Elfenbein, N. L. Richards, A. B. Davis, and J. Thomas, "Early Sexual Activity of Delinquent Adolescents," *Journal of Adolescent Health Care* 10 (1989): 398–403.

66. K. Hein and M. I. Cohen, "Age at First Intercourse Among Homeless Adolescent Females," *Journal of Pediatrics* 93 (1978): 147–48.

67. C. D. Hayes, ed., *Risking the Future: Adolescent Sexuality, Pregnancy, and Childbearing* (Washington, D.C.: National Academy Press, 1987).

68. D. K. Berger, G. Perez, J. Bistritz, M. Menendez, M. Kelly, and M. Pincus, "Hepatitis B. Markers and Persistent Antigenemia in Adolescents," *Journal of Adolescent Health Care* 9, no. 5 (1988): 374–77.

69. M. J. Alter, P. J. Coleman, W. J. Alexander, E. Kramer, J. K. Miller, E. Mandel, S. C. Hadler, and H. S. Margolis, "Importance of Heterosexual Activity in the Transmission of Hepatitis B and Non-A, Non-B Hepatitis," *Journal of the American Medical Association* 252, no. 9 (1989): 1201–5.

70. Y. Poovorawan, S. Sanpavat, W. Pongpunlert, S. Chumderm-padetsuk, P. Sentrakul, and A. Safary, "Protective Efficacy of a Recombinant DNA Hepatitis B Vaccine in Neonates of HBe Antigen-Positive Mothers," *Journal of the American Medical Association* 261, no. 22 (1989): 3278–81.

71. Centers for Disease Control, "HIV/AIDS Surveillance Report," September 1989.

72. H. Gayle, M. Rogers, S. Manoff, et al., "Demographic and Sexual Transmission Differences Between Adolescent and Adult AIDS Patients," IV International Conference on AIDS, Stockholm, June 1988.

73. K. Hein, "AIDS in Adolescence," *Journal of Adolescent Health Care* 10, no. 3 supplement (1989): 10–35s.

74. K. Hein, "AIDS in Adolescence: Beyond Education," presented to the Presidential Commission on the HIV Epidemic, New York, February 1988: 1–20.

75. J. Kennedy and D. Martin, "Testimony Before the Presidential Commission on the HIV Epidemic," Washington, D.C.: May 17, 1988.

76. *Report of the Presidential Commission on the Human Immunodeficiency Virus Epidemic,* submitted to the President of the United States, June 24, 1988.

77. G. Kolata, "AIDS Is Spreading in Teenagers, a New Trend Alarming to Experts," *New York Times,* October 8, 1989.

78. J. Kennedy, O. Hernandez, J. Altman, and M. Arkovitz, unpublished data.

79. L. Novick, R. Stricof, J. Kennedy, and I. Weisfuse, "Sero-prevalence of Adolescents at a Homeless Facility," presented at the American Public Health Association Annual Meeting, Boston, November 1988.

80. "Update: Heterosexual Transmission of Acquired Immunodeficiency Syndrome and Human Immunodeficiency Virus Infection—United States," *Morbidity and Mortality Weekly Report* 38, no. 24 (1989): 423–34.

81. "AIDS and Human Immunodeficiency Virus Infection in the United States: 1988 Update," *Morbidity and Mortality Weekly Report* 38, no. 14 (1989): 1–38.

82. "Update: Acquired Immunodeficiency Syndrome—United States, 1981–1988," *Morbidity and Mortality Weekly Report* 38, no. 14 (1989): 229–36.

83. "Trends in Human Immunodeficiency Virus Infection Among Civilian Applicants for Military Service—United States, October 1985–March 1988," *Morbidity and Mortality Weekly Report* 37, no. 44 (1988): 677–79.

84. T. C. Quinn, D. Glasser, et al., "Human Immunodeficiency Virus Infection Among Patients Attending Clinics for Sexually Transmitted Diseases," *New England Journal of Medicine* 318, no. 4 (1988): 197–203.

85. "CDC Sees No Surge in Heterosexual Spread of AIDS," *Internal Medicine News* (September 15–30, 1989).

86. M. Goulart, family nurse practitioner, Larkin Street Youth Center, San Francisco, personal communication, September 1989.

87. F. S. Rhame and D. G. Maki, "The Case for Wider Use of Testing for HIV Infection," *New England Journal of Medicine* 320, no. 19 (1989): 1248–54.

88. H. L. Minkoff and S. H. Landesman, "The Case for Routinely Offering Prenatal Testing for Human Immunodeficiency Virus," *American Journal of Obstetrics and Gynecology* 159, no. 4 (1988): 793–96.

89. G. R. Adams and G. Munro, "Portrait of the North American Runaway: A Critical Review," *Journal of Youth and Adolescence* 8, no. 3 (1979): 359–73.

90. S. Sondheim, "Gee, Officer Krupke!" *West Side Story*, Columbia Records, 1957.

91. "Mental Disorders Measured in Young," *New York Times*, June 8, 1989.

92. R. A. Feldman, A. R. Stiffman, and K. G. Jung, "Children of Mentally Ill Parents: Risk, Behavior and Implications for Mental Health Professionals," *Practice Applications* 5, no. 4 (1988): 1–8.

93. "Suicide—United States, 1970–1980," *Morbidity and Mortality Weekly Report* 34, no. 24 (1985): 353–57.

94. M. J. Rotheram, J. Bradley, "Evaluation of Imminent Danger of Suicide Among Runaways," *The Network News* 5 (1986): 10–11.

95. K. Clay, "Trespassers Will Be Poisoned," *Natural History* (September 1989): 8–14.

96. F. H. Gawin and E. H. Ellinwood, "Cocaine and Other Stimulants: Actions, Abuse, and Treatment," *New England Journal of Medicine* 318, no. 18 (1988): 1173–82.

97. S. A. Brown, "Life Events of Adolescents in Relation to Personal and Parental Substance Abuse," *American Journal of Psychiatry* 146, no. 4 (1989): 484–89.

98. D. J. Rohsenow, R. Corbett, and D. Devine, "Molested as Children: A Hidden Contribution to Substance Abuse?" *Journal of Substance Abuse Treatment* 5, no. 1 (1988): 13–18.

99. R. C. Fowler, C. L. Rich, and D. Young, "San Diego Suicide Study. II. Substance Abuse in Young Cases," *Archives of General Psychiatry* 43, no. 10 (1986): 962–65.

100. M. Marriott, "After 3 Years, Crack Plague Only Gets Worse," *New York Times*, February 20, 1989.

101. M. H. Silbert, A. M. Pines, and T. Lynch, "Substance Abuse and Prostitution," *Journal of Psychoactive Drugs* 14, no. 3 (1982): 193–97.

102. S. Press, "Crack and Fatal Child Abuse," *Journal of the American Medical Association* 260, no. 21 (1988): 3132.

103. B. Zuckerman, D. A. Frank, R. Hingson, H. Amaro, S. M. Levenson, H. Kayne, S. Parker, R. Vinci, K. Aboagye, L. E. Fried, H. Cabral, R. Timperi, and H. Bauchner, "Original Article: Effects of Maternal Marijuana and Cocaine Use on Fetal Growth," *New England Journal of Medicine* 320, no. 12 (1989): 762–68.

104. L. L. Cregler and H. Mark, "Medical Complications of Cocaine Abuse," *New England Journal of Medicine* 315 (1986): 1495–500.

105. D. Kissner, W. Lawrence, and J. Selis, "Crack Lung: Pulmonary Disease Caused by Cocaine Abuse," *American Review of Respiratory Diseases* 136 (1987): 1250–52.

106. B. Wallace, "Psychological and Environmental Determinants of Relapse in Crack Cocaine Smokers," *Journal of Substance Abuse Treatment* 6, no. 2 (1989): 95–106.

107. G. Kolata, "Experts Finding New Hope on Treating Crack Addicts," *New York Times*, August 24, 1989.

108. K. Bishop, "Fear Grows over the Effects of a New Smokable Drug," *New York Times*, September 15, 1989.

109. G. W. Bailey, "Current Perspectives on Substance Abuse in Youth," *Journal of the American Academy of Child and Adolescent Psychiatry* 28, no. 2 (1989): 151–62.

110. K. Brower and M. Anglin, "Adolescent Cocaine Use: Epidemiology, Risk Factors, and Prevention," *Journal of Drug Education* 17, no. 2 (1987): 163–80.

111. G. M. Beschner and A. S. Friedman, "Treatment of Adolescent Drug Abusers," *International Journal of Addiction* 20, nos. 6–7 (1985): 971–73.

112. J. Gross, "Views of Wretchedness by Children Born to It," *New York Times*, September 25, 1989.

113. F. H. Gawin, D. Allen, and B. Humblestone, "Outpatient Treatment of 'Crack' Cocaine Smoking with Hupenthixol Deconoate: A Preliminary Report," *Archives of General Psychiatry* 46, no. 4 (1989): 322–25.

114. I. L. Extein and M. S. Gold, "The Treatment of Cocaine Addicts: Bromocriptine or Desipramine," *Psychiatric Annals* 18, no. 9 (1988): 535–37.

115. D. E. Rogers, "Editorial: Federal Spending on AIDS—How Much Is Enough?" *New England Journal of Medicine* 320, no. 24 (1989): 1623–24.

116. National Research Council, *Risking the Future: Adolescent Sexuality, Pregnancy, and Childbearing* (Washington, D.C.: National Academy Press, 1987).

117. A. R. Stiffman and C. E. Morse, "Adolescent Sexuality, Contraception, and Pregnancy: Problems, Programs, and Progress," *Practice Applications* 3, no. 2 (1986): 1–16.

118. E. R. McAnarney and W. R. Hendee, "Adolescent Pregnancy and Its Consequences," *Journal of the American Medical Association* 262, no. 1 (1989): 74–77.

119. S. Joseph, New York City commissioner of health, "Medical Grand Rounds," New York University Medical Center, October 4, 1989.

120. S. H. Landesman and A. Willoughby, "HIV Disease in Reproductive Age Women: A Problem of the Present," *Journal of the American Medical Association* 261, no. 9 (1989): 1326–27.

121. "CDC Sees No Surge in Heterosexual Spread of AIDS," *Internal Medicine News* (September 15, 1989).

122. Associated Press, "Cost of Teen-age Pregnancies," *New York Times,* February 20, 1986.

123. H. W. French, "For Pregnant Addicts, a Clinic of Hope," *New York Times,* September 29, 1989.

124. C. Wallis, C. Booth, M. Ludtke, and E. Taylor, "Children Having Children," *Time* (December 9, 1985).

125. G. Carrill, E. Massarelli, A. Opzoomer, et al., "Adolescents with Chronic Disease: Are They Receiving Comprehensive Health Care?" *Journal of Adolescent Health Care* 4 (1983): 261–265.

126. D. M. Siegel, "Adolescents and Chronic Illness," *Journal of the American Medical Association* 257 (1987): 3396–99.

127. J. H. Freudenberger and S. E. Torkelsen, "Beyond the Interpersonal: A System Model of Therapeutic Care for Homeless Children and Youth," *Psychotherapy* 21, no. 1 (1984).

128. B. McCormick and J. Newald, "Outreach Works in Treating Homeless Youth," *Hospitals* 60, no. 9 (1986): 162.

129. R. Deisher and J. Farrow, "Recognizing and Dealing with Alienated Youth in Clinical Practice," *Pediatric Annals* 15 (1986): 759–64.

130. M. C. Brucker and M. Muellner, "Nurse-Midwifery Care of Adolescents," *Journal of Nurse Midwifery* 30, no. 5 (1985): 277–79.

131. E. J. Burns, "Report to the Board of Directors of Covenant House," New York, 1979.

132. J. M. Morrissey, A. D. Hofman, and J. C. Thorpe, *Consent and Confidentiality in the Health Care of Children and Adolescents* (New York: Free Press, 1986).

133. K. Noble, "Appeals Court Voids Statute on Informing Parents of Abortion," *New York Times,* August 27, 1987.

134. S. Taylor, "Courts Debate Judges' Role When Girls Seek Abortions," *New York Times,* February 23, 1987.

135. N. Lewis, "Florida Court Rules Against Abortion Curbs," *New York Times,* October 6, 1989.

8. Health Care for Children in Homeless Families

1. "A Report to the Secretary on the Homeless and Emergency Shelters," U.S. Department of Housing and Urban Development, 1988.

2. United States Conference of Mayors, "A Status Report on Hunger and Homelessness in America's Cities: A 27-City Survey," January 1989.

3. Committee on Health Care for Homeless People, Institute of Medicine, *Homelessness, Health and Human Needs* (Washington, D.C.: National Academy Press, 1988).

4. U.S. Bureau of Census Annual Report, 1988.

5. "Life at the Edge: The Hard Choices Facing Low-Income American Families," *Consumer Reports* (June 1987): 375.

6. L. C. Thurow, "A Surge in Inequality," *Scientific American* 256 (1987): 30–37.

7. P. Passell, *New York Times,* July 16, 1989.

8. R. I. Towber, "Characteristics and Housing Histories of Families Seeking Shelter from HRA" (New York: Human Resources Administration, October 1986).

9. K. Y. McChesney, "Families: The New Homeless," *Family Professional* 1 (1986): 13–14.

10. E. L. Bassuk, L. Ruben, and A. S. Lauriat, "Characteristics of Sheltered Homeless Families," *American Journal of Public Health* 76 (1986): 1097–101.

11. E. L. Bassuk and L. Rosenberg, "Why Does Family Homelessness Occur? A Case Control Study," *American Journal of Public Health* 78, no. 7 (1988): 783–88.

12. J. Anthony and C. Chiland, *The Child in His Family* (New York: John Wiley, 1978): 5:39–53.

13. L. Roth and E. Fox, "Children of Homeless Families: Health Status and Access to Health Care," presentation at the 116th Annual Meeting of the American Public Health Association, Boston, November 14, 1988.

14. United States Conference of Mayors, "A Status Report on Homeless Families in America's Cities: A 29-City Survey," May 1987.

15. D. Kindig and H. Movassaghi, "Small Rural Areas Falling Behind," *Rural Health Care: The Newsletter of the National Rural Health Association* 9, no. 5 (1987): 10.

16. I. Redlener, director of New York Children's Health Project, personal communication, 1988.

17. D. S. Miller and E. H. V. Liro, "Children in Sheltered Homeless Families: Reported

Health Status and Use of Health Services,"
Pediatrics 81 (1988): 668–73.
18. G. Alperstein, C. Rappaport, and J. M.
Flanigan, "Health Problems of Homeless
Children in New York City," *American
Journal of Public Health* 78 (1988): 1232–
33.
19. K. Haught, "Health Status of Homeless
Children Versus Domiciled Children," personal communication, 1989.
20. L. Egbuonu and B. Starfield, "Child Health
and Social Status," *Pediatrics* 69 (1982): 550–
57.
21. J. D. Wright and E. Weber, *Homelessness
and Health: A Special Report* (New York:
McGraw-Hill, 1988).
22. D. Weber-Burdin and J. D. Wright, "The
Robert Wood Johnson Foundation and the
Pew Memorial Trust Health Care for
the Homeless Program, 5th Report," February 1987.
23. J. D. Wright, "Poverty, Homelessness,
Health, Nutrition and Children," presentation at the National Conference on Homeless
Children and Youth, Washington, D.C.,
1989.
24. G. W. Rutherford, "Medical Status of Children in Family Shelters and Hotels," New
York City Department Health, 1983.
25. R. B. Haynes, "A Critical Review of the
Determinants of Patient Compliance with
Therapeutic Regimens," in *Compliance in
Health Care,* ed. R. B. Haynes, D. W. Tay-
lor, and D. L. Sackett (Baltimore: Johns
Hopkins University Press, 1979).
26. D. Meichenbaum, *Facilitating Treatment
Adherence: A Practitioner's Guidebook* (New
York: Plenum Press, 1987).
27. W. Chavkin, A. Kristal, C. Seabron and P.
Guigli, "The Reproductive Experience of
Women Living in Hotels for the Homeless in
New York City," *New York State Journal of
Medicine* 87, no. 1 (1987): 10–13.
28. G. Alperstein, C. Rappaport, and J. Flani-
gan, "Health Problems of Homeless Chil-

dren in New York City," presentation before
the Conference on Research and Homeless
Families: Implications for Public Policy,
1987.
29. Citizens' Committee for Children of New
York, "7,000 Homeless Children: The Crisis
Continues," Third Report on Homeless
Families with Children in Temporary Shel-
ters, October 1984.
30. K. Benker and A. De Havenon, "The Tyr-
anny of Indifference: A Study of the Health
Problems of 818 Hungry and Homeless
Families in New York City in 1988–1989"
(in press).
31. M. A. Lee, "Clinical Issues and Models in
Caring for Homeless Children," read before
the Academy of Pediatrics, San Francisco,
October 1988.
32. P. Acher, A. Fierman, and B. Dreyer,
"Health: An Assessment of Parameters of
Health and Nutrition in Homeless Children,"
American Journal of Diseases of Children
14, no. 4 (1987): 388.
33. *U.S. Public Health Service National Ambulatory Medical Care Survey: Background and
Methodology. Vital and Health Statistics,*
series 2 (61) (Washington, D.C.: Government Printing Office, 1979).
34. B. Dryer, "Homeless Children and Families," presentation before the American
Academy of Pediatrics, San Francisco, May
1988.
35. I. Redlener, "Caring for Homeless Children:
Special Challenges for the Pediatrician,"
Today's Child II (Winter 1988–1989): 4.
36. R. Yip, K. M. Walsh, and M. G. Goldfarb,
"Declining Prevalence of Anemia in Children in Middle Class Settings: A Pediatric
Success Story," *Pediatrics* 80 (1987): 330–
34.
37. American Academy of Pediatrics Committee
on Community Health Services, "Health
Needs of Homeless Children," *Pediatrics* 82
(1988): 938–40.

9. Health Concerns of Homeless Women

1. M. R. Stoner, "The Plight of Homeless
Women," *Social Service Review* (December
1983): 565–80.
2. J. L. Hagen, "The Heterogeneity of Homelessness," *Social Casework: The Journal of
Contemporary Social Work* (October 1987):
451–57.
3. L. L. Bachrach, "Homeless Women: A Context for Health Planning," *Milbank Memorial Fund Quarterly* 65, no. 3 (1987): 371–
97.
4. J. L. Hagen, "Gender and Homelessness,"
Social Work (July–August 1987): 312–16.
5. J. D. Wright and E. Weber, *Homelessness
and Health* (Washington, D.C.: McGraw-
Hill, 1987).
6. P. W. Brickner, L. K. Scharer, B. Conanan,
A. Elvy, and M. Savarese, *Health Care of
Homeless People* (New York: Springer,
1985).

7. "With Neither Home Nor Health," *Emergency Medicine* 21, no. 4 (1989): 21–46.
8. W. Chavkin, A. Kristal, C. Seabron, and P.
Guigli, "The Reproductive Experience of
Women Living in Hotels for the Homeless in
New York City," *New York State Journal of
Medicine* 87 (1987): 10–13.
9. M. Winick, "Nutrition and Vitamin Deficiency States," in *Health Care of Homeless
People,* loc. cit.
10. J. Emmons and P. Courter, "Towards Control of Chlamydial Infections," *Nurse Practitioner* 10, no. 11 (1985): 15–22.
11. J. T. Kelly, "Trauma: With the Example of
San Francisco's Shelter Programs," in *Health
Care of Homeless People,* loc. cit.
12. K. Hirsch, "The Sanctuary of Shelter, the
Horror of Home," *Boston Globe Magazine*
(March 26, 1989).
13. M. C. King and J. Ryan, "Abused Women:

Dispelling Myths and Encouraging Intervention," *Nurse Practitioner* 14, no. 5 (1989): 47–58.

14. S. V. McLeer and R. A. Anwar, "The Role of the Emergency Physician in the Prevention of Domestic Violence," *Annals of Emergency Medicine* 16, no. 10 (1987): 1155–61.

15. G. NiCarthy, *The Ones Who Got Away* (Seattle: Seal Press, 1987).

16. P. E. Mullen, S. E. Romans-Clarkson, V. E. Walton, and G. P. Herbison, "Impact of Sexual and Physical Abuse on Women's Mental Health," *Lancet* 8590 (1988): 841–45.

17. L. B. Heinrich, "Care of the Female Rape Victim," *Nurse Practitioner* 12, no. 11 (1987): 9–27.

18. S. L. Shearer and C. A. Herbert, "Long-term Effects of Unresolved Sexual Trauma," *American Family Physician* 36, no. 4 (1987): 169–75.

19. G. P. Lenehan, B. N. McInnes, D. O'Donnell, and M. Hennessey, "A Nurses' Clinic for the Homeless," *American Journal of Nursing* 85, no. 11 (1985): 1236–40.

20. E. K. Koranyi, "Morbidity and Rate of Undiagnosed Physical Illnesses in a Psychiatric Clinic Population," *Archives of General Psychiatry* 35, no. 4 (1974): 414–19.

21. M. Buda, M. T. Tsuang, and J. A. Fleming, "Causes of Death in DSM-III Schizophrenics and Other Psychotics," *Archives of General Psychiatry* 45, no. 4 (1988): 283–85.

10. The Homeless Elderly

1. U.S. Department of Housing and Urban Development, *Report to the Secretary on the Homeless and Emergency Shelters* (Washington, D. C.: Government Printing Office, 1984).

2. D. Roth, J. Bean, N. Lust, and T. Saveano, "Homelessness in Ohio: A Study of People in Need," statewide report, Ohio Department of Mental Health, Office of Program Evaluation and Research, February 1985.

3. P. J. Fischer, "Health and Social Characteristics of Baltimore's Homeless Persons," presented at the 92d annual convention of the American Psychological Association, Toronto, Candada, August 24–28, 1984.

4. J. D. Wright and E. Weber, *Homelessness and Health* (Washington, D.C.: McGraw-Hill, 1987).

5. J. O'Connell and J. Valentine, "Mortality Among Boston's Homeless, 1986," unpublished data.

6. S. M. Keigher, "The City's Responsibility for the Homeless Elderly in Chicago," Illinois Department on Aging and the Chicago Department of Aging and Disability, Chicago, Illinois, 1987.

7. S. M. Keigher, R. Berman, and S. Greenblatt, "Relocation, Residence and Risk: A Study of Housing Risks and Causes of Homelessness Among the Urban Elderly," Metropolitan Chicago Coalition on Aging, Chicago, Illinois, 1989.

8. J. O'Connell and M. Miletsky, "The Homeless Elderly: A Prospective Study of Thirty Cases," in *Elders at Risk* (Massachusetts Health Data Consortium, March 1989): 91–96.

9. *Boston's Homeless: Taking the Next Step,* City of Boston and United Community Planning Corporation Report, 1986.

10. P. H. Rossi and J. D. Wright, "The Determinants of Homelessness," Health Affairs 6 (Spring 1987): 1.

11. A. Pifer, "The Public Policy Response to Population Aging," *Daedalus* 115 (1986): 373–95.

12. M. Whitcomb, "Health Care for the Poor: A Public Policy Imperative," *New England Journal of Medicine* 315 (1986): 1220–22.

13. H. J. Cohen and K. W. Lyles, "Geriatrics," *Journal of the American Medical Association* 261 (1989): 2847–48.

14. P. J. Bloom, "Alcoholism After Sixty," *American Family Physician* 28, no. 2 (1983): 111–13.

15. K. Hesse and J. Savitsky, "The Elderly," in *Alcoholism: A Guide for the Primary Care Physician,* ed. H. N. Barnes, M. D. Aronson, and T. L. DelBanco (New York: Springer, 1987).

16. R. J. Glynn, G. R. Bouchard, J. S. LoCastro, and N. M. Laird, "Aging and Generational Effects on Drinking Behaviors in Men: Results from the Normative Aging Study," *American Journal of Public Health* 75 (1985): 1413–19.

17. D. Deykin, P. Janson, and L. McMahon, "Ethanol Potentiation of Aspirin-Induced Prolongation of the Bleeding Time," *New England Journal of Medicine* 306 (1982): 852–54.

18. C. G. Olsen-Noll and M. F. Bosworth, "Alcohol Abuse in the Elderly," *American Family Physician* 39 (1989): 173–79.

19. S. Zimberg, "Alcoholism in the Elderly: A Serious But Solvable Problem," *Postgraduate Medicine* 74, no. 1 (1983): 165–73.

20. L. L. Bachrach, "Interpreting Research on the Homeless Mentally Ill: Some Caveats," *Hospital and Community Psychiatry* 35 (1984): 914–17.

21. C. I. Cohen, J. Teresi, and D. Holmes, "The Mental Health of Old Homeless Men," *Journal of the American Geriatric Society* 36 (1988): 492–501.

22. Aging Health Policy Center, "The Homeless Mentally Ill Elderly," working paper, University of California at San Francisco, 1985.

23. "Crowded Out: Homelessness and the Elderly Poor in New York City," Coalition for the Homeless, 1984.

24. A. M. Clarfield, "The Reversible Dementias: Do They Reverse?" *Annals of Internal Medicine* 109 (1988): 476–86.

25. L. Z. Rubenstein, K. R. Josephson, and
G. D. Wieland, "Effectiveness of a Geriatric
Evaluation Unit," *New England Journal of
Medicine* 311 (1984): 1664.

26. E. W. Campion, A. Jette, and B. Beckman,
"An Interdisciplinary Geriatric Consultation
Service," *Journal of the American Geriatric
Society* 31 (1983): 792–96.

27. J. T. Brown and B. S. Hulka, "Screening
Mammography in the Elderly: A Case-Con-
trol Study," *Journal of General Internal
Medicine* 3 (1988): 126–31.

28. Consensus Conference, "Urinary Incontinence," *Journal of the American Medical Association* 261 (1989): 2685–90.

29. T-W Hu, "The Economic Impact of Urinary
Incontinence," *Clinical Geriatric Medicine*
2 (1986): 673–87.

30. N. M. Resnick, S. V. Yalla, and E. Laurino,
"The Pathophysiology of Urinary Inconti-
ence Among Institutionalized Elderly Per-

sons," *New England Journal of Medicine* 320
(1989): 1–7.

31. T-W Hu, J. F. Igou, D. L. Kaltreider, et al.,
"A Clinical Trial of a Behavioral Therapy to
Reduce Urinary Incontinence in Nursing
Homes: Outcome and Implications," *Jour-
nal of the American Medical Association* 261
(1989): 2656–62.

32. A. Lauriat and P. McGerigle, "More Than
Shelter: A Community Response to Homelessness" (Boston: United Community Planning Corporation and Massachusetts
Association for Mental Health, 1983).

33. J. Doolin, "Planning for the Special Needs
of the Homeless Elderly," *Gerontologist* 26
(1986): 229–31.

34. J. Doolin, "America's Untouchables: The
Elderly Homeless," *Perspective on Aging*
(March–April 1985): 8–11.

35. J. Gunn, "Prisons, Shelters, and Homeless
Men," Psychiatry Quarterly 48 (1974): 510.

11. Convalescence: For Those Without a Home— Developing Respite Services in Protected Environments

1. K. H. Dockett, *Street Homeless People in the
District of Columbia: Characteristics and
Service Needs* (Washington, D.C.: Center for
Applied Research and Urban Policy, UDC,
March 1989).

2. K. H. Dockett, *Homelessness in the District
of Columbia* (Washington, D.C.: Center for
Applied Research and Urban Policy, UDC,
November 1986).

3. P. R. Torrens, "Hospice Care: What Have We
Learned?" *Annual Review of the American
Journal of Public Health* (Washington, D.C.:
American Public Health Association, 1985),
vol. 6: 65–83.

4. H. Miller and J. Knowlton, *Assessment of the
Implementation of Grants to Provide Health
Services to the Homeless* (Maryland: Center
for Policy Studies, May 1989): 7.

5. N. G. Milburn, J. A. Booth, and S. E. Miles,
*Is Drug Abuse a Serious Problem Among
Homeless Shelter Users?* (Washington, D.C.:
Institute for Urban Affairs and Research,
Howard University, August 1989).

6. *The Cutting Edge of Homeless in New York
City: A Survival Plan for People with AIDS*
(New York: Partnership for the Homeless,
January 1989): 6–9.

12. Psychiatric and Mental Health Services

1. E. Susser, S. Conover, and E. L. Struening,
"Problems of Epidemiologic Method in As-
sessing the Type and Extent of Mental Illness
Among Homeless Adults," *Hospital and
Community Psychiatry* 40 (1989): 261–65.

2. C. D. Cowan, W. R. Breakey, and R. J.
Fischer, "The Methodology of Counting the
Homeless," Appendix B, in Institute of
Medicine, *Homelessness, Health, and Hu-
man Needs* (Washington, D.C.: National
Academy Press, 1988): 169–82.

3. J. P. Morrissey and I. S. Levine, "Researchers Discuss Latest Findings, Examine Needs
of Homeless Mentally Ill Persons (Conference Report)," *Hospital and Community
Psychiatry* 38 (1987): 811–12.

4. Institute of Medicine, *Homelessness, Health,
and Human Needs* (Washington, D.C.: National Academy Press, 1988).

5. P. J. Fischer and W. R. Breakey, "Homelessness and Mental Health: An Overview,"
International Journal of Mental Health 14,
no. 4 (1986): 6–41.

6. W. R. Breakey, P. J. Fischer, M. Kramer,
G. Nestadt, et al., "Health and Mental Health
Problems of Homeless Men and Women in
Baltimore," *Journal of the American Medi-
cal Association* 262 (1989): 1352–57.

7. M. McMurray-Avila and R. Hammond,
"Results of Mental Health Screening Study
Done at Albuquerque Health Care for the
Homeless, 1989," unpublished.

8. L. L. Bachrach, "Geographic Mobility and
the Homeless Mentally Ill," *Hospital and
Community Psychiatry* 38 (1987): 27–28.

9. L. Appleby and P. N. Desai, "Documenting
the Relationship Between Homelessness and
Psychiatric Hospitalization," *Hospital and
Community Psychiatry* 36 (1985): 732–37.

10. E. L. Bassuck and H. R. Lamb, "Homelessness and the Implementation of Deinstitutionalization," in *The Mental Health Needs
of Homeless Persons: New Directions for
Mental Health Services,* no. 30, ed. E. L.
Bassuk (San Francisco: Jossey-Bass, June
1986): 7–14.

11. B. Pepper, "A Public Policy for the Long-term Mentally Ill: A Positive Alternative to Reinstitutionalization," *American Journal of Orthopsychiatry* 57 (1987): 452–57.

12. R. A. Dorwart, "A Ten-Year Follow-up Study of the Effects of Deinstitutionalization," *Hospital and Community Psychiatry* 39 (1988): 287–91.

13. P. Brown, *The Transfer of Care: Psychiatric Deinstitutionalization and Its Aftermath* (London: Routledge, 1988).

14. H. M. Visotsky, "The Great American Roundup" (correspondence), *New England Journal of Medicine* 317 (1987): 1662–63.

15. H. R. Lamb, "Deinstitutionalization and the Homeless Mentally Ill," *Hospital and Community Psychiatry* 35 (1984): 899–907.

16. J. Belcher and B. G. Toomey, "Relationship Between the Deinstitutionalization Model, Psychiatric Disability, and Homelessness," *Health and Social Work* (Spring 1988): 145–53.

17. L. Gelberg, L. S. Linn, and B. D. Leake, "Mental Health, Alcohol and Drug Use, and Criminal History Among Homeless Adults," *American Journal of Psychiatry* 145 (1988): 191–96.

18. A. Gralnick, "Build a Better State Hospital: Deinstitutionalization Has Failed," *Hospital and Community Psychiatry* 36 (1985): 738–41.

19. J. Zusman, R. M. Friedman, and B. L. Levin, "Moving Treatment into the Community: Implications for Psychiatry," *Psychiatric Quarterly* 59 (1988): 140–49.

20. N. K. Worley and B. J. Lowery, "Deinstitutionalization: Could the Process Have Been Better for Patients?" *Archives of Psychiatric Nursing* 2 (1988): 126–33.

21. D. A. Bigelow, D. L. Cutler, L. J. Moore, et al., "Characteristics of State Hospital Patients Who Are Hard to Place," *Hospital and Community Psychiatry* 39 (1988): 181–85.

22. J. R. Belcher, "Are Jails Replacing the Mental Health System for the Homeless Mentally Ill?" *Community Mental Health Journal* 24 (1988): 185–95.

23. P. J. Fischer, "Criminal Activity Among the Homeless: A Study of Arrests in Baltimore," *Hospital and Community Psychiatry* 39 (1988): 46–51.

24. C. T. Mowbray, V. S. Johnson, and A. Solarz, "Homelessness in a State Hospital Population," *Hospital and Community Psychiatry* 38 (1987): 880–82.

25. E. Susser, E. L. Struening, and S. Conover, "Childhood Experiences of Homeless Men," *American Journal of Psychiatry* 144 (1987): 1599–601.

26. E. L. Bassuk and L. Rosenberg, "Why Does Family Homelessness Occur? A Case-Control Study," *American Journal of Public Health* 78 (1988): 783–88.

27. D. Baumann and C. Grigsby, *Understanding the Homeless: From Research to Action* (Austin: Hogg Foundation for Mental Health, University of Texas, 1988).

28. P. J. Fischer, B. S. Shapiro, W. R. Breakey, et al., "Mental Health and Social Characteristics of the Homeless: A Survey of Mission Users," *American Journal of Public Health* 76 (1986): 519–24.

29. I. S. Levine, A. D. Lezak, and H. H. Goldman, "Community Support Systems for the Homeless Mentally Ill," in *The Mental Health Needs of Homeless Persons: New Directions for Mental Health Services*, no. 30, loc. cit.: 27–41.

30. United States Conference of Mayors, "Local Responses to the Needs of Homeless Mentally Ill Persons," May 1987.

31. H. R. Lamb and J. A. Talbott, "The Homeless Mentally Ill: The Perspective of the American Psychiatric Association," *Journal of the American Medical Association* 256 (1986): 498–501.

32. A. Frances and S. M. Goldfinger, " 'Treating' a Homeless Mentally Ill Patient Who Cannot Be Managed in the Shelter System," *Hospital and Community Psychiatry* 37 (1986): 577–79.

33. W. R. Breakey, "Mental Health Services for Homeless People," in *Homelessness: A National Perspective*, ed. M. J. Robertson and M. Greenblatt (New York: Plenum, in press).

34. F. L. J. Ball and B. E. Havassy, "A Survey of the Problems and the Needs of Homeless Consumers of Acute Psychiatric Services," *Hospital and Community Psychiatry* 35 (1984): 917–21.

35. "Recommendations of APA's Task Force on the Homeless Mentally Ill," *Hospital and Community Psychiatry* 35 (1984): 908–9.

36. M. Rosnow and J. Donohue, "Homeless Persons' Views of Street Outreach: Milwaukee's Street Outreach Program, Milwaukee Health Care for the Homeless Program, Milwaukee, Wisconsin, January 1989.

37. E. A. Erkel, "The Implications of Cultural Conflict for Health Care," *Health Values* 4, no. 2 (1980): 51–57.

38. "A National Directory of Homeless Health Care Projects (Section 340 of the Public Health Service Act)," National Association of Community Health Centers, Inc., January 1989.

39. L. L. Bachrach, "Chronic Mentally Ill Women: Emergence and Legitimation of Program Issues," *Hospital and Community Psychiatry* 36 (1985): 1063–69.

40. R. F. Ryback and E. L. Bassuk, "Homeless Battered Women and Their Shelter Network," in *The Mental Health Needs of Homeless Persons: New Directions for Mental Health Services*, no. 30, loc. cit.: 55–61.

41. E. M. Steindler, "Alcoholic Women in Medicine: Still Homeless" (editorial), *Journal of the American Medical Association* 257 (1987): 2954–55.

42. P. Koegel, "Ethnographic Perspectives on Homeless and Homeless Mentally Ill Women," proceedings of workshop sponsored by the Division of Education and Service Systems Liaison, National Institute of Mental Health, October 30–31, 1986.

43. S. P. Damrosch, P. A. Sullivan, A. Scholler, et al., "On Behalf of Homeless Families,"

Maternal and Child Nursing 13 (1988): 259–63.

44. R. A. Torres, P. Lefkowitz, C. Kales, and P. W. Brickner, "Homelessness Among Hospitalized Patients with the Acquired Immunodeficiency Syndrome in New York City" (letter to the editor), *Journal of the American Medical Association* 258 (1987): 779–80.

45. G. R. Adams, T. Gullotta, and M. A. Clancy, "Homeless Adolescents: A Descriptive Study of Similarities and Differences Between Runaways and Throwaways," *Adolescence* 20 (1985): 715–24.

46. C. L. M. Caton, "The Homeless Experience in Adolescent Years," in *The Mental Health Needs of Homeless Persons: New Directions for Mental Health Services*, no. 30, loc. cit.: 63–70.

47. E. Bassuk and L. Rubin, "Homeless Children: A Neglected Population," *American Journal of Orthopsychiatry* 57 (1987): 279–86.

48. S. Damrosch and J. A. Strasser, "The Homeless Elderly in America," *Journal of Gerontological Nursing* 14, no. 10 (1988): 26–29.

49. N. Scheper-Hughes, "Dilemmas in Deinstitutionalization: A View from Inner-City Boston," *Journal of Operational Psychiatry* 12 (1981):90.

50. M. I. Bennett, J. E. Gudeman, L. Jenkins, et al., "The Value of Hospital-Based Treatment for the Homeless Mentally Ill," *American Journal of Psychiatry* 145 (1988): 1273–76.

51. L. L. Bachrach, "Service Delivery in Juneau," *Hospital and Community Psychiatry* 37 (1986): 669–70.

52. M. Zanditon, "Housing for the Mentally Ill: How to Find It, Fund It, and Fight for It," in *Serving the Chronically Mentally Ill in an Urban Setting: New Directions for Mental Health Serives*, no. 39, ed. M. F. Shore and J. E. Gudeman (San Francisco: Jossey-Bass, Fall 1988): 89–99.

53. M. Earls and G. Nelson, "The Relationship Between Long-term Psychiatric Clients' Psychological Well-being and Their Perceptions of Housing and Social Support," *American Journal of Community Psychology* 16 (1988): 279–93.

54. F. R. Lipton, S. Nutt, and A. Sabatini, "Housing the Homeless Mentally Ill: A Longitudinal Study of a Treatment Approach," *Hospital and Community Psychiatry* 39 (1988): 40–45.

55. E. Baxter and K. Hopper, "Shelter and Housing for the Homeless Mentally Ill," in *The Homeless Mentally Ill*, ed. H. R. Lamb (Washington, D.C.: American Psychiatric Association, 1984).

56. J. Leach and J. Wing, *Helping Destitute Men* (London: Tavistock Publishers, 1980).

57. D. L. Cutler, "Community Residential Options for the Chronically Mentally Ill," *Community Mental Health Journal* 22 (1986): 61–73.

58. J. L. Louks and J. R. Smith, "Homeless: Axis I Disorders" (letter to the editors), *Hospital and Community Psychiatry* 39 (1988): 670–71.

59. H. H. Goldman and J. P. Morrissey, "The Alchemy of Mental Health Policy: Homelessness and the Fourth Cycle of Reform," *American Journal of Public Health* 75 (1985): 727–31.

60. A. A. Arce and M. J. Vergare, "Homelessness, the Chronic Mentally Ill and Community Mental Health Centers," *Community Mental Health Journal* 23 (1987): 242–49.

13. Alcoholism and Substance Abuse

1. Case study reported by the Cleveland Health Care for the Homeless Project, August 1, 1988.

2. L. Stark, "A Century of Alcohol and Homelessness," *Alcohol Health and Research World* II, no. 3 (Spring 1987).

3. R. Straus, "Alcohol and Homeless Men," *Quarterly Journal on Studies of Alcohol* 7 (1946): 360–404.

4. P. Joegel and A. Burman, "The epidemiology of Alcohol Abuse and Dependence Among Homeless Individuals: Finds from the Inner City of Los Angeles," January 1987.

5. J. D. Wright and J. W. Knight, "Alcohol Abuse in the National 'Health Care for the Homeless' Client Population," a Report to the National Institute on Alcohol Abuse and Alcoholism, April 1987.

6. S. Sadd and D. Young, "Non Medical Treatment of Indigent Alcoholics: A Review of Recent Findings," *Alcohol Health and Research World* II, no. 3 (Spring 1987).

7. Case study reported to the Cleveland Health Care for the Homeless Project, January 1, 1989.

8. N. K. Kaufman, "Access to Housing for Homeless Substance Abusers," prepared for NIAAA/UCSD National Conference on Homelessness, Alcohol and Other Drugs, February 1989.

9. *Oxford House Manual,* Oxford House, Inc., Silver Springs, Md.: 1988.

14. Homelessness and AIDS

1. New York Department of Health, Bureau of Health Statistics Analysis, 1986.

2. Centers for Disease Control, "Update: Acquired Immunodeficiency Syndrome—United States, 1981–1988," *Morbidity and Mortality Weekly Report* 38 (1989): 229–36.

3. D. P. Andrulis, V. B. Weslowski, and L. S. Gage, "The 1987 U.S. Hospital AIDS Sur-

vey," *Journal of the American Medical Association* 262 (1989): 787–94.

4. J. D. Wright and E. Weber, *Homelessness and Health* (Washington, D.C.: McGraw-Hill, 1987).

5. G. A. Stiers, "Aids and Homelessness in America," master's dissertation, University of Massachusetts, September 1988.

6. H. Joseph and H. Roman-Ney, "The Homeless Intravenous Drug User and the AIDS Epidemic," monograph, National Institute of Drug Abuse, 1989.

7. Partnership for the Homeless, "Assisting the Homeless in New York City: A Review of the Last Year and Challenges for 1988," New York Partnership for the Homeless, 1988.

8. Partnership for the Homeless, news release, December 1, 1986.

9. R. Todedo, "The Assessment of Heroin Abuse Among Residents of the 3rd Street Men's Shelter: A Needs Assessment Study," (Internal Report) Bureau of Research and Evaluation, Ethnography Section, New York State Division of Substance Abuse Services, April 1989.

10. R. A. Torres, S. Mani, J. Altholz, and P. W. Brickner, "HIV Infection in Homeless Men in a New York City Shelter," V International Conference on AIDS, Montreal, Canada, 1989.

11. R. Avery, Boston Health Care for the Homeless Project, personal communication, June 1989.

12. Office of the Mayor, "Beyond Shelter: A Homeless Plan for San Francisco," San Francisco, August 1989.

13. G. L. Yates, "Health Risk Profile Comparison of Runaway and Non-Runaway Youths," *American Journal of Public Health* 78, no. 37 (1988): 820–21.

14. AIDS Surveillance Update, New York City Department of Health, March 29, 1989.

15. J. Kennedy, Covenant House, personal communication, June 1989.

16. P. W. Brickner, R. A. Torres, M. Barnes, R. G. Newman, D. C. Des Jarlais, D. Whalen, and D. Rogers, "Recommendations for Control and Prevention of Human Immunodeficiency Virus Infection in Intravenous Drug Users," *Annals of Internal Medicine* 110 (1989): 833–37.

17. S. Kiyasu, Seattle Health Care for the Homeless Project, personal communication, July 1989.

18. G. Froner, "AIDS and Homelessness," *Journal of Psychoactive Drugs* 20, no. 2 (1988): 197–202.

19. Chicago Department of Health, AIDS Activity Office, "AIDS and the Homeless—Overnight / Drop-in Shelters & Transitional Shelters," January 1989.

20. Centers for Disease Control, "Guidelines for Prevention of Transmission of Human Immunodeficiency Virus and Hepatitis B Virus to Health Care and Public Safety Workers," *Morbidity and Mortality Weekly Report* 38 (1989): 1–30.

21. L. Moskowitz, G. T. Hensley, J. C. Chen, et al.: "Immediate Causes of Death in Acquired Immunodeficiency Syndrome," *Archives of Pathology and Laboratory Medicine* 109 (1985): 735.

22. K. Welch, W. Finkbeiner, C. Alpers, et al., "Autopsy Findings in the Acquired Immunodeficiency Syndrome," *Journal of the American Medical Association* 252 (1984): 1152.

23. Centers for Disease Control, "Update: Acquired Immunodeficiency Syndrome—United States," *Morbidity and Mortality Weekly Report* 35 (1986): 757–60, 765–66.

24. M. A. Fischl, G. M. Dickinson, and L. LaVoie, "Safety and Efficiency of Sulfamethoxazole and Trimethoprim Chemoprophylaxis for Pneumocystis Carinii Pneumonia in AIDS," *Journal of the American Medical Association* 259 (1988): 1185–89.

25. M. S. Gottlieb, S. Knight, R. Mitsuyasu, J. Weisman, M. Roth, and L. S. Young, "Prophylaxis of Pneumocystis Carinii Infection in AIDS with Pyrimethamine-Sulfadoxine," *Lancet* 2 (1984): 389–99.

26. C. E. Metroka, M. Lane, N. Braun, M. O'Sullivan, H. Josefberg, and D. Jacobson, "Successful Chemoprophylaxis for Pneumocystis Carinii Pneumonia with Dapsone in Patients with AIDS and ARC," IV International Conference on AIDS, Stockholm, Sweden, 1988.

27. J. A. Golden, D. Chernoff, H. Hollander, D. Feigal, and J. A. Conte, "Prevention of Pneumocystis Carinii Pneumonia by Inhaled Pentamidine," *Lancet* 1, no. 8639 (1989): 654–57.

28. R. E. Chaisson and G. Slutkin, "Tuberculosis and Human Immunodeficiency Virus Infection," *Journal of Infectious Diseases* 159 (1989): 96–100.

29. G. Sunderam, R. J. McDonald, T. Maniatis, et al., "Tuberculosis as a Manifestation of the Acquired Immunodeficiency Syndrome," *Journal of the American Medical Association* 256 (1986): 256, 362–66.

30. A. E. Pitchenik, C. Cole, B. W. Russell, M. A. Fischl, T. J. Spira, and D. E. Snider, "Tuberculosis, Atypical Mycobacteriosis, and the Acquired Immunodeficiency Syndrome Among Haitian and Non-Haitian Patients in South Florida," *Annals of Internal Medicine* 256 (1984): 362–66.

31. A. E. Pitchenik and H. A. Rubinson, "The Radiographic Appearance of Tuberculosis in Patients with the Acquired Immunodeficiency Syndrome (AIDS) and Pre-AIDS," *American Review of Respiratory Diseases* 131 (1985): 393.

32. P. A. Selwyn, D. Hartel, V. A. Lewis, et al., "A Prospective Study of the Risk of Tuberculosis Among Intravenous Drug Users with Immunodeficiency Virus Infection," *New England Journal of Medicine* 320 (1989): 546–52.

33. M. S. Iseman, "Is Standard Chemotherapy Adequate in Tuberculosis Patients Infected with HIV?" (editorial), *American Review of Respiratory Diseases* 136 (1987): 1326.

34. R. S. Klein, C. A. Harris, C. B. Small, et al., "Oral Candidiasis in High Risk Patients

as the Initial Manifestation of the Acquired Immunodeficiency Syndrome," *New England Journal of Medicine* 311 (1984): 354.

35. P. W. Brickner, L. K. Scharer, B. Conanan, A. Elvy, and M. Savarese, eds., *Health Care of Homeless People* (New York: Springer, 1985).

36. R. A. Torres, P. Lefkowitz, C. Kales, and P. W. Brickner, "Homelessness Among Hospitalized Patients with Acquired Immunodeficiency Syndrome in New York City" (letter to the editor), *Journal of the American Medical Association* 258, no. 6 (1987): 779–80.

37. Centers for Disease Control, "Guidelines for Prophylaxis Against Pneumocystis Carinii Pneumonia for Persons Infected with Human Immunodeficiency Virus," *Morbidity and Mortality Weekly Report* 38 (1989): (S-5) 1–9.

38. A. S. Abdul-Quader, S. R. Friedman, D. C. Des Jarlais, M. M. Marmor, R. Maslansky, and S. Bartelme, "Methadone Maintenance and Behavior by Intravenous Drug Users That Can Transmit AIDS," *Contemporary Drug Problems* 3 (Fall 1987): 425–34.

39. V. P. Dole and H. Joseph, "Long-term Outcomes of Patients Treated with Methadone Maintenance," *Annals of New York Academy of Sciences* 311 (1978): 181–89.

40. J. C. Ball, R. W. Lange, C. P. Myers, and S. R. Friedman, "Reducing the Risk of AIDS Through Methadone Maintenance Treatment," *Journal of Health and Social Behavior* 29 (1988): 214–26.

41. C. Butkus Small, G. Laper, and L. Ricci, "Homelessness in Patients with Acquired Immunodeficiency Syndrome" (abstract), IV International Conference on AIDS, Stockholm, Sweden, 1988: 197.

42. E. Drucker, J. Rothschild, B. Poust, B. Dunsmoir, A. Pivnick and P. Vine, "Intravenous Drug Users (IVDU) Hospitalized with AIDS in New York City: A Baseline Study of Children, Housing and Drug Treatment Needs" (abstract, III International Conference on AIDS, 1987.

15. Tuberculosis in the Homeless: A National Perspective

1. P. F. Wehrle and F. H. Top, Sr., eds., *Communicable and Infectious Diseases* (St. Louis: CV Mosby, 1981): 671.

2. G. W. Comstock, "Epidemiology of Tuberculosis," *American Review of Respiratory Diseases* 125, no. 3, pt. 2 (1982): 8–15.

3. H. L. Rieder, G. M. Cauthen, G. D. Kelley, A. B. Bloch, and D. E. Snider, "Tuberculosis in the United States," *Journal of the American Medical Association* 262 (1989): 385–89.

4. New York City Department of Health, "Tuberculosis Among the Homeless," *City Health Information* 8, no. 7 (1989): 1–3.

5. E. Reilly and B. McInnis, "Boston, Massachusetts: The Pine Street Inn Nurses' Clinic and Tuberculosis Program," in *Health Care of Homeless People*, ed. P. W. Brickner, L. K. Scharer, B. Conanan, E. Elvy, and M. Savarese (New :York: Springer, 1985): 291–99.

6. J. Bernardo, "Drug Resistant Tuberculosis Among the Homeless—Boston," *Morbidity and Mortality Weekly Report* 34 (1985): 429–31.

7. M. A. Barry, L. Shirley, et al., "The Changing Epidemiology of Tuberculosis in the Homeless—Boston," abstract presented at the American Thoracic Society Annual Meeting, Cincinnati, May 1989.

8. American Thoracic Society / Centers for Disease Control, "Treatment of Tuberculosis and Tuberculous Infection in Adults and Children," *American Review of Respiratory Diseases* 134 (1986): 355–63.

9. M. N. Sherman, P. W. Brickner, M. S. Schwartz, C. Vitarella, S. L. Wobido, C. Vickery, et al., "Tuberculosis in Single-Room-Occupancy Hotel Residents: A Persisting Focus of Disease," *New York Medical Quarterly* (Fall 1980): 39–41.

10. J. M. McAdam, P. W. Brickner, L. L. Scharer, J. A. Crocco, and A. E. Duff, "The Spectrum of Tuberculosis in a New York City Men's Shelter Clinic," *Chest* 97 (1990): 798–805.

11. H. M. Ginzburg, S. H. Weiss, M. G. MacDonald, and R. L. Hubbard, "HTLV-III Exposure Among Drug Users," *Cancer Research* 45 (1985): 4605s–8s.

12. G. H. Friedland, C. Harris, C. Butkus-Small, D. Shine, B. Moll, W. Darrow, et al., "Intravenous Drug Abusers and the Acquired Immunodeficiency Syndrome (AIDS)," *Archives of Internal Medicine* 145 (1985): 1413–17.

13. M. Guroff-Robert, S. H. Weiss, J. A. Giron, A. M. Jennings, H. M. Ginzburg, I. B. Margolis, et al., "Prevalence of Antibodies to HTLV-I, -II, -III in Intravenous Drug Abusers from an AIDS Endemic Region," *Journal of the American Medical Association* 255 (1986): 3133–37.

14. R. E. Chaisson, A. R. Moss, R. Onishi, D. Osmond, and J. R. Carlson, "Human Immunodeficiency Virus Infection in Heterosexual Intravenous Drug Users in San Francisco," *American Journal of Public Health* 77 (1987): 169–72.

15. "Update: Acquired Immunodeficiency Syndrome Associated with Intravenous Drug Use—United States, 1988," *Morbidity and Mortality Weekly Report* 38 (1989): 165–70.

16. E. E. Schoenbaum, D. Hartel, P. A. Selwyn, R. S. Klein, K. Davenny, M. Rogers, et al., "Risk Factors for Human Immunodeficiency Virus Infection in Intravenous Drug Users," *New England Journal of Medicine* 321 (1989): 874–79.

17. L. B. Reichman, C. P. Felton, and J. R. Edsall, "Drug Dependence, a Possible New Risk Factor for Tuberculous Disease," *Ar-*

chives of Internal Medicine 139 (1979): 337–39.

18. "Tuberculosis—1985—and the Possible Impact of T-lymphotropic Virus Type III/Lymphadenopathy Associated Virus Infection," Morbidity and Mortality Weekly Report 35 (1986): 74–76.

19. New York City Department of Health, "Tuberculosis and Acquired Immunodeficiency Syndrome (AIDS) in New York City," City Health Information 7 (1988): 3. Available from the New York City Department of Health, 125 Worth Street, New York, NY 10013.

20. P. A. Selwyn, D. Hartel, V. A. Lewis, E. E. Schoenbaum, S. H. Vermund, R. S. Klein, et al., "A Prospective Study of the Risk of Tuberculosis Among Intravenous Drug Users with Human Immunodeficiency Virus Infection," New England Journal of Medicine 320 (1989): 545–50.

21. D. C. Des Jarlais, S. R. Friedman, D. M. Novick, M. A. Sotheran, P. Thomas, S. R. Yancovitz, et al., "HIV-1 Infection Among Intravenous Drug Users in Manhattan, New York City, from 1977 through 1987," Journal of the American Medical Association 261 (1989): 1008–12.

22. R. E. Chaisson, P. Bacchetti, D. Osmond, B. Brodie, M. A. Sande, and A. R. Moss, "Cocaine Use and HIV Infection in Intravenous Drug Users in San Francisco," Journal of the American Medical Association 261 (1989): 561–65.

23. S. H. Weiss, "Links Between Cocaine and Retroviral Infection" (editorial), Journal of

the American Medical Association 261 (1989): 607–8.

24. Table 2: Tuberculosis Cases by Form of Disease States, 1986, Tuberculosis in the United States, 1985–1986, p. 6. Available from Centers for Disease Control, Atlanta, GA 30333.

25. Table 23: Tuberculosis Cases by Form of Disease, Cities of 250,000 or More Population, 1986, Tuberculosis in the United States 1985–1986, p. 29.

26. Table 11: Tuberculosis Cases by Age, States, 1986, Tuberculosis in the United States 1985–1986, p. 15.

27. Table 8: Tuberculosis Cases in the United States by Race and Sex, States, 1986, Tuberculosis in the United States 1985–1986, p. 12.

28. R. L. Riley, "Disease Transmission and Contagion Control," American Review of Respiratory Diseases 125 (1982): 16–19.

29. R. M. Des Prez and R. A. Goodwin, "Mycobacterium Tuberculosis," in Principles and Practice of Infectious Disease, 2d ed., ed. G. L. Mandell, R. G. Douglas, and J. E. Bennett (New York: Wiley, 1985): 1386.

30. M. E. Teller, The Tuberculosis Movement (New York: Greenwood Press, 1988): 13, 101–2.

31. L. B. Reichman and R. O'Day, "Tuberculosis in a Large Urban Population," American Review of Respiratory Diseases 117 (1978): 705–12.

32. D. Wlodarczyk, San Francisco Department of Public Health, personal communication.

16. Hypertension Screening and Treatment in the Homeless

1. The Joint National Committee on Detection, Education and Treatment of High Blood Pressure, "The 1984 Report of the Joint National Committee," Archives of Internal Medicine 144 (1984): 1045–57.

2. T. R. Dawber, The Framingham Study (Cambridge, MA: Harvard University Press, 1980).

3. J. Conmoni-Huntley, A. Z. LaCroix, and R. J. Havlich, "Race and Sex Differences in the Impact of Hypertension in the United States: The National Health and Nutrition Examination Survey I Epidemiologic Follow-Up Study," Archives of Internal Medicine 149 (April 1989): 780–88.

4. M. Moser, "A Decade of Progress in the Management of Hypertension," Hypertension 5 (1983): 808.

5. R. Byington, A. R. Dyer, D. Garside, K. Liu, P. Moss, J. Stamler, and Y. Tsong, "Recent Trends of Major Coronary Risk Factors and CHD Mortality in the United States and Other Industrialized Countries," in Proceedings of the Conference on the Decline of Coronary Heart Disease Mortality, ed. R. J. Havlik et al. (Bethesda, Md.: DHEW/NIH, 1979): 340–80.

6. R. Cooper, J. Stamler, A. Dyer, and D. Garside, "The Decline in Mortality from Coro-

nary Heart Disease, USA, 1968–1975," Journal of Chronic Diseases 31 (1978): 709–20.

7. J. D. Wright, E. Weber-Burdin, R. C. Tessler, C. E. Stewart, M. Geronimo, and J. Lam, "Health and Homelessness," The Social and Demographic Research Institute, University of Massachusetts, Amherst, 1985.

8. J. D. Wright and E. Weber, Homelessness and Health (Washington, D.C.: McGraw-Hill, 1987).

9. R. H. Ropers and R. Boyer, "Perceived Health Status Among the New Urban Homeless," Social Service Medicine 24, no. 8 (1987): 669–78.

10. T. Filardo, "Chronic Disease Management in the Homeless," in Health Care of Homeless People, ed. P. W. Brickner, L. K. Scharer, B. Conanan, A. Elvy, and M. Savarese (New York: Springer, 1985): 19–29.

11. "Progress in Chronic Disease Prevention Mortality Trends—United States, 1986–1988," Morbidity and Mortality Weekly Report 38 (March 3, 1989): 117–23.

12. U.S. Department of Health, Education, and Welfare, Health Services and Mental Health Administration, Health and Nutrition Survey 1971–1974. Advance Data: Vital and Health Statistics of the National Center for Health

Statistics (Washington, D.C.: Government Printing Office, 1976): no. 1.

13. J. H. Pratt, J. J. Jones, J. Z. Miller, M. A. Wagner, and N. S. Fineberg, "Racial Differences in Aldosterone Excretion and Plasma Aldosterone Concentrations in Children," *New England Journal of Medicine* 321, no. 17 (October 26, 1989): 1152–57.

14. "Black / White Comparisons of Premature Mortality for Public Health Program Planning—District of Columbia," *Morbidity and Mortality Weekly Report* 38, no. 3 (January 27, 1989): 34–37.

15. United States Conference of Mayors, "The Continued Growth of Hunger, Homelessness and Poverty in American Cities," Washington, D.C., 1986.

16. "Mary Lasker Heart and Hypertension Program," New York State Department of Health, 1983–1988.

17. P. Amadio, Jr., D. M. Cummings, and P. B. Amadio, "Tailoring the Antihypertensive Drug Regimen," *American Family Physician* 34, no. 2 (August 1986): 157–70.

18. E. Braunwald, K. J. Isselbacher, R. G. Petersdorf, J. D. Wilson, J. B. Martin, and A. S. Fauci, eds., *Harrison's Principles of Internal Medicine,* 11th ed. (New York: McGraw-Hill, 1987): 1030–35.

19. F. R. Kellogg, O. Piantieri, B. Conanan, P. Doherty, W. J. Vicic, and P. W. Brickner, "Hypertension: A Screening and Treatment

Program for the Homeless," in *Health Care of Homeless People,* loc. cit.: 114.

20. M. Moser and J. Lunn, "Comparative Effects of Pindolol and Hydrochlorthiazide in Black Hypertensive Patients," *Angiology* 32 (1981): 561–66.

21. S. Popli, J. T. Davirdas, B. Neubauer, B. Hochenberry, J. E. Hano, and T. S. Ing, "Transdermal Clonidine in Mild Hypertension," *Archives of Internal Medicine* 146 (1986): 2140–44.

22. M. Michael and S. Brammer, "Medical Treatment of Homeless Hypertensives," *American Journal of Public Health* (1988): 78–94.

23. P. W. Brickner, B. C. Scanlon, B. Conanan, A. Elvy, J. McAdam, K. L. Scharer, and W. J. Vicic, "Homeless Persons and Health Care," *Annals of Internal Medicine* 104 (1986): 405–9.

24. D. D. Buff, J. F. Kenny, and D. Light, "Health Problems of Residents in Single-Room-Occupancy Hotels," *New York State Journal of Medicine* 80 (1980): 2000–10.

25. D. MacIntyre, "Medical Care for the Homeless: Some Experiences in Glasgow," *Scottish Medical Journal* 24 (1979): 240–45.

26. M. Michael, T. M. Boyce, and A. W. Wilcox, *Biomedical Bestiary: Flaws and Fallacies in the Biomedical Literature* (Boston: Little, Brown, 1985): 59–63.

17. Governance, Program Control, and Authority

1. "The Citizen Board in Voluntary Agencies," United Way of America, 1979.

2. R. Smith, "Now What Should I Do?: Service on a Nonprofit's Board of Directors," *Non-Profit Times* 3, no. 1 (April 1989).

3. R. Chait and B. Taylor, "Charting the Territory of Nonprofit Boards," *Harvard Business Review* (January–February 1989).

4. J. Weber, "Managing the Board of Directors," Greater New York Fund, New York, 1975.

18. Staff Organization, Retention, and Burnout

1. K. Sellick, "Interdisciplinary Health Teams: A Question of Attitude," *Journal of Advances in Nursing* 3, no. 1 (September–November 1985).

2. A. J. Ducanis and A. K. Golin, *The Interdisciplinary Health Care Team* (Germantown, Md.: Aspen Systems Corp, 1979).

3. I. M. Rubin, M. S. Plovnick, and R. E. Fry, *Improving the Coordination of Care: A Program for Health Team Development* (Cambridge, MA: Ballinger, 1976).

4. H. J. Knopke and N. L. Dickelmann, *Approaches to Teaching Primary Health Care* (St. Louis: C. V. Mosby, 1981).

5. S. Gross, "The Truth about Non-Profit Managers," *Foundation News* (September–October 1988).

6. M. Savarese, "Transcript for Workshop on Interdisciplinary Teams," Conference on Health Issues in Care for the Homeless, New York, October 1983.

7. M. Savarese, B. Conanan, W. Vicic, et al.,

"Transcript for Conference on Value of Team Approach in Working with Homeless People," St. Vincent's Hospital, Department of Community Medicine, New York, August 1985.

8. E. Baxter and K. Hopper, "The New Mendicancy: Homeless in New York City," *American Journal of Orthopsychiatry* 52 (1982): 393–407.

9. S. M. Goldfinger and L. Chafetz, "Developing a Better Service Delivery System for the Homeless Mentally Ill," in *The Homeless Mentally Ill,* ed. H. R. Lamb (Washington, D.C.: American Psychiatric Association, 1984).

10. B. Conanan and M. J. O'Brien, "New York City: The St. Vincent's SRO and Shelter Programs," in *Health Care of Homeless People,* ed. P. W. Brickner, L. K. Scharer, B. Conanan, A. Elvy, and M. Savarese (New York: Springer, 1985).

11. H. B. Gleicher and M. Savarese, "Staffing

Survey: Working with the Homeless," survey of Baltimore and St. Vincent's (New York) Health Care for the Homeless Programs project staff, internal document. Available from St. Vincent's Hospital (New York) Health Care for the Homeless Program.

12. P. W. Brickner, *Home Health Care for the Aged* (New York: Appleton-Century-Crofts, 1978): 28.

13. C. Shannon and D. Saleebey, "Training Child Welfare Workers to Cope with Burnout," *Child Welfare* 59 (1980): 463–68.

14. F. Fuller and J. Jackson, "Burnout Special

and Patterns for Reviving a Sick Organization," Baltimore, 1989, unpublished.

15. H. Wise, R. Beckhard, I. Rubin, and A. Kyte, *Making Health Teams Work* (Cambridge, MA: Ballinger, 1974).

16. P. Moulder, A. Staal, and M. Grant, "Making the Interdisciplinary Team Approach Work," *Rehabilitation Nursing* (November–December 1988).

17. W. Menninger, "Dealing with Staff Reactions to Perceived Lack of Progress by Chronic Mental Patients," *Hospital and Community Psychiatry* (August 1984).

19. Case Management

1. C. Singer and E. A. Underwood, *A Short History of Medicine*, 2d ed. (New York: Oxford University Press, 1962).

2. D. Rog, C. D. Andranovich, and S. Rosenblum, *Intensive Case Management for Persons Who Are Homeless and Mentally Ill*, prepared under Contract #278-86-0014, with funding from the Division of Education and Service Systems Liaison of the National Institute of Mental Health (Washington, D.C.: Cosmos Corp, May 1987): I.

3. J. P. Sullivan, "Case Management," in *The Chronic Mentally Ill: Treatment, Programs, Systems*, ed. J. A. Talbott (New York: Human Sciences Press, 1981).

4. N. V. Lourie, "Case Management," in *The Chronic Mental Patient: Problems, Solutions and Recommendations for a Public Policy*, ed. J.A. Talbott (Washington, D.C.: American Psychiatric Association, 1978).

5. D. Mechanic, "The Challenge of Chronic Mental Illness: A Retrospective and Prospective View," *Hospital and Community Psychiatry* 37, no. 9 (September 1986), 891–96.

6. F. R. Lipton and A. Sabatini, "Constructing Support Systems for Homeless Chronic Patients," in *The Homeless Mentally Ill*, ed. H. R. Lamb (Washington, D.C.: American Psychiatric Association, 1984).

7. F. J. Ingelfinger, "Management Medicine: The Doctor's Job Today," in *Great Ideas Today* (Chicago: Encyclopaedia Britannica, 1978).

8. J. Noble, C. H. DeFriese, F. D. Pickard, and A. R. Meyers, "Concepts of Health and Illness," in *Textbook of General Medicine and Primary Care*, ed. J. Noble (Boston: Little, Brown, 1987).

9. F. Baker and R. S. Weiss, "The Nature of Case Manager Support," *Hospital and Community Psychiatry* 35, no. 9 (September 1984): 925–28.

10. N. Hansell, M. Wodarczyk, and H. M. Visotsky, "The Mental Health Expediter," *Archives of General Psychiatry* 18 (April 1968): 392–99.

11. R. B. Granet and J. A. Talbott, "The Continuity Agent: Creating a New Role to Bridge the Gaps in the Mental Health System (Open

Forum)," *Hospital and Community Psychiatry* 29, no. 2 (February 1978): 132–33.

12. K. Fisher, ed., "Quality Assurance Update: Case Management," *Quality Review Bulletin* 13, no. 8 (August 1987): 287–90.

13. S. Sherwood and J. N. Morris, "The Pennsylvania Domiciliary Care Experiment: Impact on Quality of Life," *American Journal of Public Health* 73, no. 6 (June 1983): 646–53.

14. P. N. Goering, D. A. Wasylenki, M. Farkas, W. J. Lancee, and R. Ballantyne, "What Difference Does Case Management Make?" *Hospital and Community* Psychiatry 39, no. 3 (March 1988): 272–76.

15. J. L. Franklin, B. Solovitz, N. Mason, J. R. Clemons, and G. E. Miller, "An Evaluation of Case Management," *American Journal of Public Health* 77, no. 6 (June 1987): 674–78.

16. M. Baier, "Case Management with the Chronically Mentally Ill," *Journal of Psychosocial Nursing* 25, no. 6 (1987): 17–20.

17. L. L. Bachrach, "Asylum and Chronically Ill Psychiatric Patients," *American Journal of Psychiatry* 141, no. 8 (August 1984): 875–78.

18. *World Health Organization Basic Document*, 35th ed. (Geneva: World Health Organization, 1985).

19. E. Bandman and B. Bandman, *Nursing Ethics in the Life Span* (Norwalk, CT: Appleton-Century Crofts, 1985).

20. C. Edleman and C. L. Mandle, *Health Promotion Throughout the Life Span* (St. Louis: C. V. Mosby, 1986).

21. D. Mechanic, *Symptoms, Illness, Behavior and Help Seeking* (New Brunswick, N. J.: Rutgers University Press, 1982).

22. F. Walsh, *Normal Family Processes* (New York: Guilford Press, 1982).

23. E. J. Anthony and C. Chiland, *The Child in His Family: Children and Their Parents in a Changing World* New York: John Wiley, 1978), vol. 5.

24. G. Caplan, *Support Systems and Community Mental Health* (New York: Behavioral Publications, 1974).

25. J. Intagliata, B. Willer, and G. Egri, "Role of the Family in Case Management of the

Mentally Ill," *Schizophrenia Bulletin* 12, no. 4 (1986): 699–708.

26. H. R. Lamb and R. Peele, "The Need for Continuing Asylum and Sanctuary," *Hospital and Community Psychiatry* 35, no. 8 (August 1984): 798–802.

27. J. A. Talbott, *The Death of the Asylum: A Critical Study of State Hospital Management, Services, and Care* (New York: Grune and Stratton, 1978).

28. Institute of Medicine Committee on Health Care for Homeless People, *Homelessness, Health, and Human Needs* (Washington, D.C.: National Academic Press, 1988).

29. S. M. Goldfinger and L. Chafetz, "Developing a Better Service Delivery System for the Homeless Mentally Ill," in *The Homeless Mentally Ill,* loc. cit.

30. E. Baxter and K. Hopper, "The New Mendicancy: Homeless in New York City," *American Journal of Orthopsychiatry* 52 (1982): 393–407.

31. P. W. Brickner, "Health Issues in Care of the Homeless," in *Health Care of Homeless People,* loc. cit.

32. S. P. Segal, J. Baumohl, and E. Johnson, "Falling Through the Cracks: Mental Disorder and Social Margin in a Young Vagrant Population," *Social Problems* 24 (1977): 387–400.

33. F. L. J. Ball and B. E. Havassy, "A Survey of the Problems and Needs of Homeless Consumers of Acute Psychiatric Services," *Hospital and Community Psychiatry* 35, no. 9 (September 1984): 917–21.

34. K. Hopper quote in J. O'Connor, ed., "Advocacy and Services for the Homeless Examined at St. Elizabeth's Convocation," *Hospital and Community Psychiatry* 35, no. 9 (September 1984): 948.

35. J. Fernandez quote in H. R. Lamb, "Deinstitutionalization and the Homeless Mentally Ill," *Hospital and Community Psychiatry* 35, no. 9 (September 1984): 900.

36. L. L. Bachrach, "Research on Services for the Homeless Mentally Ill" (conference report), *Hospital and Community Psychiatry* 35, no. 9 (September 1984): 910–13.

37. J. K. Wing, "Who Becomes Chronic?" *Psychiatric Quarterly* 50, no. 3 (1978): 178–90.

38. C. I. Cohen and J. Sokolovsky, "Toward a Concept of Homelessness Among Aged Men," *Journal of Gerontology* 38 (1983): 81–89.

39. E. L. Bassuk, L. Rubin, and A. Lauriat, "Characteristics of Sheltered Homeless Families," *American Journal of Public Health* (September 1986): 1097–1107.

40. A. Frances and S. M. Goldfinger, "Treating a Homeless Mentally Ill Patient Who Cannot Be Managed in the Shelter System," *Hospital and Community Psychiatry* 37, no. 6 (June 1986): 577–79.

41. S. T. Boyd, "Psychological Reactions of Disaster Victims," *South African Medical Journal* 60 (1981): 744–48.

42. "Recommendations of the American Psychiatric Association's Task Force on the Homeless Mentally Ill," *Hospital and Community Psychiatry* 35, no. 9 (September 1984): 908–9.

43. H. R. Lamb and J. A. Talbott, "The Homeless Mentally Ill: The Perspective of the American Psychiatric Association," *Journal of the American Medical Association* 256, no. 4 (July 25, 1986): 498–501.

44. L. D. Ozarin, "The Pros and Cons of Case Management," in *The Chronic Mental Patient: Problems, Solutions, and Recommendations of a Public Policy,* loc. cit.

45. E. M. Gruenberg, "The Social Breakdown Syndrome—Some Origins," *American Journal of Psychiatry* (June 1967).

46. E. Pellegrino, "Protection of Patients' Rights and the Doctor-Patient Relationship," in *Matters of Life and Death,* ed. J. E. Thomas (Toronto: Samuel Stevens, 1978).

47. "Guidelines for Use of Intensive Case Management (ICM) Service Dollars: Intensive Case Management Initiative," New York State Office of Mental Health, April 12, 1989.

48. J. R. Greenley, "Social Factors, Mental Illness, and Psychiatric Care: Recent Advances from a Sociological Perspective," *Hospital and Community Psychiatry* 35, no. 8 (August 1984): 813–20.

49. M. Savarese, "Health Care Teams in Work with the Homeless," in *Health Care of Homeless People,* loc. cit.

50. K. Sellick, "Interdisciplinary Health Teams: A Question of Attitude," *Australian Journal of Advanced Nursing* 3, no. 1 (September–November 1985).

51. A. J. Ducanis and A. K. Colin, *The Interdisciplinary Health Care Team* (Germantown, MD: Aspen Systems Corp, 1979).

52. C. D. Austin, "Case Management in Long-Term Care: Options and Opportunities," *Health and Social Work* (1983): 16–30.

53. Robert Wood Johnson Foundation / Pew Memorial Trust, "Health Care for the Homeless Program Requests for Proposal," The Robert Wood Johnson Foundation, Princeton, N. J., 1984.

54. "Making America Work. Productive People, Productive Policies. Bringing Down the Barriers," National Governors Association Center for Policy Research, 1987.

55. H. R. Lamb, *Treating the Long-Term Mentally Ill* (San Francisco: Jossey-Bass, 1982).

20. Entitlements

1. C. O'Shaughnessy, R. Price, and J. Griffith, *Financing and Delivery of Long-Term Care Services For the Elderly;* and Office of the Actuary, HCFA (August 1985), Health Care Financing Program Statistics: Analysis of State Medicaid Program Characteristics (Baltimore, MD: U.S. Department of Health and Human Services, 194).

2. T. W. Maloney and R. J. Blendon, "Report on the Forum," in *New Approaches to the Medicaid Crisis,* ed. R. J. Blendon and T. W. Maloney (New York: F and S Press, 1982).

3. W. A. MacAdam and D. S. Piktialis, "Mechanisms of Access and Coordination," in *Older Veterans,* ed. T. Wetle and J. Rowe (Cambridge, MA: Harvard University Press, 1984): 159–203; and G. Georgeson, "The Veterans Administration Nurse-Administered Unit," in *Medicare and Extended Care,* ed. B. Vladeck and G. Alfano (Owings Mills, MD: National Health Publishing, 1987): 79–83.

4. J. D. Wright and E. Weber, *Homelessness and Health* (Washington, D.C.: McGraw-Hill, 1987): 4.

5. E. Fox, S. Axelrod, and J. Loeb, *Homelessness in Philadelphia: People, Needs, Services* (Philadelphia Health Management Corporation, October 1985).

6. Physicians Task Force on Hunger in America, "Increasing Hunger and Declining Help: Barriers to Participation in the Food Stamp Program," Harvard School of Public Health, Boston, 1986.

7. Public Assistance P.A.E.M. 1987; (iii): 505,4 (H)–(L).

8. M. Harrington, *The New American Poverty* (New York: Macmillan, 1985).

9. Philadelphia Housing Voucher Program, Philadelphia, July 1988.

10. W. J. Wilson, *The Truly Disadvantaged: The Inner City, the Underclass and Public Policy* (Chicago: University of Chicago Press, 1987).

21. Education and Training

1. G. A. Paccione, E. Cohen, and C. E. Schwartz, "From Forms to Focus: A New Teaching Model in Ambulatory Care," *Archives of Internal Medicine* 149 (1989): 2407–11.

2. J. D. Gooson, "Physician Training Outside the Hospital: Who Pays for the Future?" (editoral), *Annals of Internal Medicine* 107 (1987): 415–17.

3. S. A. Schroeder, J. A. Showstack, and G. Gerbert, "Residency Training in Internal Medicine: Time for a Change?" *Annals of Internal Medicine* 104 (1986): 554–56.

4. Special Requirements for Residency Training Programs in Internal Medicine, American Board of Internal Medicine, Philadelphia, Pennsylvania.

5. S. M. Mellinkoff, "The Medical Clerkship," *New England Journal of Medicine* 317 (1987): 1089–91.

6. D. J. Leizman, W. L. Stewart, T. F. Dodson, W. W. Hitzig, and G. J. Schiller, individual letters to the "Medical Clerkship" article cited above, *New England Journal of Medicine* 318 (1988): 1133–34.

7. Collected students comments, St. Vincent's Hospital, W. Vicic, preceptor.

8. G. Smithwick, "Introduction to the Homeless Population," presented at the University of North Carolina School of Public Health Conference of Nurse Educators, May 21, 1986.

9. J. Noble (project director), "Final Report. Assessment of the Development and Support of Primary Care Residency Training," *General Internal Medicine and Pediatrics* NTIS No. HRP-0907161. U.S. Department of Health and Human Services, Public Health Service, Division of Medicine, Bureau of

Health Professions, Health Resources and Services Administration, Boston University Medical Center, September 30, 1985–September 30, 1987.

10. O. G. Barnett and J. E. Midtling, "Public Policy and the Supply of Primary Care Physicians," *Journal of the American Medical Association* 262 (1989): 2864–68.

11. D. L. Goldenberg, J. T. Pozen, and A. S. Cohen, "The Effect of a Primary-Care Pathway on Internal Medicine Residents Career Plans," *Annals of Internal Medicine* 91 (1979): 271–74.

12. New York State Council on Graduate Medical Education, "First Annual Report," Albany, N.Y., 1988: 6.

13. A. M. Lindsey, "Health Care for the Homeless," *Nursing Outlook* 37, no. 2 (1989): 78–81.

14. G. P. Lenehan, B. N. McInnis, D. O'Donnell, and M. Hennessey, "A Nurses' Clinic for the Homeless," *American Journal of Nursing* 85 (November 1985): 11.

15. J. O'Connell, "On the Fringe of Society," *Harvard Medical School Bulletin* (Spring 1988).

16. E. Reilly and B. McInnis, "Boston, Massachusetts: The Pine Street Inn Nurses' Clinic and Tuberculosis Program," in *Health Care of Homeless People,* ed. P. W. Brickner, L. K. Scharer, B. Conanan, A. Elvy, and M. Savarese (New York: Springer, 1985).

17. D. Stasior, "Mixed Company," *Harvard Medical School Bulletin* (Spring 1988).

18. J. D. Wray, "Undergraduate and Graduate Education in Community Medicine," in *Community Medicine,* ed. W. Lathen and A. Newbery (New York: Appleton-Century-Crofts, 1970): 12.

22. Outreach

1. H. R. Lamb, ed., *The Homeless Mentally Ill* (Washington, D.C.: American Psychiatric Association, 184).

2. Clearinghouse on Homelessness Among Mentally Ill People. "Notes" from *CHAMP* (April 1987).

3. G. Morse, "Conceptual Overview of Mobile Outreach for Persons Who Are Homeless and Mentally Ill," presented at the American Public Health Association, New Orleans, October 1987: 18–22.
4. W. G. Smillie, *Public Health: Its Promise for the Future* (New York: Macmillan, 1955).
5. E. B. G. Hebenstreit, "Principles of the Science of Medical Police," in *From Medical Police to Social Medicine: Essays on the History of Health Care,* ed. G. Rosen (New York: Science History Publications, 1974): 145.
6. *From Medical Police to Social Medicine: Essays on the History of Health Care,* loc. cit.: 176–200.
7. Ibid.: 304.
8. M. E. Clark, R. M. Neal, S. L. Neibacher, and S. L. Wobido, "A Flexible Approach to Health Services for the Homeless," presented at the American Public Health Association, Washington, D.C., November 1985.
9. F. Lipton, Clearinghouse on Homelessness Among Mentally Ill People, Notes from Opening Address, *CHAMP* (April 1987).
10. H. R. Lamb, "Deinstitutionalization and the Homeless Mentally Ill," in "Engaging Homeless Persons with Mental Illnesses into Treatment," ed. D. J. Roy, presented at the National Mental Health Association, June 1988: 18.
11. A. Frances and L. Goldfinger, "Treating a Homeless Mentally Ill Patient Who Cannot Be Managed in the Shelter System," ibid.
12. K. Minkoff, "Beyond Deinstitutionalization: A New Ideology for the Postinstitutional Era," ibid.: 19.
13. M. Test, "Effective Community Treatment of the Chronically Mentally Ill: What Is Necessary," ibid.
14. J. F. Putnam, N. L. Cohen, and A. M. Sullivan, "Innovative Outreach Services for the Homeless Mentally Ill," ibid.
15. L. Stein and R. J. Diamond, "A Program for Difficult-to-Treat Patients," ibid.
16. D. J. Roy, G. D. Andranovich, and L. Rosenblum, "Intensive Care Management for Persons Who Are Homeless and Mentally Ill: A Review of Community Support Program and Human Resource Development Program Efforts, NIMH," ibid.: 20.
17. S. M. Barrow and A. M. Lovell, "The Referral of Outreach Clients to Mental Health Services: Community Support Systems Evaluation Program, New York," ibid.
18. E. Baxter and K. Hopper, "Shelter and Housing for the Homeless Mentally Ill," ibid.
19. S. E. Axelroad and G. Toff, "Outreach Services for Homeless Mentally Ill People, a Report Summarizing the First in a Series of Four Meetings Held by the Clearinghouse on Homelessness Among Mentally Ill People," *CHAMP* (March 1987): 3, 25, 29, 30.
20. S. E. Axelroad and G. Toff, "Outreach Services for Homeless Mentally Ill People," in "Engaging Homeless Persons with Mental Illnesses into Treatment," loc. cit.: 21, 22,.
21. M. Keshy-Wolff, S. Matthews, F. Kalibat, and L. R. Mosher, "Crossing Place: A Residential Model for Crisis and Intervention," ibid.: 21.
22. M. Breton, "A Drop-in Program for Transient Women: Promoting Competence Through the Environment," ibid.
23. R. Stern and K. Minkoff, "Paradoxes in Programming for Chronic Patients in a Community Clinic," ibid.: 22.
24. L. Van Tosh, "Discussion in D. J. Roy Workshop on Enjoying Homeless Individuals with Mental Illness in Treatment," ibid.: 23.

23. A Public-Private Partnership in Health Care for the Homeless

1. R. Trobe, "Request for Proposals and Applications, New York City" (Human Resources Administration of the City of New York, 1984): 2, 27, 45.
2. G. Brager, H. Specht, and J. Torczynek, *Community Organizing* (New York: Columbia University Press, 1983): 196.
3. E. Baxter and K. Hopper, "The New Mendicancy: Homeless in New York City," *American Journal of Orthopsychiatry* 52, no. 3 (1982): 393–408; K. Hopper et al., "One Year Later, the Homeless Poor in New York City," Community Service Society, June 1982; E. Baxter and K. Hopper, *Private Lives / Public Places* (New York: Community Service Society, 1984); and K. Hopper and J. Hamberg, *The Making of America's Homeless from Skid Row to New Poor* (New York: Community Service Society, 1984).
4. G. Brager and S. Holloway, *Changing Human Service Organizations* (New York: Free Press, 1978): 181–83.
5. R. O. York, *Human Service Planning: Concepts, Tools, and Methods* (Chapel Hill, N.C.: University of North Carolina Press, 1982): 7, 14, 30, 34–35.
6. G. Schneider, memo to Homeless Project Steering Committee, "Summary of Additional Information Requested by RWJ Evaluation Team," September 25, 1984.
7. Minutes of New York City Coalition for Health Care for the Homeless, January 31, 1985.
8. B. E. Collins and H. Guetzkow, *A Social Psychology of Group Processes for Decision Making* (New York: John Wiley, 1964).
9. New York City Coalition for Health Care for the Homeless, Program Mission Statement.

24. A Twenty-Year Experience in Health Care of the Homeless: The St. Vincent's Hospital (New York) Program

1. Verbal report, New York City Human Resources Administration, June 1989.
2. A. Kaufman, verbal report, 1969.
3. P. W. Brickner, D. Greenbaum, A. Kaufman, F. O'Donnell, J. T. O'Brian, R. Scalice, J. Scanizzo, and T. Sullivan, "A Clinic for Male Derelicts," *Annals of Internal Medicine* 77 (1972): 565–69.
4. J. D. Wright, *Address Unknown: The Homeless in America* (New York: Aldine de Gruyter, 1989): 46.
5. J. D. Wright, P. H. Rossi, J. W. Knight, E. Weber-Burdin, R. C. Tessler, C. E. Stewart, M. Geronimo, and J. Lam, "Health and Homelessness in New York City," research report to the Robert Wood Johnson Foundation, January 1985.
6. "National Ambulatory Medical Care Survey (NAMCS), United States, 1979 Summary" (Washington, D.C.: U.S. Public Health Service, 1979).
7. A. Elvy, "Access to Care," in *Health Care of Homeless People,* ed. P. W. Brickner, L. K. Scharer, B. Conanan, A. Elvy, and M. Savarese (New York: Springer, 1985).
8. E. Erkel, "The Implication of Cultural Conflict for Health Care," *Health Values* 4 (1980): 51–57.
9. *Webster's Ninth New Collegiate Dictionary,* 1985: 979.
10. H. R. Huessy, "The Chronic Psychiatric Patient in the Community: Highlights from a Boston Conference," *Hospital and Community Psychiatry* 28 (1977): 287.
11. Personal communication from a nurse in the SRO / Homeless Program, 1984.
12. Personal communication from an ambulatory care unit, staff member, 1982.
13. P. W. Brickner, R. A. Torres, M. Barnes,

R. G. Newman, D. C. Des Jarlais, D. P. Whalen, and D. E. Rogers, "Recommendations for Control and Prevention of Human Immunodeficiency Virus (HIV) Infection in Intravenous Drug Users," *Annals of Internal Medicine* 110 (1989): 833–37.
14. E. Luder, E. Boey, B. Buchalter, and C. Martinez-Weber, "Assessment of the Nutritional Status of Urban Homeless Adults," *Public Health Reports* 104 (1989): 451–57.
15. C. Martinez-Weber, "The Homeless Person with Diabetes: A Diagnostic and Therapeutic Challenge," *Postgraduate Medicine* 81 (1987): 289–98.
16. J. M. McAdam, P. W. Brickner, L. Scharer, J. Crocco, and A. E. Duff, "The Spectrum of Tuberculosis in a New York City Men's Shelter Clinic (1982–1988)," *Chest* 97 (1990): 798–805.
17. R. A. Torres, P. Lefkowitz, C. Kales, and P. W. Brickner, "Homelessness Among Hospitalized Patients with the Acquired Immunodeficiency Syndrome in New York City" (letter to the editor), *Journal of the American Medical Association* 258 (1987): 779–80.
18. V. Taylor, W. W. Stead, G. Schecter, M. Skinner, M. A. Barry, E. A. Nardell, P. W. Brickner, M. Hansen, S. Schultz, and A. Vennema, "Tuberculosis Control Among Homeless Populations," *Morbidity and Mortality Weekly Report* 36 (1987): 257–60.
19. R. K. Kellogg, O. Piantieri, B. Conanan, P. Doherty, W. Vicic, and P. W. Brickner, "Hypertension: A Screening and Treatment Program for the Homeless," in *Health Care of Homeless People,* loc. cit.: 109–20.
20. W. Vicic, "Sum of the Parts: A Memory of a Homeless Man," *Psychotherapy Patient* 2, no. 4 (1986): 147–52.

25. Assuring Good-Quality Care

1. A. Donabedian, *Explorations in Quality Assessment and Monitoring,* volume 1, *The Definition of Quality and Approaches to Its Assessment* (Ann Arbor, Mich.: Health Administration Press, 1988).
2. J. LoGerfo and R. Brook, "The Quality of Health Care," in *Introduction to Health Services,* 3d ed., ed. S. J. Williams and P. R. Torrens (New York: John Wiley, 1988).
3. O. R. Bowen, "What Is Quality Care?" *New England Journal of Medicine* 316 (1987): 1578–80.
4. U.S. Congress, Office of Technology Assessment, *The Quality of Medical Care: Information for Consumers* (Washington, D.C.: Government Printing Office, 1988), OTA-H-386.
5. L. K. Demlo, "Assuring Quality of Health Care: An Overview," *Evaluation and Health Professions* 6 (1983): 161–96.
6. H. Vuori, *Quality Assurance of Health Ser-

vices: Concepts and Methodology* (Copenhagen: Regional Office for Europe World Health Organization, 1982).
7. K. Lohr and R. Brook, *Quality Assurance in Medicine: Experience in the Public Sector* (Santa Monica, CA: Rand, 1984), #R3193HHS.
8. H. Palmer and M. C. Reilly, "Individual and Institutional Variables Which May Serve as Indicators of Quality of Care," *Medical Care* 17 (1979): 693–717.
9. B. Gerbert, G. Stone, M. Stulbarg, D. S. Gullion, and S. Greenfield, "Agreement Among Physician Assessment Methods: Searching for the Truth Among Fallible Methods," *Medical Care* 26 (1988): 513–35.
10. M. R. Chassin, J. Kosecoff, D. H. Solomon, and R. H. Brook, "How Coronary Angiography Is Used: Clinical Determinants of Appropriateness," *Journal of the American*

Medical Association 258 (1987): 2543–47.

11. J. E. Wennberg, "The Paradox of Appropriate Care," *Journal of the American Medical Association* 258 (1987): 2568–69.

12. E. Wall, "Continuity of Care and Family Medicine: Definition, Determinants and Relationship to Outcome," *Journal of Family Practice* 13 (1981): 655–64.

13. R. H. Brook, A. Davies-Avery, S. Greenfield, et al., "Assessing the Quality of Care Using Outcome Measures: An Overview of the Method," *Medical Care* 15 (suppl): 1–165.

14. J. W. Williamson, S. Aronovitch, L. Simonson, C. Ramirez, and D. Kelly, "Health Accounting: An Outcome-Based System of Quality Assurance: Illustrative Application to Hypertension," *Bulletin of the New York Academy of Medicine* 51 (1975): 727–44.

15. J. E. Ware, Jr., "The Assessment of Health Status," in *Applications of Social Science to Clinical Medicine,* ed. L. Aiken and D. Mechanic (New Brunswick, N.J.: Rutgers University Press, 1986).

16. M. Bergner and M. L. Rothman, "Health Status Measures: An Overview and Guide for Selection," *Annual Review of Public Health* 8 (1987): 191–210.

17. J. G. Roberts and P. Tugwell, "Comparison of Questionnaires Determining Patient Satisfaction with Medical Care," *Health Services Research* 22 (1987): 637–54.

18. J. E. Ware, A. Davies-Avery, and A. L. Stewart, "The Measurement and Meaning of Patient Satisfaction," *Health and Medical Care Services Review* 1 (1978): 3–15.

19. J. W. Williamson, "Evaluating Quality of Patient Care: A Strategy Relating Outcome and Process Assessment," *Journal of the American Medical Association* 218 (1971): 564–69.

20. R. H. Brook and K. N. Lohr, "Efficacy, Effectiveness, Variations, and Quality: Boundary-Crossing Research," *Medical Care* 23 (1985): 710–22.

21. A. Donabedian, op. cit., volume 2, *The Criteria and Standards of Quality,* loc. cit.

22. R. H. Brook and F. A. Appel, "Quality-of-Care Assessment: Choosing a Method for Peer Review," *New England Journal of Medicine* 288 (1973): 1323–29.

23. S. Greenfield, S. Cretin, L. G. Worthman, F. J. Dorey, N. E. Solomon, and G. A. Goldberg, "Comparison of a Criteria Map to a Criteria List in Quality of Care Assessment for Patients with Chest Pain: The Relation of Each to Outcome," *Medical Care* 19 (181): 255–72.

24. R. H. Fletcher, M. S. O'Malley, J. A. Earp, et al., "Patients' Priorities for Medical Care," *Medical Care* 21 (1983): 234–42.

25. Department of Clinical Epidemiology and Biostatistics, McMaster University Health Sciences Center, "How to Read Clinical Journals: VI. To Learn About the Quality of Clinical Care," *Canadian Medical Association Journal* 130 (1984): 377–81.

26. F. Baker, "Data Sources for Health Care Quality Evaluation," *Evaluation and Health Professions* 6 (1983): 263–81.

27. J. E. Wennberg, N. Roos, L. Sola, A. Schori, and R. Jaffe, "Use of Claims Data Systems to Evaluate Health Care Outcomes," *Journal of the American Medical Association* 257 (1987): 933–36.

28. L. Wyszewianski and A. Donabedian, "Equity in the Distribution of Quality of Care," *Medical Care* 19 (1981): 28–56.

29. R. H. Palmer and H. R. Nesson, "A Review of Methods for Ambulatory Medical Care Evaluations," *Medical Care* 20 (1982): 758–81.

30. J. M. Eisenberg and S. V. Williams, "Cost Containment and Changing Physicians' Practice Behavior," *Journal of the American Medical Association* 246 (1981): 2195–201.

31. P. J. Sanazaro, "Determining Physicians' Performance: Continuing Medical Education and Other Interacting Variables," *Evaluation and Health Professions* 6 (1983): 197–210.

32. R. B. Haynes, D. A. Davis, A. McKibbon, and P. Tugwell, "A Critical Appraisal of the Efficacy of Continuing Medical Education," *Journal of the American Medical Association* 251 (1984): 61–64.

33. C. J. McDonald, S. L. Hui, D. M. Smith, et al., "Reminders to Physicians from an Introspective Computer Medical Record," *Annals of Internal Medicine* 100 (1984): 130–38.

34. Joint Commission on the Accreditation of Hospitals, *Quality Assurance in Ambulatory Care* (Chicago: Joint Commission on the Accreditation of Hospitals, 1987).

35. Joint commission on the Accreditation of Hospitals, "Monitoring and Evaluation of the Quality and Appropriateness of Care: A Hospital Example," *Quality Review Bulletin* 12 (1986): 326–30.

36. Joint Commission on the Accreditation of Hospitals, "Monitoring and Evaluation of the Quality and Appropriateness of Care: An Ambulatory Health Care Example," *Quality Review Bulletin* 13 (1987) 26–30.

37. Joint Commission on the Accreditation of Hospitals, "Quality Assurance Standards Revised," *JCAH Perspectives* 4 (1984): 2–3, 16–21.

38. Joint Commission on the Accreditation of Healthcare Organizations, *Sample Indicators for Evaluating Quality in Ambulatory Care* (Chicago: Joint Commission on the Accreditation of Healthcare Organizations, 1987).

39. R. W. Dubois, W. H. Rogers, J. H. Moxley, D. Draper, and R. H. Brook, "Hospital Inpatient Mortality: Is It a Predictor of Quality?" *New England Journal of Medicine* 317 (1987): 1674–80.

40. M. S. Kramer, L. Arsenault, and I. B. Pless, "The Use of Preventable Adverse Outcomes to Study the Quality of Child Health Care," *Medical Care* 22 (1984): 223–30.

41. D. D. Rutstein, W. Berenberg, T. C. Chalmers, C. G. Child, A. P. Fishman, and E. B. Perrin, "Measuring the Quality of Medical Care: A Clinical Method," *New England Journal of Medicine* 294 (1976): 582–88.

42. T. L. Panniers and J. Newlander, "The Ad-

verse Patient Occurrences Inventory: Validity, Reliability and Implications," *Quality Review Bulletin* 11 (1986): 311–15.
43. D. M. Berwick, "Continuous Improvement as an Ideal in Health Care," *New England Journal of Medicine* 320 (1989): 53–56.
44. Joint Commission on the Accreditation of Healthcare Organizations, *Accreditation Manual for Hospitals. Ambulatory Health Care Standards Manual. Consolidated Standards Manual* (psychiatric and substance abuse facilities, facilities offering services to the mentally retarded / developmentally disabled, facilities offering community mental health services). *Long Term Care Standards Manual. Hospice Standards Manual. Standards for the Accreditation of Home Care* (Chicago: Joint Commission on the Accreditation of Healthcare Organizations, 1987–1989).
45. M. S. Thompson, R. H. Palmer, J. K. Rothrock, R. Strain, L. H. Brachman, and E. A. Wright, "Resource Requirements for Evaluating Ambulatory Health Care," *American Journal of Public Health* 74 (1984): 1244–84.
46. M. M. Jackson and P. Lynch, "Applying an Epidemiological Structure to Risk Management and Quality Assurance Activities," *Quality Review Bulletin* 11 (1986): 306–12.
47. J. W. Williamson, H. R. Braswell, S. D. Horn, and S. Lohmeyers, "Priority Setting in Quality Assurance: Reliability of Staff Judgments in Medical Institutions," *Medical Care* 17 (1978): 931–40.
48. M. S. Torres, "Quality Assurance of Brokered Services," *Quality Review Bulletin* 14 (1988): 187–92.
49. J. D. Wright and E. Weber, *Homelessness and Health* (Washington, D.C.: McGraw-Hill, 1987).
50. H. S. Luft and S. S. Hunt, "Evaluating Individual Hospital Quality Through Outcome Statistics," *Journal of the American Medical Association* 255 (1986): 2780–84.
51. M. S. Blumberg, "Risk-Adjusting Health Care Outcomes: A Methodologic Review," *Medical Care Review* 43 (1986): 351–93.
52. L. I. Iezzoni, "Case Classification and Quality of Care: Issues to Consider Before Making the Investment," *Quality Review Bulletin* 13 (1987): 135–39.
53. W. L. Roper, W. Winkenwerder, G. M. Hackbarth, and H. Krakauer, "Effectiveness in Health Care: An Initiative to Improve Medical Practice," *New England Journal of Medicine* 319 (1988): 1197–202.
54. W. E. Deming, *Out of the Crisis* (Cambridge, Mass.: Massachusetts Institute of Technology, Center for Advanced Engineering Study, 1986).

26. Program Sustainment

1. Action memo, National Association of Community Health Centers, Washington, D.C., June 30, 1989.
2. P. Wolfe, Memorandum, Washington, (D.C.) Health Care for the Homeless Program, Washington, D.C., 1989.
3. H. Gleicher, Memorandum, Baltimore Health Care for the Homeless Program, Baltimore, Md., 1989.

Index

Page numbers in *italics* refer to illustrations.